SURGICAL TECHNIQUES IN OTOLARYNGOLOGY HEAD AND NECK SURGERY

Series Editor: **Robert T Sataloff** MD DMA FACS

OTOLOGIC AND NEUROTOLOGIC SURGERY

SURGICAL TECHNIQUES IN
OTOLARYNGOLOGY
HEAD AND NECK SURGERY

Series Editor: **Robert T Sataloff** MD DMA FACS

OTOLOGIC AND NEUROTOLOGIC SURGERY

Authors

Michael J LaRouere MD

President and Fellowship Director, Michigan Ear Institute
Co-Director of Neurosciences, Providence Hospital and Medical Centers
Clinical Associate Professor, Wayne State University
Clinical Professor, Oakland University William Beaumont School of Medicine
Clinical Professor, Michigan State University
Farmington Hills, Michigan, USA

Seilesh C Babu MD

Chief Financial Officer, Michigan Ear Institute
Clinical Associate Professor, Wayne State University
Clinical Professor, Oakland University William Beaumont School of Medicine
Clinical Professor, Michigan State University
Farmington Hills, Michigan, USA

Dennis I Bojrab MD

CEO and Director of Research, Michigan Ear Institute
Director of Skull Base Surgery and Co-Director of Neurosciences, Providence Hospital and Medical Centers
Clinical Professor, Wayne State University
Clinical Professor, Michigan State University
Clinical Professor, Oakland University William Beaumont School of Medicine
Farmington Hills, Michigan, USA

JAYPEE *The Health Sciences Publisher*

New Delhi | London | Philadelphia | Panama

Jaypee Brothers Medical Publishers (P) Ltd

Headquarters
Jaypee Brothers Medical Publishers (P) Ltd.
4838/24, Ansari Road, Daryaganj
New Delhi 110 002, India
Phone: +91-11-43574357
Fax: +91-11-43574314
E-mail: jaypee@jaypeebrothers.com

Overseas Offices

J.P. Medical Ltd.
83, Victoria Street, London
SW1H 0HW (UK)
Phone: +44-20 3170 8910
Fax: +44(0)20 3008 6180
E-mail: info@jpmedpub.com

Jaypee-Highlights Medical Publishers Inc.
City of Knowledge, Bld. 237, Clayton
Panama City, Panama
Phone: +1 507-301-0496
Fax: +1 507-301-0499
E-mail: cservice@jphmedical.com

Jaypee Medical Inc.
The Bourse
111 South Independence Mall East
Suite 835
Philadelphia, PA 19106, USA
Phone: +1 267-519-9789
E-mail: jpmed.us@gmail.com

Jaypee Brothers Medical Publishers (P) Ltd.
17/1-B, Babar Road, Block-B, Shaymali
Mohammadpur, Dhaka-1207
Bangladesh
Mobile: +08801912003485
E-mail: jaypeedhaka@gmail.com

Jaypee Brothers Medical Publishers (P) Ltd.
Bhotahity, Kathmandu, Nepal
Phone: +977-9741283608
E-mail: kathmandu@jaypeebrothers.com

Website: www.jaypeebrothers.com
Website: www.jaypeedigital.com

Inquiries for bulk sales may be solicited at: jaypee@jaypeebrothers.com

Surgical Techniques in Otolaryngology—Head and Neck Surgery: Otologic and Neurotologic Surgery

First Edition: **2015**

ISBN: 978-93-5152-463-2

Printed at: Ajanta Offset & Packagings Ltd., New Delhi

Dedication

The book is dedicated to our loving families.
Janice, Jacqueline, Stephen and Jessica LaRouere
Abbey, Kavan, Kethan, Karun and Kareena Babu
Andria, Dennis, Adrianna and Andrew Bojrab

Contributors

Seilesh C Babu MD
Chief Financial Officer
Michigan Ear Institute
Clinical Associate Professor
Wayne State University
Clinical Professor
Oakland University William Beaumont
School of Medicine
Clinical Professor
Michigan State University
Farmington Hills, Michigan, USA

Brent J Benscoter MD
Neurotology Fellow
Michigan Ear Institute
Farmington Hills, Michigan, USA

Dennis I Bojrab MD
CEO and Director of Research
Michigan Ear Institute
Director of Skull Base Surgery and
Co-Director of Neurosciences
Providence Hospital and Medical Centers
Clinical Professor
Wayne State University
Clinical Professor
Michigan State University
Clinical Professor
Oakland University William Beaumont
School of Medicine
Farmington Hills, Michigan, USA

Eleanor Y Chan MD
Attending Physician
Michigan Ear Institute
Associate Professor
Oakland University William Beaumont
School of Medicine
Farmington Hills, Michigan, USA

Peter Y Chen MD FACR
Professor
Oakland University William Beaumont
School of Medicine
Department of Radiation Oncology
Medical Director, Gamma Knife Center
William Beaumont Hospital
Farmington Hills, Michigan, USA

Adam Folbe MD
Associate Professor
Wayne State University
Assistant Professor
Oakland University William Beaumont
School of Medicine
Southfield, Michigan, USA

Robert S Hong MD PhD
Attending Physician
Michigan Ear Institute
Assistant Professor
Department of Otolaryngology
Wayne State University
Farmington Hills, Michigan, USA

Jack M Kartush MD
Professor Emeritus
Michigan Ear Institute
Clinical Professor
Wayne State University
Clinical Professor
Oakland University William Beaumont
School of Medicine
Farmington Hills, Michigan, USA

Michael J LaRouere MD
President and Fellowship Director
Michigan Ear Institute
Co-Director of Neurosciences
Providence Hospital and Medical Centers
Clinical Associate Professor
Wayne State University
Clinical Professor
Oakland University William Beaumont
School of Medicine
Clinical Professor
Michigan State University
Farmington Hills, Michigan, USA

Ann Maitz PhD MSc
Director
Gamma Knife Center Physics
Senior Physicist
William Beaumont Hospital
Farmington Hills, Michigan, USA

Ilka C Naumann MD
Attending Physician
Michigan Ear Institute
Assistant Professor
Michigan State University
Farmington Hills, Michigan, USA

Daniel R Pieper MD
Associate Professor of Neurosurgery
Oakland University William Beaumont
School of Medicine
Farmington Hills, Michigan, USA

Eric W Sargent MD FACS
Attending Physician, Michigan Ear Institute
Clinical Associate Professor
Wayne State University
Clinical Associate Professor
Oakland University William Beaumont
School of Medicine
Farmington Hills, Michigan, USA

Robert T Sataloff MD DMA
Professor and Chairman
Department of Otolaryngology and
Head & Neck Surgery
Senior Associate Dean for Clinical
Academic Specialties
Drexel University College of Medicine
Philadelphia, Pennsylvania, USA

Dan Sdrulla MD PhD
Neurotology Fellow
Michigan Ear Institute
Farmington Hills, Michigan, USA

Pradeep Setty DO
Resident Section of Neurosurgery
St John Providence Health System
Michigan State University
Southfield, Michigan, USA

Otologic and Neurotologic Surgery

Eric L Slattery MD
Neurotology Fellow
Michigan Ear Institute
Farmington Hills, Michigan, USA

Emily Z Stucken MD
Neurotology Fellow
Michigan Ear Institute
Farmington Hills, Michigan, USA

John J Zappia MD
Attending Physician
Michigan Ear Institute
Clinical Associate Professor
Wayne State University
Associate Professor
Oakland University William Beaumont
School of Medicine
Farmington Hills, Michigan, USA

Foreword

Surgical Techniques in Otolaryngology—Head and Neck Surgery is a six-volume compendium. In addition to being an integral component of the compendium, each volume was written to stand alone, as well. The volumes in this work include Atlases of Otologic and Neurotologic Surgery, Rhinologic and Sinus Surgery, Laryngeal Surgery, Facial Plastic and Reconstructive Surgery, Pediatric Otolaryngologic Surgery, and Head and Neck Surgery. The authors of each volume have included not only background information and step-by-step details of surgical technique, but also "pearls" gleaned through vast experience. Each volume contains extensive illustrations and intraoperative photographs that illustrate and simplify the techniques described.

Surgical Techniques in Otolaryngology—Head and Neck Surgery is intended to provide clinicians with thorough, accessible and clinically useful details of surgery for nearly all disorders cared for by otolaryngologists. The work also serves as a companion to Sataloff's six-volume *Comprehensive Textbook of Otolaryngology—Head and Neck Surgery,* which was written simultaneously with the compendium on surgical techniques. Hopefully, *Surgical Techniques* will prove useful for otolaryngologists by making it easier to provide (and teach) state-of-the-art otolaryngologic surgery.

Robert T Sataloff MD DMA FACS
Series Editor
Professor and Chairman
Department of Otolaryngology—Head and Neck Surgery
Senior Associate Dean for Clinical Academic Specialties
Drexel University College of Medicine
Philadelphia, Pennsylvania, USA

Preface

Otologic and Neurotologic Surgery is based on the experience gained in teaching otology and neurotology fellows at Michigan Ear Institute over the past 25 years. It has been created as a practical resource for otolaryngology residents, otology fellows, and practicing otolaryngologists who perform otologic surgery.

Each chapter reviews the most up-to-date information pertaining to specific otologic and neurotologic disorders. Step-by-step surgical techniques, accompanied by intraoperative photos, are then presented with an emphasis on surgical "pearls" practiced at the Michigan Ear Institute. Complications related to each surgical procedure are outlined. Newer surgical procedures such as over-under tympanoplasty, repair of superior semicircular canal dehiscence, endoscopic retrosigmoid vestibular nerve section, and endoscopic retrosigmoid tumor removal are presented.

It is hoped that this atlas will provide the otologic surgeon with much of the knowledge that we try to pass on to our fellows in training to allow them to become outstanding otologic and neurotologic practitioners and thus provide their patients with the most optimal outcomes.

Michael J LaRouere MD
Seilesh C Babu MD
Dennis I Bojrab MD

Acknowledgments

We would like to acknowledge the many authors, including our partners, our neurosurgeons and current fellows at Michigan Ear Institute who have spent numerous hours preparing each chapter. We would also like to thank our office and operating room staff and in particular Cheryl Thrushman at Providence Park Hospital and Alison Devine at Michigan Ear Institute who have dedicated their time towards this atlas.

Finally we would like to acknowledge the emeritus physicians at Michigan Ear Institute who have dedicated their careers to teaching otologic and neurotologic surgery. These include Drs. Ted McGee, Malcolm Graham and Jack Kartush. We would be remiss if we did not thank the nearly 50 fellows who have kept us on our "A" game over the past 25 years.

Contents

CHAPTER 1

General Considerations in Otologic and Neurotologic Surgery

Michael J LaRouere

INTRODUCTION

Performing otologic and neurotologic surgery requires attention to the most minute details. This is ever so apparent in the operating room. In order to achieve the best results, otologic surgeons find that routine is of utmost importance. Variations from a routine may lead to errors and poor outcomes.

Operating room personnel include the surgeon, experienced scrub and circulating nurses who have a thorough understanding of otologic instrumentation and an anesthesiologist familiar with neuroanesthesia and nerve monitoring. Additional personnel can include a neuromonitoring team who has good rapport with the surgeon. Finally, a good surgical team consisting of a neurotologist and neurosurgeon who have a thorough understanding of each other's role in the particular procedure is essential.

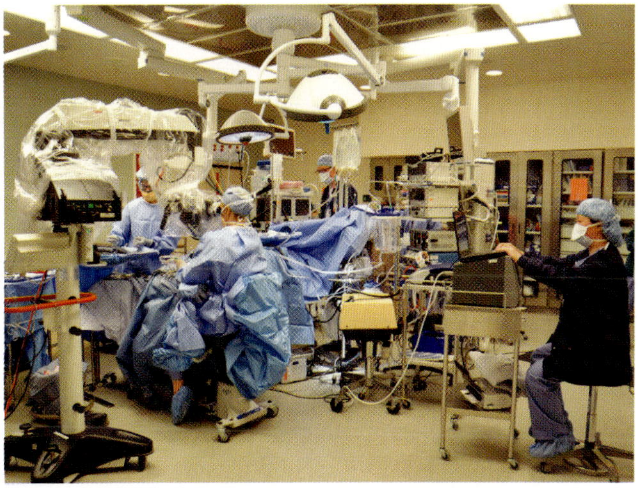

Fig. 1.1: Panoramic view of an otology room setup. The table is rotated 180°. The surgeon is opposite the scrub nurse. The operating microscope is at the head of the patient, anesthesia at the foot. An intraoperative monitor is located behind the surgeon, giving real-time feedback regarding facial nerve stimulation

OPERATING ROOM EQUIPMENT

The operating room table is unique to otology. The bed is usually rotated 180° away from anesthesia with the patients head at the foot of the table. This allows the surgeon to be seated with his legs under the table (Fig. 1.1). Being able to rotate the bed side to side allows for optimal visualization of the surgical field through the microscope. Important for the operating surgeon is a chair with a back and arm rests. This allows for arm support, thereby decreasing fatigue (and also decreases the likelihood of neck, arm, and shoulder problems in the future) (Fig. 1.2).

The operating microscope is positioned at the head of the bed. The microscope should be freely moveable yet able to lock in position to prevent drift (Fig. 1.1).

Our experience scrub nurses control suction and irrigation. The surgeon controls fine suction with his thumb over the control hole. Our scrub nurses also control the on and off function of the otologic drill responding to the surgeons voice. This allows the surgeon to concentrate on the procedure and eliminates the need for the surgeon to control the drill with his feet. The scrub nurse is routinely positioned across the head from the surgeon, making the passing of instruments straight forward.

Monitoring

Facial nerve, auditory brainstem-evoked recordings and lower cranial nerve monitoring have become routine in otologic and neurotologic surgery.[1,2] Having a thorough understanding of the specific monitoring technique is of the utmost importance. Poor monitoring is worse than no monitoring at all.[3] We stress the importance of intraoperative stimulation (active monitoring as opposed to passive monitoring) to assess the function of both the equipment as well as the nerve. This involves electrically stimulating the nerve as early as possible in all cases in which monitoring is used. Currently, we use a constant current facial nerve monitor with the EMG recording displayed both visually and audibly (Medtronic) (Fig. 1.3).

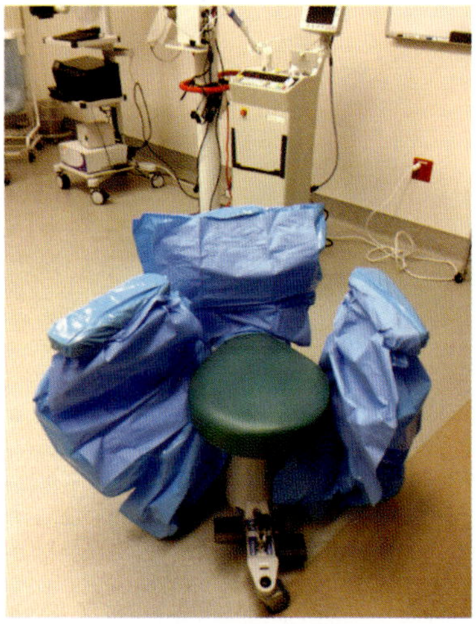

Fig. 1.2: An otology operating chair with arms is sterilely draped. Arm rests allow for continuous arm support

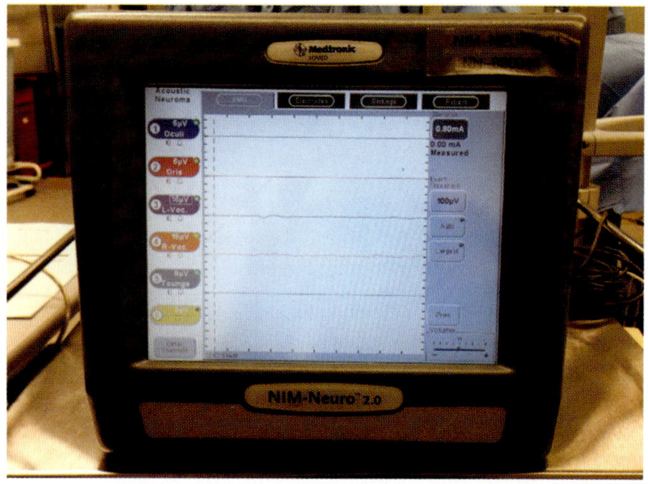

Fig. 1.3: A constant current facial monitor is shown that allows both visual and auditory feedback

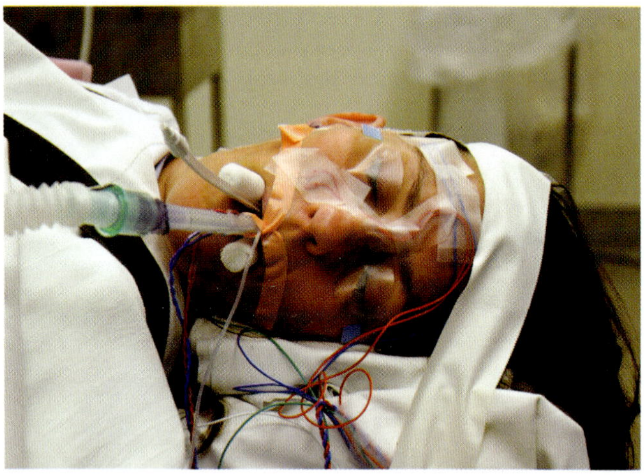

Fig. 1.4: Electrodes are placed in a bipolar montage. Two channels are generally used: one based above the brow (orbicularis oculi) and the other in the orbicularis oris. A ground electrode is placed over the sternum and an anode electrode is also placed over the sternum to allow for monopolar stimulation. This patient has a monitoring endotracheal tube in place

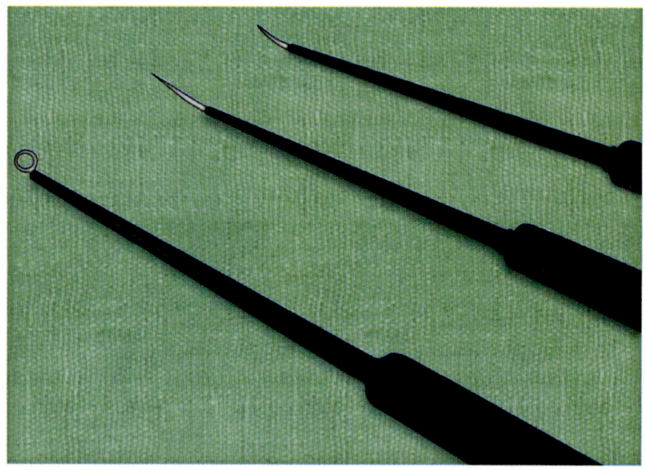

Fig. 1.5: Kartush stimulating dissectors are shown. These are insulated to just before the tip and allow for simultaneous dissection and stimulation

Electrode placement for otologic and neurotologic surgery is done in a two-channel montage. A pair of needle electrodes are placed in the orbicularis oculi and orbicularis oris muscles. We place a ground electrode over the sternum in addition to an anode electrode for monopolar nerve stimulation (Fig. 1.4).

Several steps should then be followed to ensure adequate facial nerve monitoring:

Step 1: After insertion check electrode impedance (<5k Ohms).

Step 2: Confirm current flow back to the monitor.

Step 3: Obtain an early baseline response (active monitoring). This is usually done over the tympanic segment of the nerve.

Unique to motor nerve (facial, lower cranial nerve) monitoring in our practice is the use of intraoperative stimulus dissectors. Developed by Dr Jack Kartush, the stimulus dissectors are insulated to near the tip (Fig. 1.5), allowing for simultaneous stimulation and surgical dissection. These instruments have proved to be invaluable in tumor dissection and also in chronic ear surgery when cholesteatoma and granulation tissue surround the facial nerve.

Errors in monitoring usually result in false negative responses or a lack of response. Rarely a false positive response can occur—usually due to current spread from using too high a current level. False negative responses can occur with current going through CSF or blood. Lack of a response can be due to nerve injury, anesthesia, faulty setup or lack of sufficient current.

Intraoperative auditory brainstem evoked recordings have proven to be useful in several neurotologic procedures when hearing preservation is a goal. Acoustic tumor surgery, vestibular nerve section, and microvascular decompression surgery are the major procedures in which intraoperative ABR monitoring is routinely used. As with facial nerve monitoring, electrode placement is critical. The insert earphone should be placed securely in the ear canal after the canal is cleaned of wax and prep solution. Baseline recordings should be established prior to beginning the surgical procedure.

ABR changes are not related to depth of anesthesia. Increased latencies/decreased amplitudes are seen with eighth nerve injury and injury to the internal auditory artery. Other causes of ABR changes include fluid in the middle ear and opening the dura prior to any intervention near the nerve.

In the majority of cases, loss of the ABR signal altogether signifies poor postoperative hearing. This does not always correlate however as we have seen normal postoperative hearing results with marked intraoperative ABR changes.

ANESTHESIA

Unique to otologic and neurotologic surgery is the relationship of the surgeon to the anesthesiologist or nurse anesthetist. This is especially important in conscious sedation cases where patient movement at a critical juncture of the procedure can be met with poor results. Also important is the choice of anesthetic agents during cases in which motor nerve (i.e. facial) monitoring is used. The absence of long-term paralyzing agents while keeping the patient still needs to be communicated to the anesthetic team. Short-acting paralytic agents are routinely used for intubation, and a train of four testing is done to ensure the effect of these agents has dissipated prior to beginning the surgical procedure.

Local anesthetic injections need to be monitored closely by the operating surgeon. Inadvertent infiltration of the facial nerve can render facial nerve monitoring useless. This is why active monitoring of the facial nerve during all otologic and neurotologic procedures is critical.

Further the use of agents to help with brain relaxation (decreased $PaCO_{2,}$ Mannitol, Lasix, Hypertonic Saline) need to be appropriately timed by both the surgical and anesthetic team.

REFERENCES

1. Heman-Ackah SE, Gupta S, Lalwani AK. Is facial nerve integrity monitoring of value in chronic ear surgery? Laryngoscope. 2013;123(1):2-3.
2. National Institutes of Health. Consensus Statement; Acoustic Neuroma. Presented at the NIH Consensus Development Conference, Bethesda, MD, 1991.
3. Porter R, Kartush J. Diagnosis, evaluation and treatment of facial nerve disorders (Chapter 30). In: Sanna M, Kirtane MV, Devaiah A, DeSouza C (Eds). Otology Neurotology. New York: Thieme Publishers; 2013.

CHAPTER

2 Eustachian Tube Surgery

Seilesh C Babu, Emily Z Stucken

INTRODUCTION

The eustachian tube functions to equalize pressure between the middle ear space and atmospheric pressure via its connection to the nasopharynx. Anatomically, the lateral third of the eustachian tube is bony; this transitions to a cartilaginous tube at the medial two thirds. The eustachian tube is collapsed at rest; it opens briefly with swallowing, yawning, or other movements performed to equalize middle ear pressure. Eustachian tube disorders may result from inadequate opening of the eustachian tube, termed eustachian tube dysfunction (ETD), or from abnormal patency of the eustachian tube, known as patulous eustachian tube.

DISORDERS OF THE EUSTACHIAN TUBE

Patients with ETD commonly present with a sensation of plugged ears and may develop middle ear effusions. Chronic ETD may lead to chronic otitis media with or without the formation of cholesteatoma. The most commonly employed treatment for ETD is the placement of pressure equilibration (PE) tubes; however, PE tubes provide temporary aeration of the middle ear space at best. More permanent tubes are often fraught with problems including bacterial colonization and chronic otorrhea, plugging, or tube dysfunction.

A patulous eustachian tube often produces symptoms of ear fullness and autophony. A patient may be bothered by hearing their own breath sounds. Symptoms are temporarily ameliorated by placing the head in a dependent position; however, symptoms return when the head is returned upright. The onset of symptoms may be related to rapid or pronounced weight loss, or pregnancy. Initial therapy involves the use of topical estradiol nasal drops. Topical therapy is rarely tolerated longer than several months, however, as many patients experience a burning sensation in the nasopharynx with use of the drops.

SURGERY FOR EUSTACHIAN TUBE DYSFUNCTION

Initial attempts at surgical repair of ETD focused on widening the bony eustachian tube at the isthmus and entryway into the middle ear.[1-4] It was noted, however, that these techniques posed a risk of injury to the neighboring carotid canal. Recently, it has been proposed that many cases of ETD result from a functional rather than strictly anatomic defect and that the affected region is the cartilaginous portion of the eustachian tube.[5] The portion of the cartilaginous eustachian tube just medial to the bony junction is referred to as the valve. The valve region dilates when the eustachian tube is engaged to equalize middle ear pressure. Poe et al. have proposed that ETD results from faulty opening of the eustachian tube valve, anatomic obstruction caused by mucosal edema, or dysfunction of the tensor veli palatini and/or levator veli palatini muscles.[5] Accordingly, surgical techniques have been developed to address these factors. The first described procedures to address the cartilaginous portion of the eustachian tube used a laser to ablate mucosa, soft tissue, and cartilage at the nasopharyngeal orifice.[5-7] Others have used a powered microdebrider to remove hypertrophied mucosa from the posterior eustachian tube cushion.[8] Another technique involves dilation of the cartilaginous eustachian tube with a balloon catheter.[9-14] Results have been generally favorable, though criteria for success and follow-up are inconsistent among studies. Symptomatic improvement has been described approximately 70% of patients.[8,12] The same proportion were found to be free of effusion at 6-month time.[5]

Surgical Technique: Balloon Dilation of the Eustachian Tube

Anesthesia

Balloon dilation of the eustachian tube is often performed under general anesthesia, though it may be possible to perform under local anesthesia in the clinic setting.

Step 1

Pledgets soaked with oxymetazoline or topical 4% cocaine are placed into the nasal cavity for approximately 5 minutes to provide topical vasoconstriction and anesthesia.

Step 2

A 30° 4 mm endoscope is used to survey the nasal cavity and assure adequate access to the nasopharynx and allow visualization of the eustachian tube (Fig. 2.1). The choice of endoscope is dependent on the patient's anatomy and surgeon preference.

Step 3

An angled sinus balloon measuring 5–7 mm in diameter and 15 mm in length is introduced into the nasal cavity and positioned at the eustachian tube orifice.

Step 4

If the balloon system has a lighted guidewire, this can be used to confirm proper placement of the balloon system. In this case, a second 0° endoscope and video tower is used. The second telescope is positioned in the ear canal to visualize the tympanic membrane. The room lights are dimmed, and the lighted guidewire is positioned in the nasopharynx and advanced through the eustachian tube until the light is just visualized in the middle ear space on the second video monitor. If the balloon system does not have a lighted guidewire, the guidewire should not be used for this procedure, as the wire will not have adequate markings and may be threaded blindly into the middle ear space, placing the ossicles at risk.

Step 5

The balloon is advanced into the eustachian tube orifice (Fig. 2.2). The guidewire (if used) is withdrawn.

Step 6

The balloon is inflated with saline to 8 atm and held for 30 seconds (Fig. 2.3). If the balloon herniates into the nasopharynx, saline is withdrawn and the balloon is repositioned then reinflated.

Step 7

After 30 seconds, the balloon is deflated and withdrawn from the nasal cavity.

Step 8

The eustachian tube office is assessed with the endoscope for degree of dilation and any signs of injury such as bleeding or mucosal disruption.

Surgical Technique: Microdebrider Eustachian Tuboplasty

Anesthesia

The procedure is performed under general anesthesia.

Step 1

Pledgets soaked with oxymetazoline or topical 4% cocaine are placed into the nasal cavity for approximately 5 minutes to provide topical vasoconstriction and anesthesia.

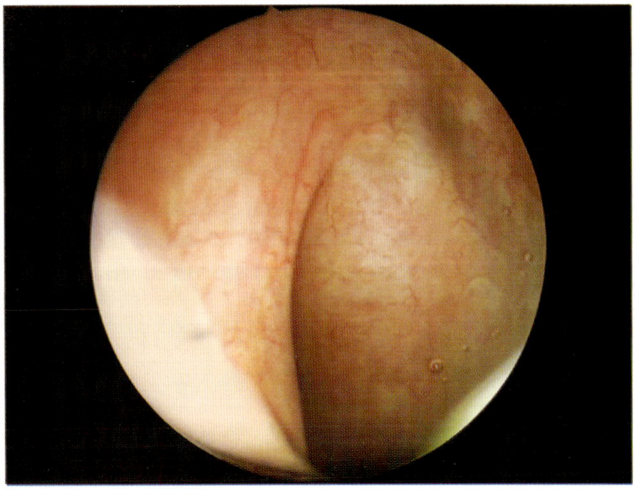

Fig. 2.1: The eustachian tube is visualized using a 30° sinus endoscope.

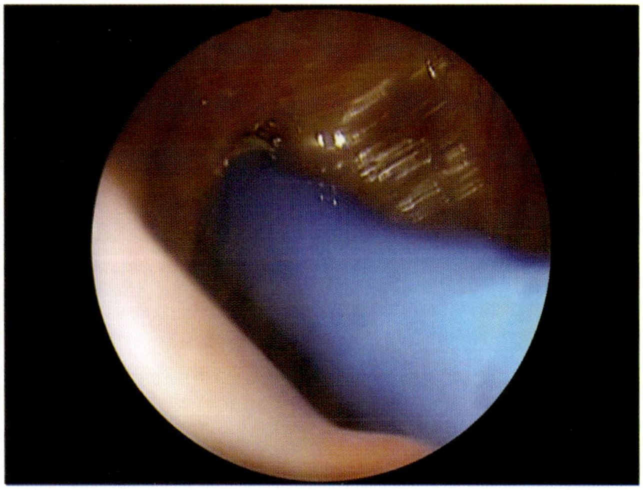

Fig. 2.2: The balloon is advanced into the eustachian tube orifice.

Step 2

A 30° 4 mm endoscope is used to survey the nasal cavity and assure adequate access to the nasopharynx and allow visualization of the eustachian tube. The choice of endoscope is dependent on the patient's anatomy and surgeon preference.

Step 3

The posterior cushion of the eustachian tube orifice is injected submucosally with 1% lidocaine with 1:100,000 epinephrine to aid in vasoconstriction. The superior portion of the anterior cushion may also be injected.

Step 4

A 4 mm microdebrider blade is introduced into the nasopharynx. An appropriate angled blade should be selected based on an individual patient's anatomy. The blade will typically be a 0°, 15°, or 30° angled blade. The open edge of the microdebrider blade should contact the posterior cushion of the eustachian tube orifice, with the guarded portion facing the anterior cushion.

Step 5

The microdebrider is engaged at the posterior cushion, and used to debride the mucosa of the posterior cushion down to, but not through, the level of the cartilage. The anterior mucosal surface is protected by the guarded side of the microdebrider blade; great care must be taken to assure that the anterior mucosa is not disrupted to prevent synechiae formation at the eustachian tube orifice.

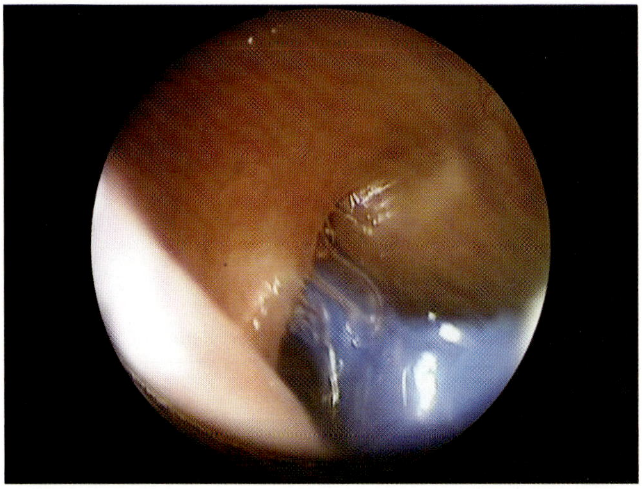

Fig. 2.3: The balloon is inflated within the eustachian tube orifice.

Step 6

Hemostasis is achieved with topical application of pledgets soaked in oxymetazoline.

Surgery for Patulous Eustachian Tube

Many procedures have been proposed to alleviate the symptoms associated with a patulous eustachian tube. Various substances have been injected submucosally at the nasopharyngeal orifice including cartilage[15] and hydroxyapatite.[16,17] Others have performed eustachian tuboplasty by either implanting cartilage or Alloderm into a submucosal pocket along the anterolateral wall of the eustachian tube,[18] or inverting the curvature of a concave tubal cartilage through laser application.[19] Several authors have described complete closure of the nasopharyngeal orifice of the eustachian tube in an effort to eliminate autophony, either with or without the concurrent placement of myringotomy tubes. This has been achieved by a combination of methods including endoluminal cauterization, fat plugging, and suture ligation.[20-22] Many of these techniques are relatively new and have only been published in small case series with limited follow-up; however, results thus far are promising.

Surgical Technique: Cartilage Pocket Eustachian Tuboplasty

Anesthesia

The procedure is performed under general anesthesia.

Step 1

Pledgets soaked with oxymetazoline or topical 4% cocaine are placed into the nasal cavity for approximately 5 minutes to provide topical vasoconstriction and anesthesia.

Step 2

A 30° 4 mm endoscope is used to survey the nasal cavity and assure adequate access to the nasopharynx and allow visualization of the eustachian tube. The choice of endoscope is dependent on the patient's anatomy and surgeon preference.

Step 3

The posterior cushion of the eustachian tube orifice is injected submucosally with 1% lidocaine with 1:100,000 epinephrine to aid in vasoconstriction. The superior portion of the anterior cushion may also be injected.

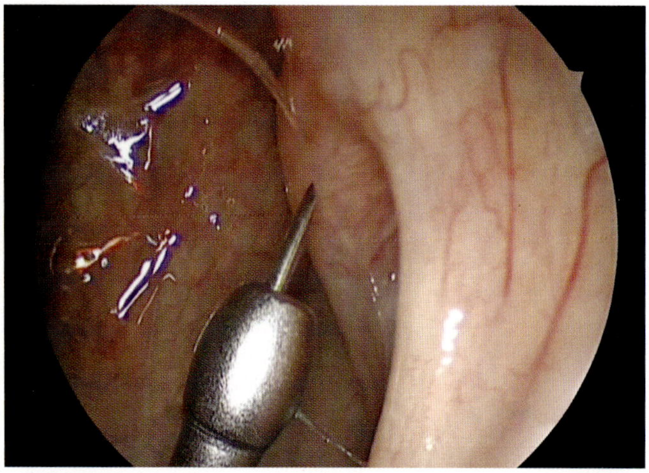

Fig. 2.4: The posterior cushion of the eustachian tube orifice is injected submucosally with 1% lidocaine with 1:100,000 epinephrine.

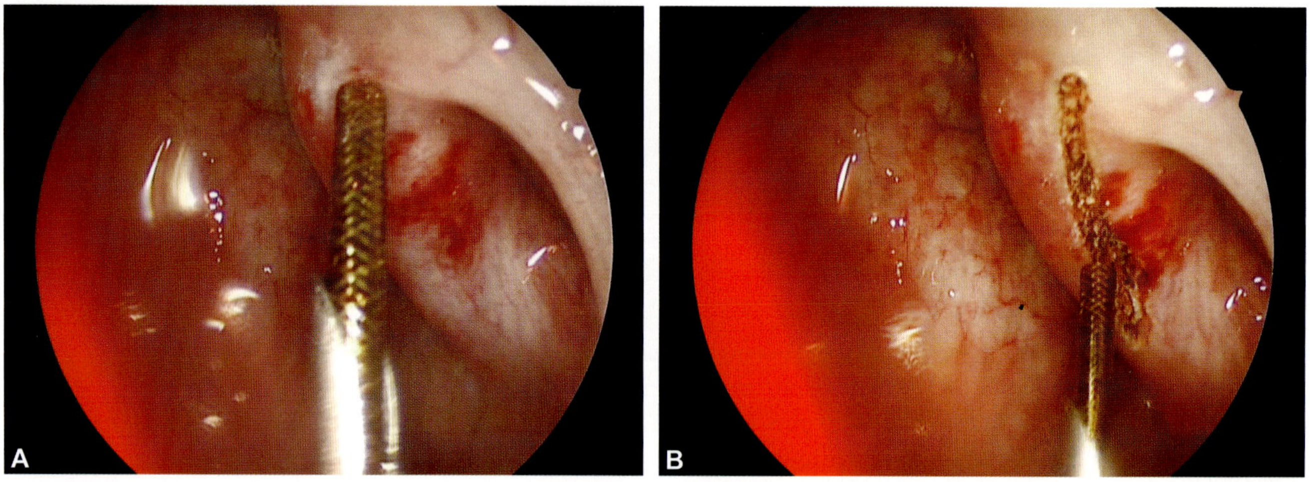

Figs. 2.5A and B: (A) The handheld CO_2 laser fiber is loaded onto an angled-tip handle and positioned at the posterior cushion of the eustachian tube. (B) The CO_2 laser is used to incise the mucosa over the posterior cushion to the level of the underlying cartilage, which is kept intact.

Injection is performed by threading a spinal needle through a curved suction tip to achieve the appropriate angle (Fig. 2.4).

Step 4

The handheld CO_2 laser fiber is loaded onto an angled-tip handle. The laser is set to 2 W. The laser is used to incise the mucosa over the posterior cushion of the eustachian tube (Figs. 2.5A and B). The mucosa is incised to the level of the underlying cartilage and Ossman's fat pad.

Step 5

The laser fiber is withdrawn. The empty laser handle or a curved suction tip is placed in the mucosal incision and used to dissect a submucosal pocket anterior to the cartilage (Figs. 2.6A and B).

Step 6

A piece of tragal cartilage is harvested measuring approximately 1 cm × 7 mm. The tragal incision is closed using 5-0 fast absorbing suture. We have found the best results when the cartilage is divided into four to five pieces each measuring 2–3 mm in size.

Step 7

The tragal cartilage is grasped with a sinonasal forceps and placed in the submucosal pocket (Figs. 2.7A and B). Four or five separate pieces of cartilage are placed in the pocket, each measuring 2–3 mm in size. The tragal cartilage is positioned on the luminal surface of the native eustachian tube cartilage.

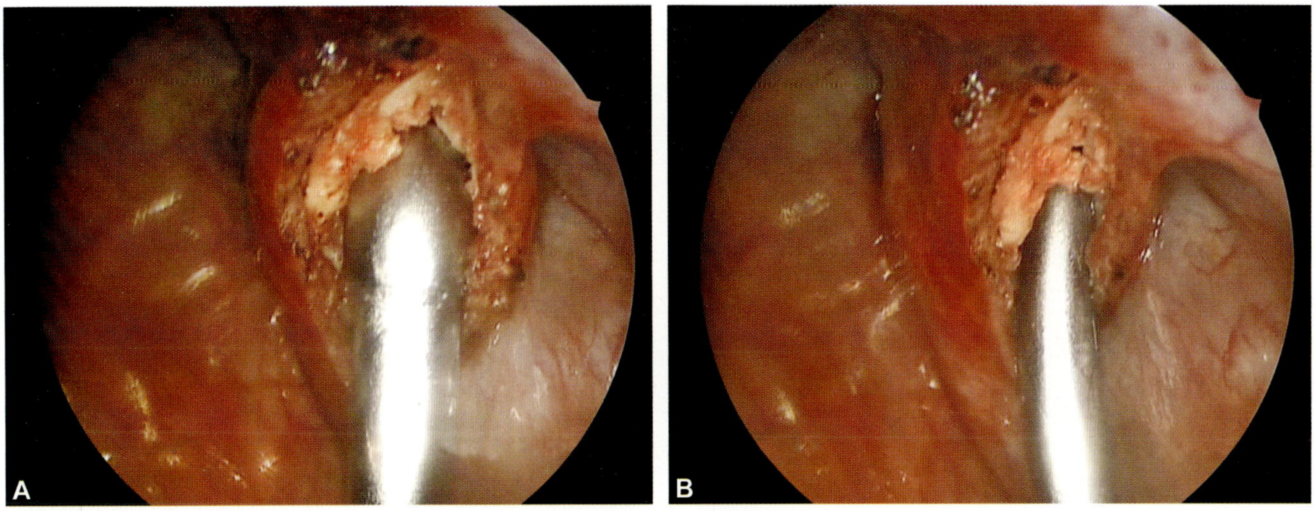

Figs. 2.6A and B: A curved suction tip is used to dissect a submucosal pocket along the anterior face of the cartilage.

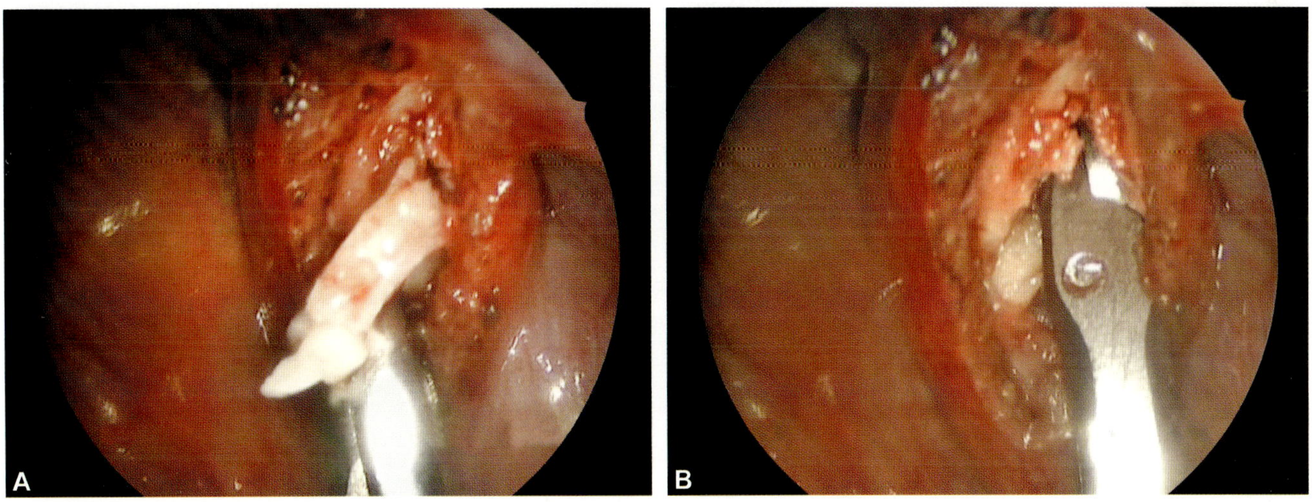

Figs. 2.7A and B: The tragal cartilage is grasped with sinonasal forceps and placed into the submucosal pocket. It is useful to have a forceps with an adjustable arm to facilitate alterations in the angle of curvature.

Step 8

Closure can be attempted with endoscopic needle passing instruments. Alternatively, fibrin glue seems to be effective for closure of the mucosal incision. It must be verified that the incision is closed in order to prevent cartilage from refluxing into the pharynx.

REFERENCES

1. Wullstein H. Eustachian tube in tympanoplasty. Arch Otolaryngol. 1960;71:408-10.
2. House WF, Glasscock ME, Miles J. Eustachian tuboplasty. Laryngoscope. 1969;79:1765-82.
3. Misurya VK. Eustachian tuboplasty. J Laryngol Otol. 1975; 89:807-13.
4. Jansen CW. Functional repair of the eustachian tube. Am J Otol. 1985;6:231-2.
5. Poe DS, Metson RB, Kujawski O. Laser eustachian tuboplasty: a preliminary report. Laryngoscope. 2003;113:583-91.
6. Kujawski O. Laser eustachian tuboplasty (LETO): 4th European Congress of EUFOS. Otorhinolaryngol Head Neck Surg. 2000;2:835-42.
7. Yanez C. Cross-hatching: a novel technique for Eustachian tuboplasty. Preliminary report. Otolaryngol Head Neck Surg. 2010;142(5):688-93.
8. Metson R, Pletcher SD, Poe DS. Microdebrider eustachian tuboplasty: a preliminary report. Otolaryngol Head Neck Surg. 2007;136(3):422-7
9. Ockermann T, Reineke U, Upile T, et al. Balloon dilation eustachian tuboplasty: a feasibility study. Otol Neurotol. 2010;31(7):1100-3.

10. Poe DS, Hanna BM. Balloon dilation of the cartilaginous portion of the eustachian tube: initial safety and feasibility analysis in a cadaver model. Am J Otolaryngol. 2011;32(2): 115-23.
11. Poe DS, Silvola J, Pyykko I. Balloon dilation of the cartilaginous Eustachian tube. Otolaryngol Head Neck Surg. 2011; 144(4):563-9.
12. Catalano PJ, Jonnalagadda S, Yu VM. Balloon catheter dilation of Eustachian tube: a preliminary study. Otol Neurotol. 2012;33(9):1549-52.
13. McCoul ED, Singh A, Anand VK, et al. Balloon dilation of the eustachian tube in a cadaver model: technical considerations, learning curve, and potential barriers. Laryngoscope. 2012;122(4):718-23.
14. Jurkiewicz D, Bien D, Szczygielski K, et al. Clinical evaluation of balloon dilation Eustachian tuboplasty in the Eustachian tube dysfunction. Eur Arch Otorhinolaryngol. 2013; 270(3):1157-60.
15. Kong SK, Lee IW, Goh EK, et al. Autologous cartilage injection for the patulous eustachian tube. Am J Otolaryngol. 2011;32(4):346-8.
16. Wolraich D, Zur KB. Use of calcium hydroxylapatite for management of recalcitrant otorrhea due to a patulous eustachian tube. Int J Pediatr Otorhinolaryngol. 2010;74(12): 1455-7.
17. Vaezeafshar R, Turner JH, Li G, et al. Endoscopic hydroxyapatite augmentation for patulous Eustachian tube. Laryngoscope. 2014;124(1):62-6.
18. Poe DS. Diagnosis and management of the patulous eustachian tube. Otol Neurotol. 2007;28(5):668-77.
19. Yañez C, Pirrón JA, Mora N. Curvature inversion technique: a novel tuboplastic technique for patulous Eustachian tube—a preliminary report. Otolaryngol Head Neck Surg. 2011; 145(3):446-51.
20. Doherty JK, Slattery WH 3rd. Autologous fat grafting for the refractory patulous eustachian tube. Otolaryngol Head Neck Surg. 2003;128(1):88-91.
21. Takano A, Takahashi H, Hatachi K, et al. Ligation of eustachian tube for intractable patulous eustachian tube: a preliminary report. Eur Arch Otorhinolaryngol. 2007;264(4):353-7.
22. Rotenberg BW, Busato GM, Agrawal SK. Endoscopic ligation of the patulous eustachian tube as treatment for autophony. Laryngoscope. 2013;123(1):239-43.

CHAPTER

3 Surgery of the Ear Canal

Eleanor Y Chan

INTRODUCTION

This chapter focuses on the surgical management of several pathologies affecting the external auditory canal (EAC), including exostoses, osteoma, keratosis obturans, EAC cholesteatoma, acquired canal stenosis, and aural atresia. The commonly encountered problems of otitis externa, foreign body impaction, dermatitis, and aural polyps are beyond the scope of this review. Cancers of the EAC will be discussed in Chapter 8 along with other temporal bone malignancies.

ANATOMY

The EAC is comprised of a cartilaginous segment that forms the outer third of the canal, and an osseous part that forms the inner two thirds. The canal is a funnel-shaped structure, and winds in a slightly superior direction for 2.5 cm to end at the tympanic membrane. The tympanic membrane forms an acute angle at the anterior sulcus, by virtue of the anteroinferior canal wall being somewhat longer than the posterosuperior canal wall. Prominence of the anterior canal convexity may make complete visualization of the tympanic membrane challenging. Posterosuperior retraction of the pinna helps to straighten the canal to aid examination.

The subcutaneous layer of the lateral cartilaginous portion contains hair follicles, apocrine, and sebaceous glands. These glands form a lipid-rich protective coating of cerumen over the skin of the lateral canal. The medial canal is formed by the bony tympanic ring devoid of any glands or hair, with firmly adherent epidermis over it. The epidermis is in continuity with the epithelial layer of the tympanic membrane. The fissures of Santorini are variably occurring dehiscences within the cartilaginous canal that may allow passage of infection or pathology to the temporomandibular joint or parotid region. Similarly, Huschke's foramen situated in the anteroinferior tympanic bone provides a direct conduit for infection or cancer to invade the preauricular and facial soft tissues.[1-3]

Sensory innervation of the EAC includes contributions from cranial nerves V, VII, IX, and X. The auriculotemporal branch of the trigeminal nerve supplies most of the anterior and superior walls of the canal, whereas the auricular branch of the vagus (Arnold's nerve) accrues fibers from the facial and glossopharyngeal nerves to supply the posterior and inferior portions of the canal. The precise boundaries of innervation are slightly variable between individuals. Arterial supply is from the external carotid artery (posterior auricular, superficial temporal, deep auricular branch from the internal maxillary artery). Venous drainage is carried by the superficial temporal (internal jugular vein) and posterior auricular (external jugular vein) veins.[1,3]

EXOSTOSES AND OSTEOMA

Exostoses and osteomas of the EAC are benign lesions of bony hyperplasia. Exostoses are commonly known as "Surfer's Ear," as they have been ascribed to repeated exposures to cold water and wind.[4,5] They are associated with aquatic sports such as swimming, surfing, kayaking, sailing, diving, or jet-skiing. Cumulative exposure to cold water followed by the evaporative cooling of wind is thought to result in a reactive periostitis that stimulates new bone growth.[4,5] Exostoses typically occur as multiple variably-sized broad-based protuberances along the anterior and posterior bony canal walls (Figs. 3.1A and B). They tend to arise bilaterally, in contrast to osteomas, which are usually unilateral and pedunculated with tendency to favor suture lines (Figs. 3.2A and B). Although the cold-induced inflammatory etiology has been proposed for osteomas as well, their occurrence is mainly attributed to a developmental anomaly of mature bone growth.[6]

Treatment of exostoses and osteomas is not necessary unless they cause symptoms. Progressive enlargement of these bony bulges eventually results in canal luminal obstruction, and may cause entrapment of cerumen, conductive hearing loss, or recurrent otitis externa.

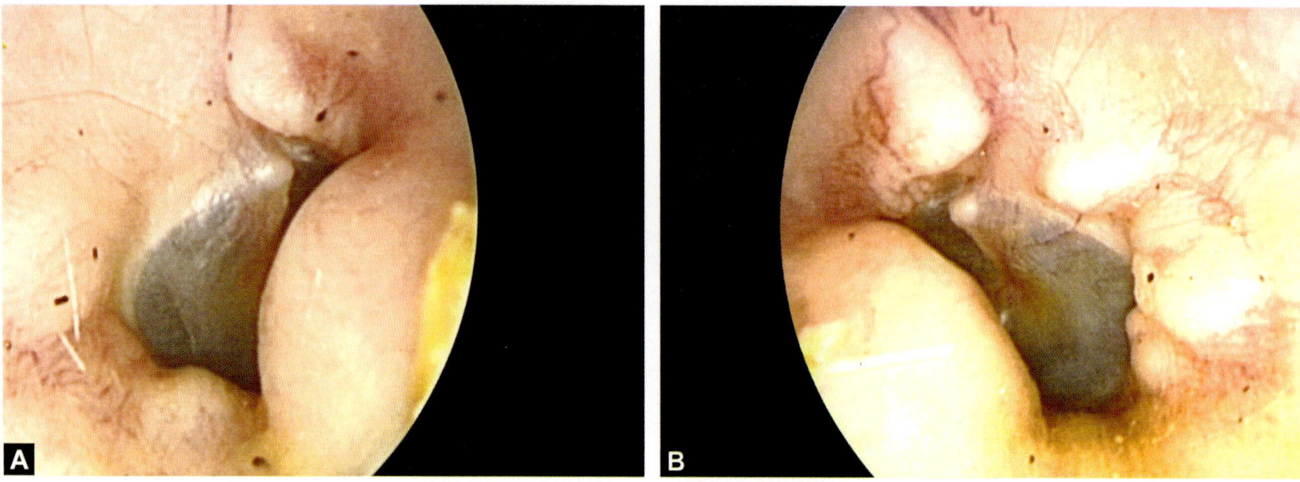

Figs. 3.1A and B: (A) Bilateral external auditory canal exostoses, right ear. (B) Bilateral external auditory canal exostoses, left ear.

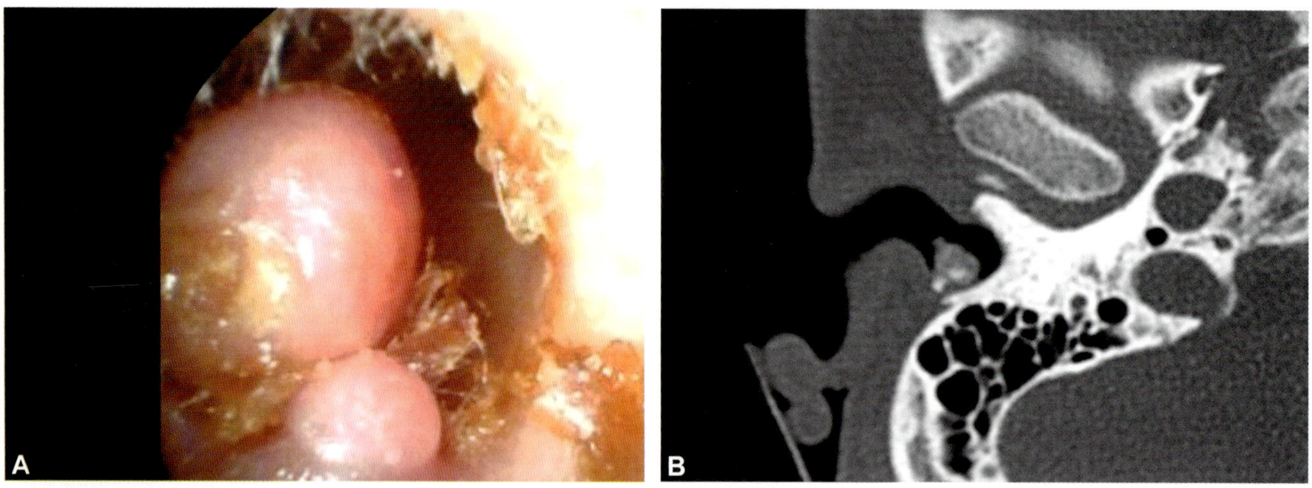

Figs. 3.2A and B: (A) Right external auditory canal osteoma. (B) Axial CT temporal bone demonstrating right external auditory canal osteoma. *Courtesy*: Seilesh Babu, MD.

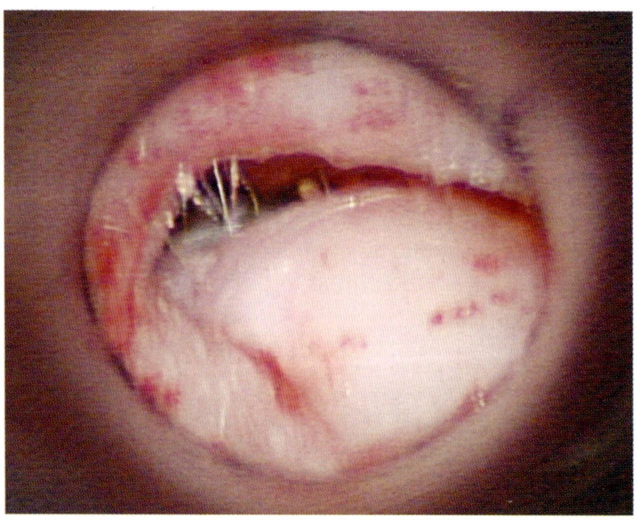

Fig. 3.3: Surgical view of right external auditory canal exostoses. Severe luminal obstruction with impaired visualization of tympanic membrane.

Avoidance of continued water exposure or cessation of the inciting activity may curtail their growth and development. Canalplasty is indicated for pathological obstruction and its sequelae.

Surgical Technique: Exostoses Removal

Step 1

Micro-otoscopic examination of the ear is performed. The severity and depth of exostoses within the canal, as well as status of the tympanic membrane are assessed (Fig. 3.3).

Step 2

The EAC is infiltrated with local anesthetic and vasoconstrictor along its four quadrants to achieve blanching

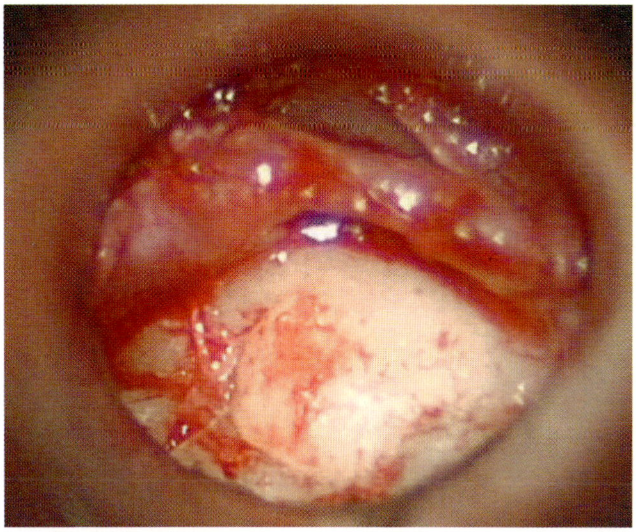

Fig. 3.4: Elevation of posterior skin flap (right ear).

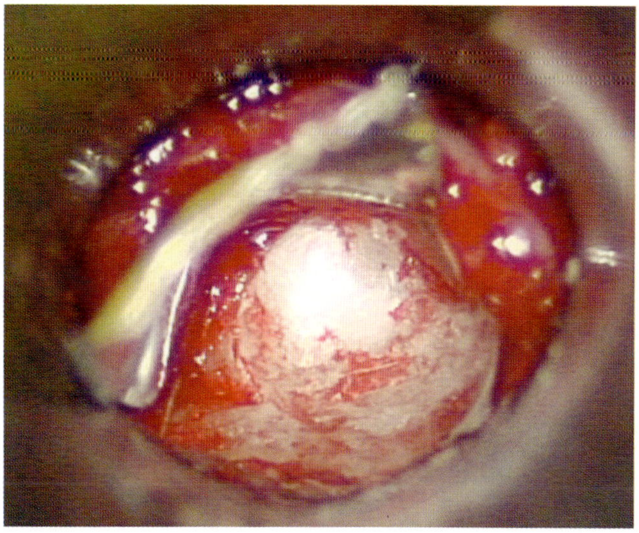

Fig. 3.5: Foil placed between skin flap and exostoses (right ear).

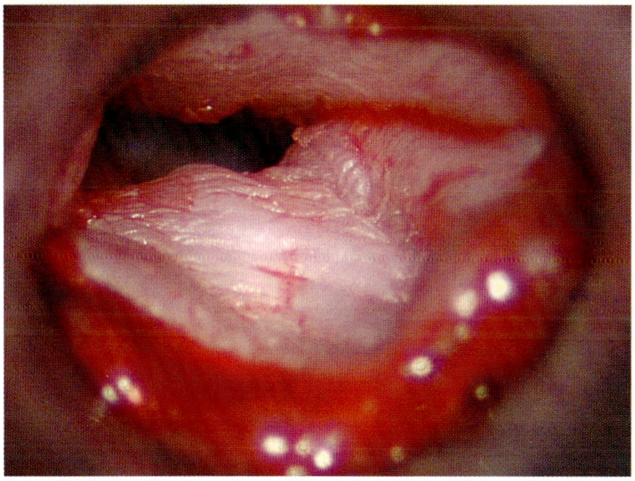

Fig. 3.6: Interim view after removal of posterior exostosis (right ear).

without causing a bleb. With exostoses already reducing the canal caliber, a bleb not only impedes visualization and dissection, but is also detrimental to the skin and subsequent healing.

Step 3

An incision is made several millimeters lateral to the exostoses to create a posterior vascular strip. Incision is made with a round knife, and extended superiorly and inferiorly around the canal to allow reflection of skin flap and adequate exposure for the anticipated drilling required to remove the exostoses.

Step 4

Skin flap is elevated over the bony prominence of the exostoses (Fig. 3.4) and drilling is begun.

Step 5

A skin flap protector made from suture foil can be placed between the exostoses and the canal skin flap to prevent inadvertent drill injury (Fig. 3.5). Use of a diamond drill can minimize risk of tearing the skin flap.

Step 6

In cases of large exostoses, skin flap elevation and drilling of exostoses may be performed in alternating fashion, i.e. as exposure is increased with drilling of exostoses, skin flap can be further elevated medially to allow more drilling (Figs. 3.6 and 3.7), until complete removal of exostoses is achieved (Fig. 3.8).

Step 7

Gelfoam packing soaked in an antibiotic-steroid solution is used to fill the canal following replacement of skin flaps. A nonadherent sheeting such as Silastic or Epifilm can be placed as an under-layer over the skin flaps prior to Gelfoam packing.

Surgical Technique: Osteoma Removal

Canalplasty for resection of osteoma is performed in a similar fashion to that described above for exostoses (Fig. 3.9).[6] Pedunculated osteomas can often be chiseled off with a curette or Freer elevator by fracturing its stalk from the canal wall, but in cases of broad-based lesions, a drill is similarly employed as for exostoses removal (Figs. 3.10 and 3.11).

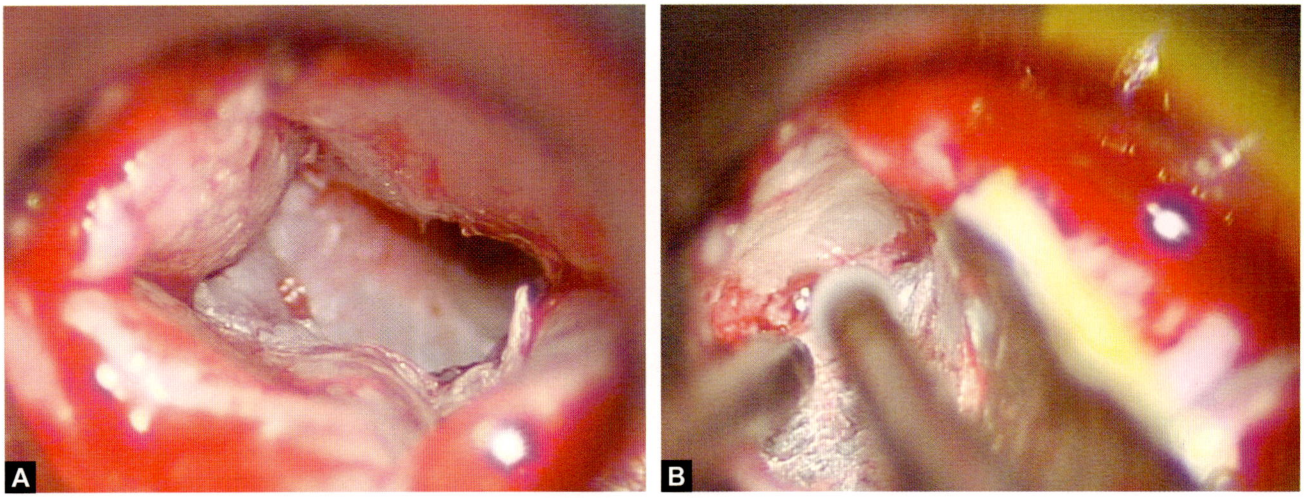

Figs. 3.7A and B: (A) Superior exostosis (right ear). (B) Drilling of superior exostosis (right ear).

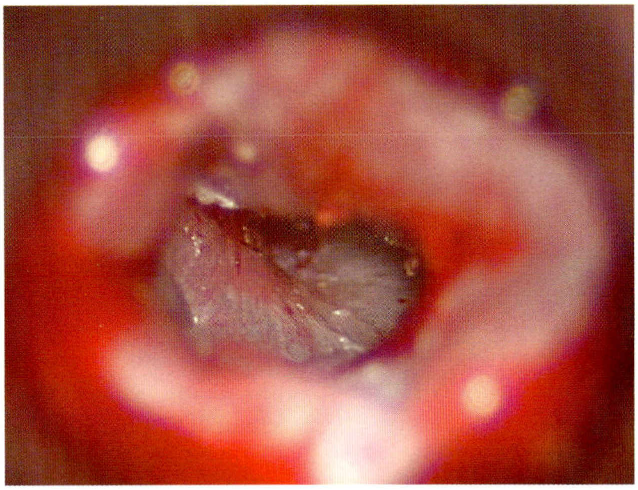

Fig. 3.8: Exostoses completely removed (right ear). Intraoperative view of tympanic membrane with canal skin flap edema.

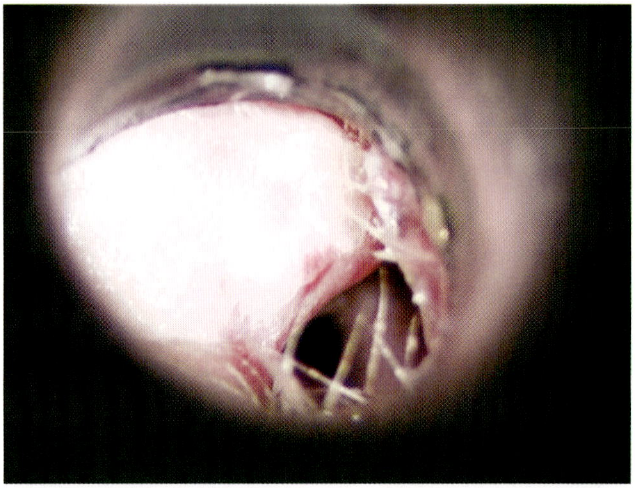

Fig. 3.9: Preoperative view of right external auditory canal osteoma. *Courtesy*: Ilka Naumann, MD.

Intraoperative Considerations and Complications: Exostoses and Osteomas

Surgical resection of osteomas and exostoses may be performed via a transcanal (Figs. 3.3 to 3.8) or postauricular (Figs. 3.9 to 3.11) approach. The postauricular technique undoubtedly provides superior access and exposure and affords familiar orientation to anatomical landmarks, and is consequently preferred in more challenging scenarios. However, safe removal of these lesions can be accomplished successfully with either approach as long as the appropriate technique is carefully chosen after a thorough preoperative assessment.

Facial nerve injury is a well-described complication of canalplasty. This usually results from excessive bone removal in the posterior and inferior direction, with inadvertent encroachment onto the mastoid portion of the facial nerve. Extra caution must be employed in transcanal canalplasty, as large lesions may cause apparent distortion of the canal to mastoid transition. Frequent verification of the location of dissection with temporal bone landmarks, as well as use of intraoperative facial nerve monitor, can help minimize this risk.

Although exostoses and osteomas are confined to the osseous canal, tympanoplasty may be required if the drum is violated during surgery. The tympanic membrane is most at risk when treating large obstructive

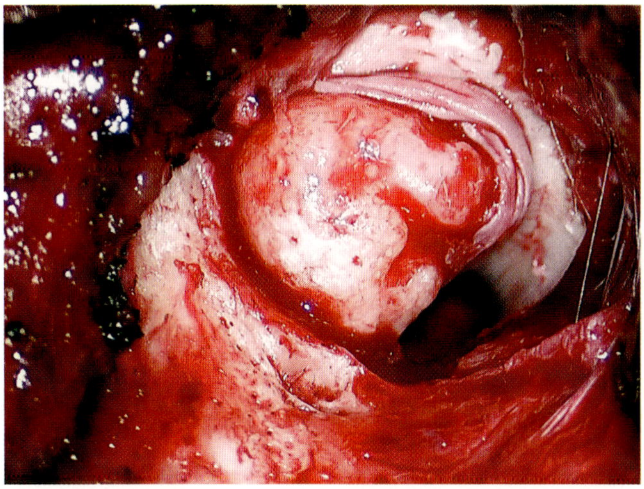

Fig. 3.10: Postauricular exposure of osteoma following skin flap elevation, right ear.
Courtesy: Ilka Naumann, MD.

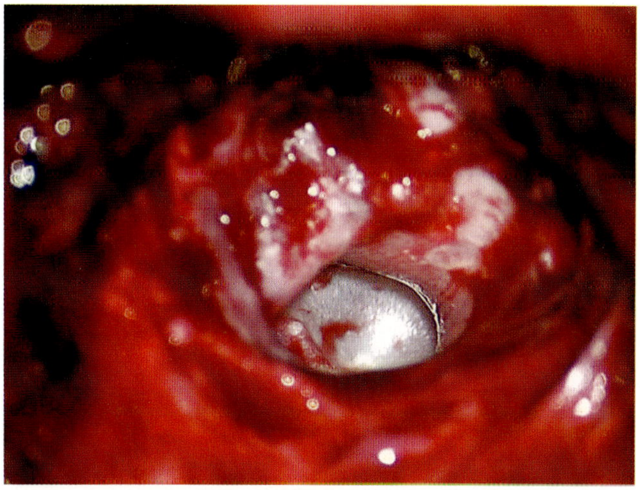

Fig. 3.11: Postresection of osteoma, right ear.
Courtesy: Ilka Naumann, MD.

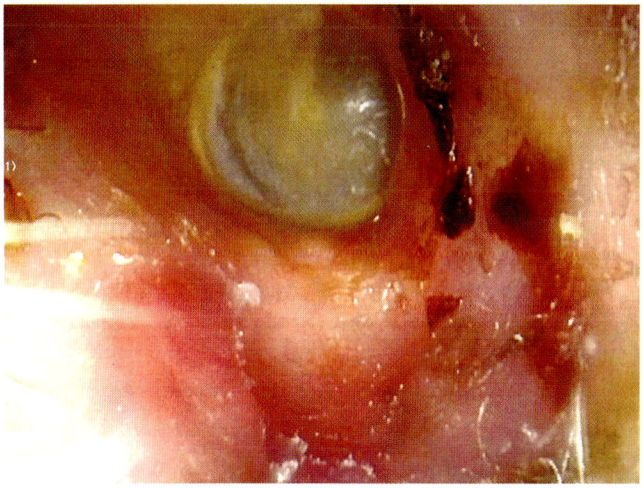

Fig. 3.12: Keratosis obturans with inferior canal wall remodeling (right ear).

lesions that abut the tympanic membrane. The depth and angle of the tympanic membrane must be kept in mind especially when dissection progresses medially. Choice of smaller drill bits aid in visualization, and appropriate use of foil protectors can help prevent iatrogenic drum perforation. Appropriate grafting should be performed if a perforation is created. Attention must also be taken not to drill onto the lateral process of the malleus, which can result in sensorineural hearing loss.

Anterior canal wall injury with prolapse of the temporomandibular joint can be avoided by careful thinning of bone with a diamond bur in this region. The anterior canal skin flap can be protected from drill injury by using a piece of suture foil as previously described. Significant areas of exposed bone that are not adequately covered by the vascular strip or skin flap should be grafted with fascia or split-thickness skin.

Postoperative Care: Exostoses and Osteomas

The patient is instructed to keep the packing moist by daily application of ototopical drops containing antibiotic and steroid, which help to prevent infection and reduce postsurgical inflammation, respectively. Dry ear precautions should be maintained. Packing is gradually removed over 4 to 6 weeks postoperatively.

KERATOSIS OBTURANS

Keratosis obturans is formed by tight compactions of desquamated keratin that result in obstruction of the bony EAC often causing acute otalgia and hearing loss. They tend to occur bilaterally and affect younger patients. A chronic inflammatory reaction develops, whereby the underlying canal skin becomes thickened and hyperplastic with increased epithelial sloughing and loss of its natural migratory ability.[7,8] Progressive accumulation of a laminar keratin plug leads to remodeling of the osseous canal with formation of a smooth-bordered crater that spares the tympanic membrane and annulus (Fig. 3.12).[8,9] Bronchiectasis and sinusitis are commonly associated conditions upon survey of past medical history.[7–9]

The mainstay of treatment consists of periodic office debridement with removal of the keratin plug and ototopicals for inflammation or infection resulting from

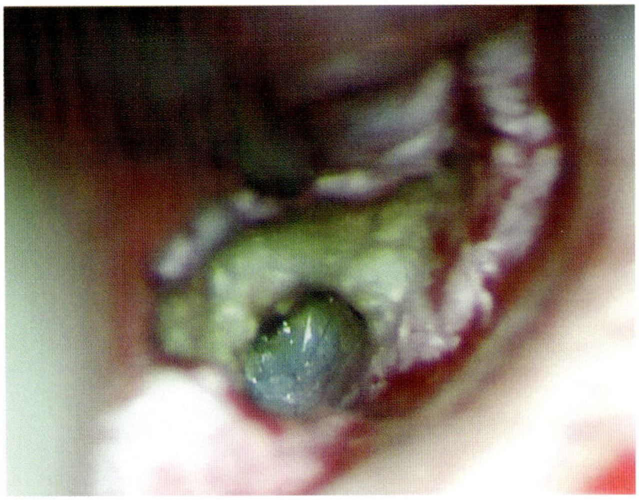

Fig. 3.13: Primary external auditory canal cholesteatoma in setting of congenital aural atresia with 1 mm lumen (left ear).

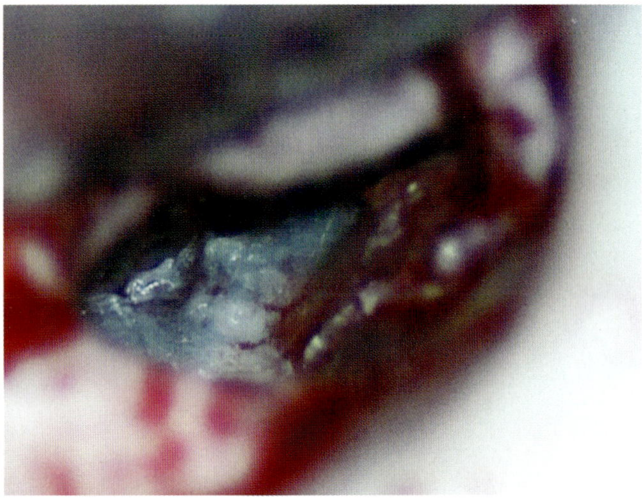

Fig. 3.14: Cholesteatoma spares drum with absence of bony erosion (left ear).

the impaction. Mineral oil is particularly useful during office cleaning, improving patient tolerance and facilitating complete removal. If severe pain precludes office management, debridement under anesthesia may be required. Home maintenance with good aural hygiene, avoidance of self-instrumentation, and irrigation with an acetic acid and alcohol solution may help keep symptoms at a controllable level. For cases resistant to conservative office treatment, canalplasty with resection of diseased epithelium and replacement with skin graft are performed. A split-thickness skin graft can be easily obtained from the posterior auricular surface with a #11 scalpel, or when a larger surface area is required, the medial upper arm or the upper lateral thigh are suitable donor sites for skin graft harvest using a dermatome. Alloderm can also be employed, and avoids donor site morbidity.

EAC CHOLESTEATOMA

Although EAC cholesteatoma is similar to keratosis obturans by virtue of accumulation of keratin debris in the canal, they are distinct clinical entities derived from different pathologic mechanisms.[9-11]Cholesteatoma arising in the ear canal can be primary or secondary. Primary canal cholesteatomas (Figs. 3.13 and 3.14) are rare, and are thought to arise from focal periostitis leading to bony sequestration and keratin entrapment. Secondary canal cholesteatomas may be caused by direct trauma or temporal bone fracture, infectious or inflammatory stenosis, or iatrogenic injury.

The keratin debris of canal cholesteatoma forms loose and flaky aggregates, as opposed to the densely packed concretions that characterize keratosis obturans.[10-12] These cholesteatomas are typically unilateral and present in older patients complaining of dull boring pain and otorrhea with conductive hearing loss.[12] Erosion of the canal wall is more common, in contrast to the smooth expansion seen with keratosis obturans.[10,12] Bony erosion may extend posteriorly into the mastoid (Figs. 3.15A and B) to involve the facial nerve. Anterior extension to the temporomandibular joint is less common. Debridement is the key treatment, with main goal of removing all the skin debris and clearing any necrotic bone. In severe cases of canal cholesteatomas, simple office debridement may be insufficient, and exteriorization with canalplasty and conchomeatoplasty may be required. Formal tympanomastoidectomy is rarely necessary.

ACQUIRED EAC STENOSIS

Acquired EAC stenosis is also known as medial canal fibrosis, whereby a circumferential plug of fibroinflammatory tissue forms and eventually obliterates the canal lumen resulting in a laterally positioned blind epithelial-lined pouch.[13,14] The condition typically results from infection or inflammation, and may be promoted by inadequate medical treatment along with an inherent predisposition to anomalous wound healing. Common causes include chronic otitis externa with or without underlying dermatopathy, ear canal instrumentation with resultant injury, temporal bone trauma, as well as prior otologic surgery leading to iatrogenic stenosis.[13-15] Prompt

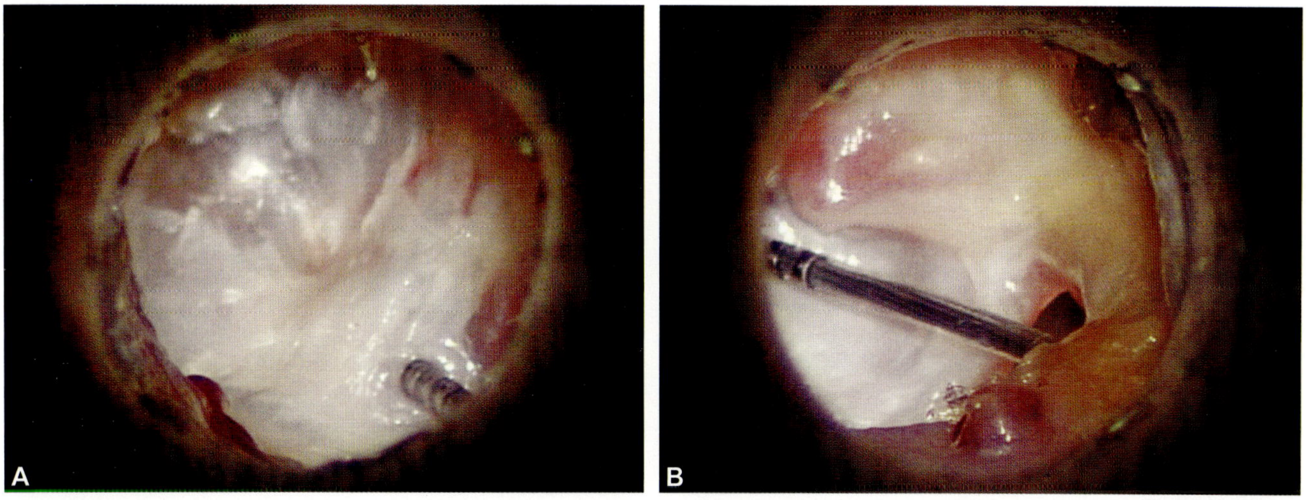

Figs. 13.5A and B: External auditory canal cholesteatoma with erosion of scutum and medial posterior canal wall resulting in exposure of cochlear implant lead (left ear).

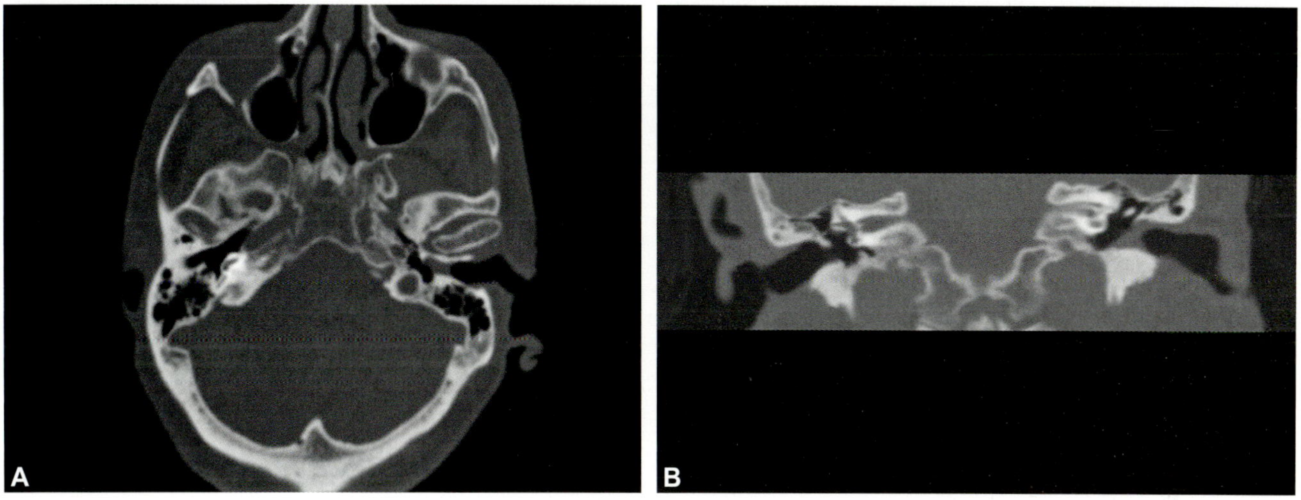

Figs. 3.16A and B: Axial and coronal CT temporal bone demonstrating acquired external auditory canal stenosis of left ear with fibroinflammatory soft-tissue plug filling the canal down to tympanic membrane. Middle ear and mastoid are spared.

treatment and atraumatic debridement of infection and raw granulation tissue are keys to prevention.

Following the acute phase, the patient often presents with conductive hearing loss and aural fullness without otorrhea or otalgia. A CT scan of the temporal bones demonstrates soft-tissue density filling the entire medial canal down to the tympanic membrane, the latter which becomes incorporated into the scar and is no longer distinguishable on imaging (Figs. 3.16A and B). Middle ear and mastoid are usually spared, unless there is concomitant cholesteatoma or chronic otitis media. Surgical treatment is performed to resect the obliterative scar to correct hearing loss and allow removal of concurrent disease.

Surgical Technique: Acquired EAC Stenosis

Step 1

Micro-otoscopic examination of the ear canal is performed. The location of the blind pouch stenosis is noted, occurring typically at or just lateral to the bony-cartilaginous junction (Fig. 3.17).

Step 2

A four-quadrant injection of the EAC is performed with local anesthetic and vasoconstrictor.

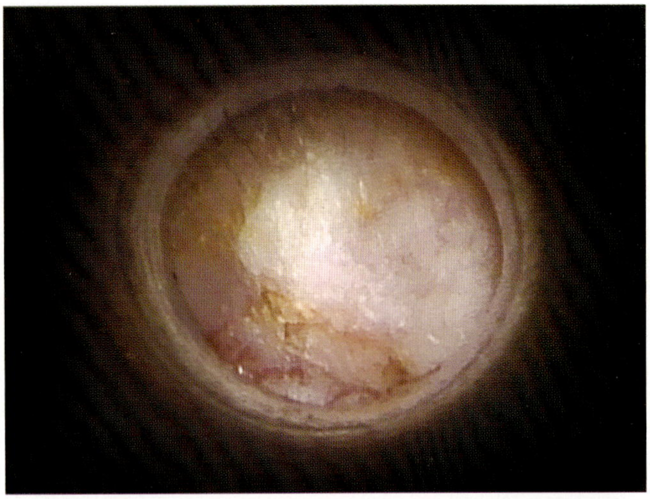

Fig. 3.17: Right external auditory canal acquired stenosis. Speculum view of blind-end pouch lined with epithelium.

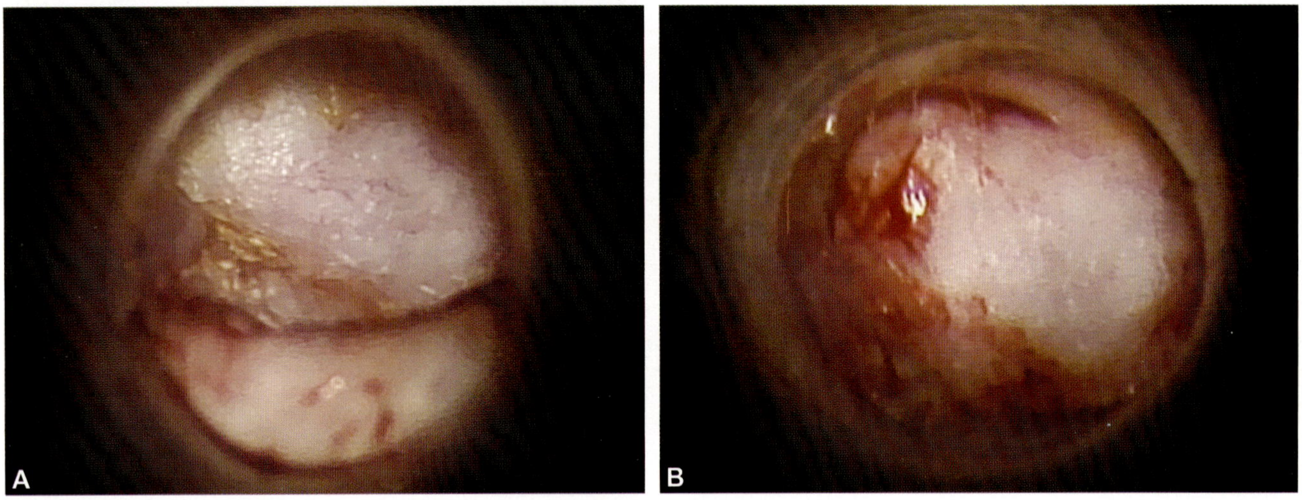

Figs. 3.18A and B: (A) Posterior canal incision is made just lateral to stenotic segment (right ear). (B) Incision is extended circumferentially around the canal (right ear).

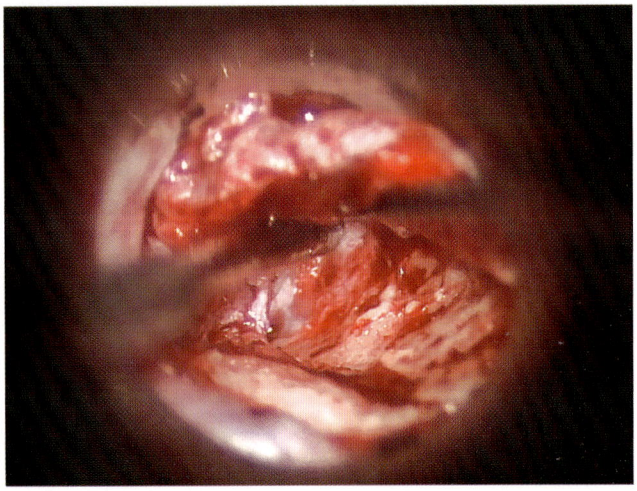

Fig. 3.19: Dissection of fibroinflammatory plug that fills medial extent of canal (right ear).

Step 3

The canal incision is made just lateral to the blindsac using a round knife and carried around circumferentially (Figs. 3.18A and B). Vascular strip is preserved.

Step 4

Dissection is carried out from the incision heading medially toward the tympanic membrane using a weapon or similar elevator (Fig. 3.19).

Step 5

The cicatrix can usually be dissected free from the medial layer of the tympanic membrane (Figs. 3.20A and B). If the scar is inseparable from the drum, the diseased portion is resected leaving a drum perforation to be repaired by tympanoplasty.

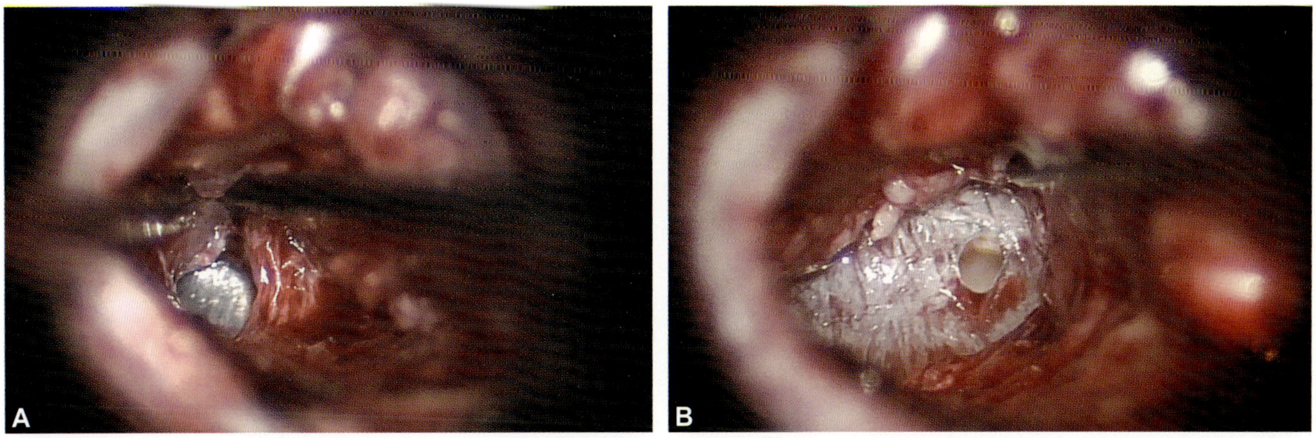

Figs. 3.20A and B: (A) Identification of tympanic membrane proper deep to fibroinflammatory plug (right ear). (B) Separation of cicatrix from the drum (right ear). A small posterior tympanic membrane perforation is revealed.

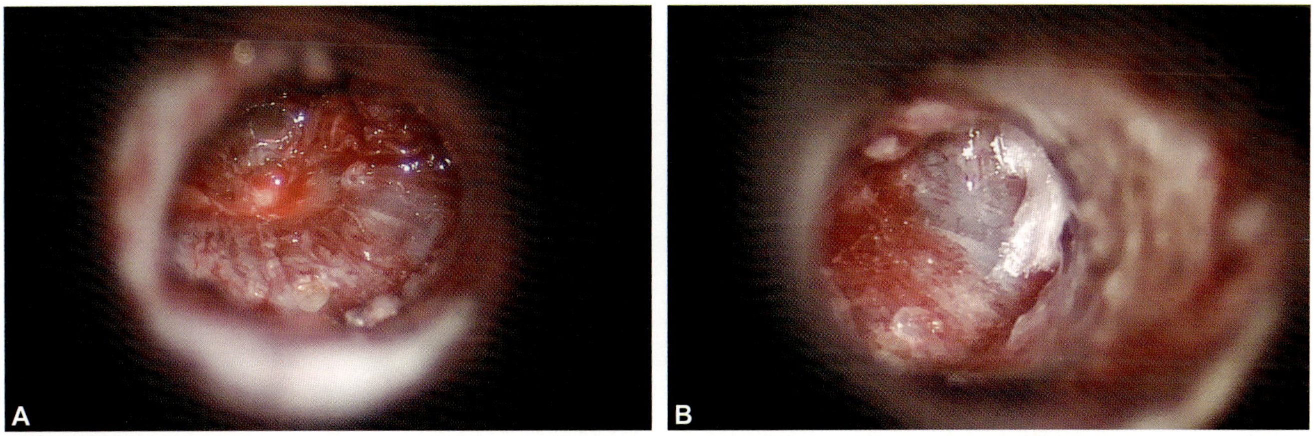

Figs. 3.21A and B: (A) Two small tympanic membrane perforations to be repaired (right ear). (B) Entrapped cholesteatoma inferiorly between drum and cicatrix (right ear).

Step 6

The drum is inspected for any perforations (Fig. 3.21A) or disease (Fig. 3.21B) that may have resulted from the inciting injury.

Step 7

Middle ear exploration is not always necessary, and should be guided by the presence of obvious or suspected disease such as infection or cholesteatoma.

Step 8

Medial or lateral grafting of the tympanic membrane is performed as needed (Fig. 3.22).

Step 9

The exposed bone of the osseous canal is lined with skin graft.

Step 10

Gelfoam packing soaked in an antibiotic-steroid solution is used to fill the canal. A nonadherent dressing such as Silastic or Epifilm can be placed as an under-layer over the skin flaps prior to Gelfoam packing.

Intraoperative Considerations and Complications: Acquired EAC Stenosis

Surgery for acquired EAC stenosis may be performed via a transcanal exposure with or without endaural extension or a postauricular incision. Choice of approach is guided by the adequacy of visualization, and can be successfully accomplished in both scenarios.

Restenosis of the canal postoperatively can be mitigated by meticulous surgical attention to several crucial steps. Full resection of the involved segment and

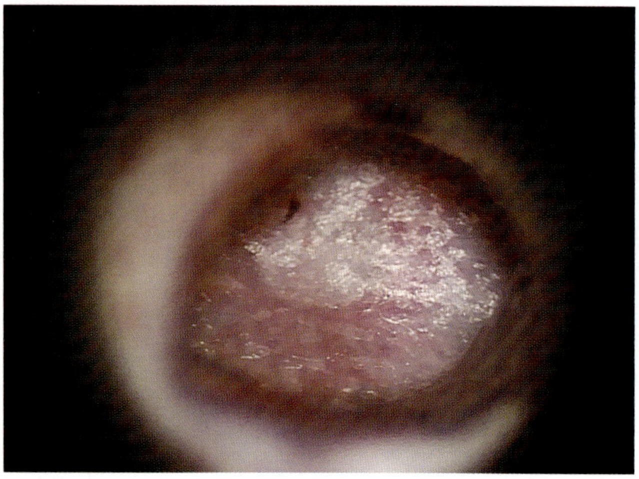

Fig. 3.22: Lateral grafting using Alloderm (right ear).

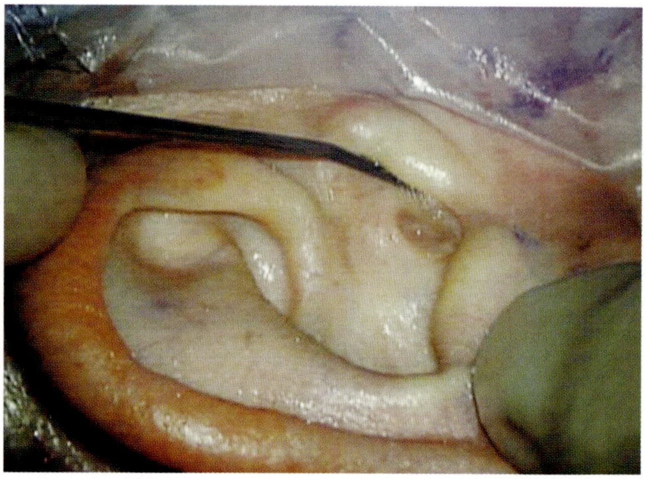

Fig. 3.23: Pit at site of atretic ear canal associated with type I microtia, right ear.
Courtesy: Eric Sargent, MD.

complete relining the canal with grafts are important. Leaving behind diseased skin with underlying inflammatory subcutaneous tissue may serve as a nidus for development of recalcitrant scarring. Bare areas of the canal should be covered with a skin graft to prevent healing by secondary intention that may promote granulation and recurrent scar. Some degree of mild restenosis from postsurgical inflammation and healing may be anticipated, and thus, canalplasty and conchomeatoplasty should be considered if necessary to establish a reasonable canal caliber.

Choice of graft material is dependent on the surgeon.[16] If concurrent tympanoplasty is required, temporalis fascia can be easily harvested in the surgical field. The EAC is lined with a split-thickness skin graft, which may be harvested from the posterior surface of the pinna or the upper lateral thigh. Alloderm is an acellular dermal matrix, and can also be used for canal coverage by applying it with dermal side down against the canal wall.

Postoperative Care: Acquired EAC Stenosis

The patient is instructed to keep the packing moist by applying ototopical drops containing antibiotic and steroid daily. Topical antibiotics help prevent infection, and the steroids aim to reduce expected postsurgical inflammation. Dry ear precautions should be maintained. Packing is gradually removed over 4 to 6 weeks postoperatively. Depending on graft take and degree of postsurgical swelling, tendency is toward slower removal of packing to ensure sufficient stenting of grafts circumferentially and prevention of restenosis during healing. Alternatively, a custom plug can be fashioned to serve as a stent to prevent circumferential restenosis during the early phase of wound healing. Close monitoring and aggressive treatment of any infection during the postoperative period is crucial to achieve optimal results. However, restenosis rates continue to be relatively high.[14-16]

CONGENITAL AURAL ATRESIA

Congenital aural atresia is a rare condition resulting from failure of canalization of the first branchial cleft during fetal development. Consequently, there is persistence of the epithelial plug and the tympanic ring remains as a bony atresia plate at the level of the tympanic membrane.[3] Severity is variable, ranging from complete absence of the EAC (Fig. 3.23) to a partially formed canal ending in a blind sac. Other times, there may be a stenotic and tortuous canal that leads to an abnormal tympanic membrane and ossicular mass (Figs. 3.24A and B).[3,17] Conductive hearing loss is caused by the varying combination of canal, drum, or ossicular malformation. In 10–47% cases, there may be concomitant sensorineural hearing loss as well.[17-19] The incidence of atresia is 1 in 10,000, and 10% are associated with identifiable syndromes. Of the nonsyndromic majority, 5% are linked to an inherited genetic defect, and the remainder are blamed on anomalous temporal bone formation during fetal development. Unilateral atresia is seven times more common than bilateral cases.[18,19]

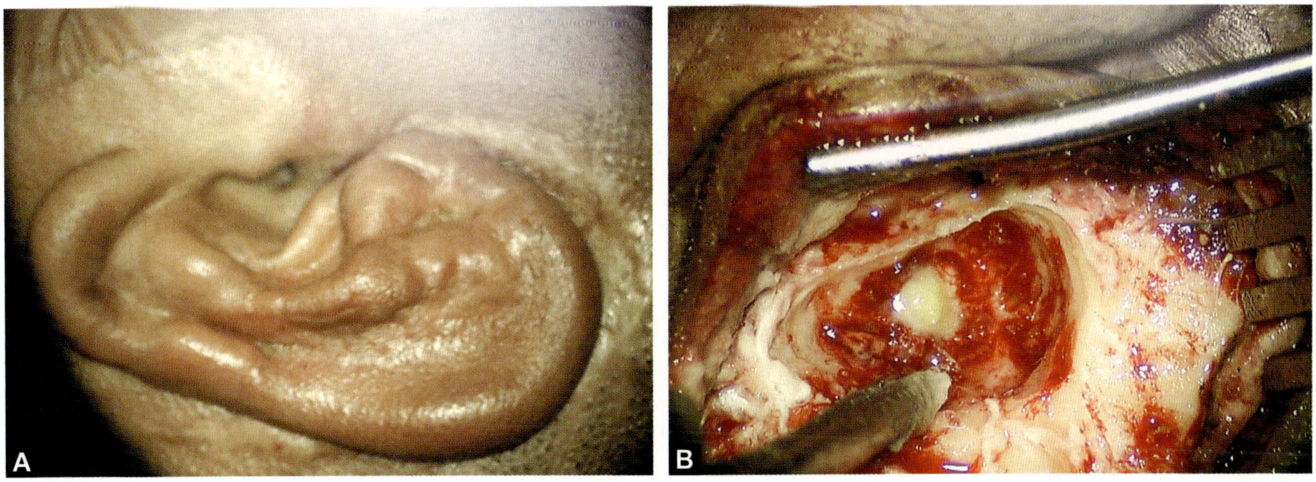

Figs. 3.24A and B: Congenital aural atresia presenting with chronic otorrhea via a pinpoint canal, with associated microtia status postauricular reconstruction (left ear).

Table 3.1: Jahrsdoerfer's preoperative grading system of candidacy for congenital aural atresia repair (1992)

Parameter	*Points*	*Rating*	*Projected Success of Repair*
Stapes present	2	10	Excellent
Oval window open	1	9	Very Good
Middle ear space	1	8	Good
Facial nerve	1	7	Fair
Malleus-incus	1	6	Marginal
Mastoid penumatized	1	≤5	Poor
Incus-stapes	1		
Round window	1		
External ear appearance	1		
Total Score	**10**		

Surgical correction aims to restore the normal ear canal and improve hearing. Challenges abound in this demanding operation; familiarity with variations in temporal bone anatomy and meticulous surgical technique are paramount to a successful outcome.[17,20-22] Preoperative CT scan of the temporal bones aids in the selection of appropriate surgical candidates. Comprehensive counseling of the patient and family should be undertaken to discuss anticipated benefits, predicted hearing outcomes, and potential complications. There is a substantially increased risk of facial nerve injury and sensorineural hearing loss compared to routine ear surgeries.[23] The facial nerve is often positioned more anteriorly and laterally than normal due to failure of the mastoid to migrate in the usual posterior and inferior direction during embryologic development. Use of intraoperative facial nerve monitoring and stimulating dissectors is critical but does not replace knowledge of anatomy and thorough preoperative planning. Insomuch as primary correction of hearing loss is desired, it is prudent to recognize the unfavorable surgical candidate where improvement is at best limited, and to offer alternative solutions to aural rehabilitation.

Jahrsdoerfer's grading system (Table 3.1)[24] is mainly based on preoperative CT temporal bone findings and provides an excellent guide for candidate selection. Presence of the stapes is given the heaviest weighting among all the parameters considered, as it plays a crucial role in determining ultimate success or failure of the procedure. If a fixed stapes is encountered, staged surgery is usually required. As in chronic ear surgery, the ability to create and maintain a well-aerated middle ear space greatly affects the hearing results. Deformity of the external ear has been correlated to the degree of middle ear abnormality. Presence of good cochlear function and lack of inner ear malformation on imaging must be established before undertaking surgical correction of atresia.[17,18,21]

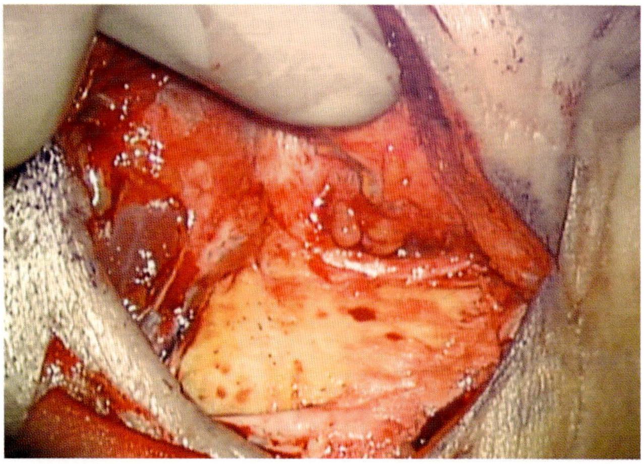

Fig. 3.25: Anterior reflection of auricle with exposure of mastoid cortex (right ear).
Courtesy: Eric Sargent, MD.

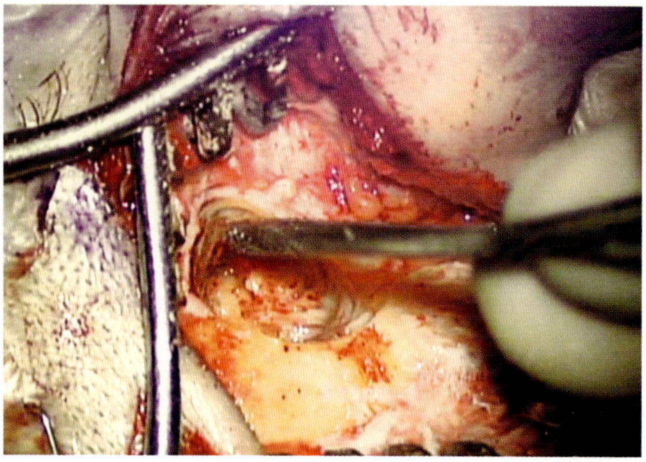

Fig. 3.26: Drilling through atretic plate (right ear).
Courtesy: Eric Sargent, MD.

Patients who score favorably (7–10) per the grading scale have a 70–80% chance of achieving normal hearing in the hands of an experienced surgeon.[17,22,24] Surgery is typically performed around 6–7 years of age, and presence of concurrent microtia is taken into consideration. It is generally agreed upon that reconstructive surgery of the auricle should precede that of atresia repair. However, exact timing of surgery is varied based on the severity of microtia, use of synthetic versus autologous materials for cosmetic reconstruction, and whether unilateral or bilateral atresia correction is undertaken. In-depth discussion of these considerations is beyond the scope of this chapter, and the reader is referred to the many excellent reviews on the subject.[17–24]

Surgical Technique: Congenital Aural Atresia

Step 1

A postauricular skin incision is made 5–10 mm behind the postauricular sulcus using a #15 scalpel. A reconstructed auricle is less pliable and must be treated with extra care.

Step 2

Incision is carried through the subcutaneous tissues staying lateral to the temporalis fascia and musculoperiosteal layer.

Step 3

A T-shaped incision is made along the temporal line, with a vertical limb perpendicular to it down toward the mastoid tip. The Bovie electrocautery is used cautiously, and should be avoided completely if there are any concerns of facial nerve anomaly.

Step 4

Musculoperiosteal flaps are elevated using a Lempert to expose the mastoid cortex (Fig. 3.25). The zygomatic root and glenoid fossa are important landmarks in atresia surgery and should be exposed by adequate anterior elevation. Weitlaner retractors are placed.

Step 5

The tympanic bone remnant is represented by a slight divot in the area of the expected EAC, and serves as a pointer to the middle ear.

Step 6

Drilling is begun at the tympanic bone remnant. If the remnant cannot be located, drilling is started in the cribriform area of the mastoid process just posterior to the glenoid fossa, staying superiorly near the linea temporalis (Fig. 3.26).

Step 7

The tegmen is first identified, and defines the superior extent of dissection.

Step 8

Drilling proceeds medially to identify the antrum. A diamond bur should be employed when approaching the deeper planes of dissection where critical anatomy is anticipated.

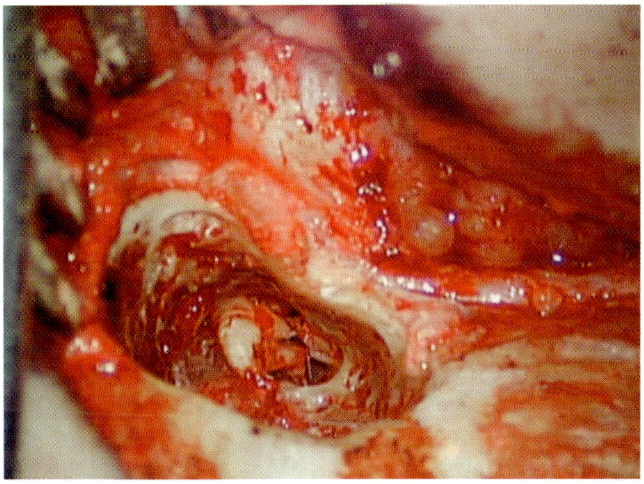

Fig. 3.27: View of incus, foreshortened malleus and stapes (right ear).
Courtesy: Eric Sargent, MD.

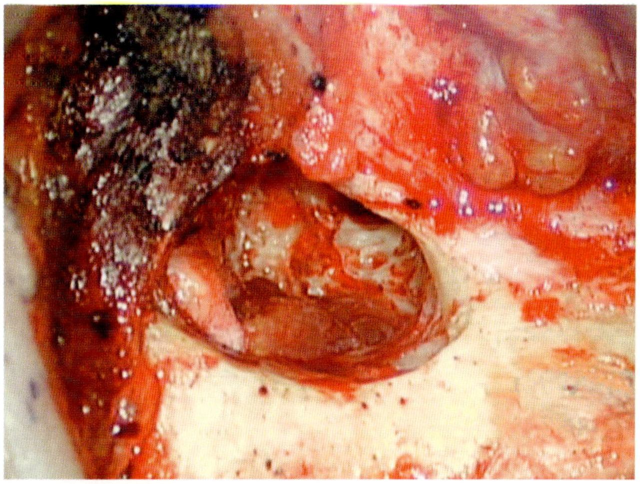

Fig. 3.28: Cartilage, bone pate and temporalis fascia are laid over the reconstructed posterior-superior canal wall (right ear).
Courtesy: Eric Sargent, MD.

Step 9

Mastoid air cells may be encountered, but dissection should be limited to the anterosuperior region with aim to open into the antrum and identify the horizontal semicircular canal and ossicles. The expected course of the facial nerve should be mapped out with stimulating instruments.

Step 10

The incus is visualized. The rest of the atretic plate is cautiously removed to define the epitympanum and remaining ossicles (Fig. 3.27).

Step 11

The iter chordae may emanate from the facial nerve in an aberrant position, but is preserved whenever possible.

Step 12

Opened mastoid air cells should be blocked off with cartilage, bone pate, or hydroxyapatite material. A piece of temporalis fascia is draped over these areas (Fig. 3.28).

Step 13

Temporalis fascia is used as a scaffold for the new tympanic membrane, and is tucked into the anterior bony annulus, brought over the ossicles and epitympanum, and draped onto the posterior canal wall. Gelfoam is placed in the middle ear around the ossicles to help support the fascia graft.

Step 14

Split thickness skin graft (STSG) is harvested from the upper lateral thigh or the medial upper arm using a dermatome to obtain a hairless reconstruction.

Step 15

Meatoplasty is performed in a similar fashion to the usual (*see* Chapter 7).

Step 16

The lateral end of the STSG is juxtaposed to the meatal skin and stabilized using 5-0 plain or chromic gut sutures. Two to three strips of STSG are typically used to line the reconstructed tympanic membrane and EAC. The thicker end of the STSG is oriented at the meatal side, with the thinner end over the drum (Fig. 3.29).

Step 17

Silastic sheeting is used along the length of the canal to line the grafts and provide a nonadherent surface to facilitate later packing removal (Fig. 3.29).Gelfoam packing soaked in ototopical antibiotic and steroid solution is placed in the canal from the neotympanic membrane out to the reconstructed meatus.

Step 18

Postauricular deep subcutaneous soft tissues and musculoperiosteal layer is closed using a 3-0 absorbable braided suture, e.g. Vicryl, to maintain an anteroinferior to posterosuperior pull to help resuspend the auricle in its natural position.

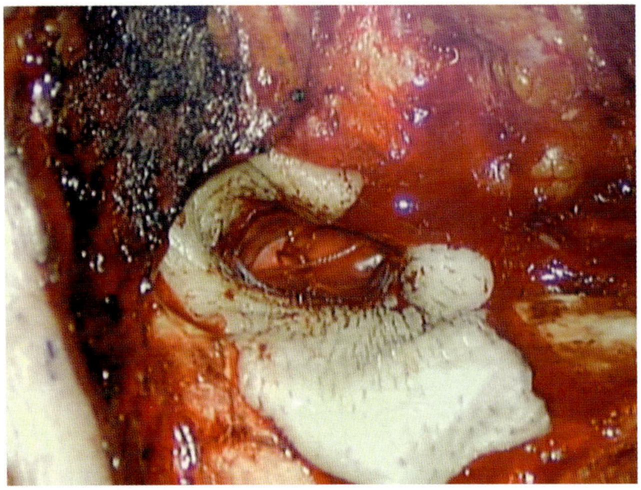

Fig. 3.29: Reconstructed tympanic membrane, with split thickness skin graft lining canal and Silastic sheeting in place (right ear). *Courtesy*: Eric Sargent, MD.

INTRAOPERATIVE CONSIDERATIONS AND COMPLICATIONS: CONGENITAL AURAL ATRESIA

Discerning the appropriate location to begin drilling may be challenging at times. Be aware that the posterior wall of the glenoid fossa may mimic the posterior bony canal wall. Soft tissues anterior to this should be gently elevated in the usual fashion. If the osseous canal is present, the normal canal skin should lift off easily from the posterior canal wall. In the absence of canal development, the thick, tougher, fibrous tissues of the temporomandibular joint capsule will be encountered when dissection is attempted. Additionally, if the glenoid fossa is mistaken for the posterior canal wall, it would be situated further anteriorly to the auricular soft tissues and the mastoid tip than expected, although these relationships may be distorted in severe atresia cases.

When creating the new EAC, avoid drilling too far posteriorly. A wide mastoidectomy is not required nor is desired, and creates need for future regular maintenance. Congenital aural atresia is not typically associated with chronic otitis media or disease except in cases of concurrent congenital cholesteatoma, or secondarily acquired cholesteatoma that may result from poor ventilation through a stenotic canal causing postobstructive infection. If the anatomy is difficult and normal landmarks are not readily identifiable, drill posteriorly to delineate the sinodural angle. Identification of the sigmoid sinus and tegmen will help orient the surgeon to the expected location of the antrum. A pneumatized cavity provides easier distinction between the mastoid cavity proper and the neocanal being drilled as air cells can serve as a guide. In sclerotic cavities, the horizontal semicircular canal and ossicles may "pop through" suddenly once the last layer of the atretic plate is removed. Care must be taken to avoid drill trauma to these structures due to the risk of resultant sensorineural hearing loss.

A variety of ossicular presentations may be encountered. The incus and malleus handle are the most easily injured due to their superficial positions and attachment to the atresia plate. To minimize drill trauma to the ossicular chain, bone of the atretic plate should be adequately thinned with the drill, leaving the last remaining layer to be removed with microinstruments such as a Rosen needle or right-angle pick.[25] The CO_2 laser can be employed to atraumatically free up any remaining connections between the ossicles and atresia plate. Occasionally, a fibrous remnant of the tympanic membrane may remain attached to the malleus handle and can be preserved.

Once the entire ossicular chain is freed, the remaining bony atretic plate should be drilled out anteriorly up to the glenoid fossa to recreate as much of the anterior sulcus as possible to minimize future blunting. Caution must be used to avoid violating the temporomandibular joint, which can cause joint prolapse and is difficult to correct.

The ossicular chain should be carefully examined and mobility confirmed. Presence of the stapes reflex upon facial nerve stimulation is an excellent sign. Correction of concomitant congenital ossicular fixation is usually deferred to a separate operation, although this is dependent on the exact findings encountered and surgeon preference. If active infection or congenital cholesteatoma is discovered during aural atresia repair, ossicular work should be staged. Silastic is sometimes used as a spacer between the ossicles and surrounding bone to minimize future risk of refixation.

The surgeon must remain cognizant of the anomalous facial nerve during dissection.[17,22-23] Drill potentials on the intraoperative monitor provide indication of facial nerve proximity. Once all the bony work is completed, the facial nerve should be restimulated to confirm proper function. It is good practice to perform periodic stimulation throughout atresia surgery, so that the integrity of the facial nerve can be monitored throughout the procedure.

The location of the external auditory meatus is often obvious in mild cases of atresia. In severe atresia with associated microtia, especially if the tragus is absent, the location of the new meatus must be carefully determined. The drilled bony anatomy is used as a reference to guide design and positioning of the meatus. Resection of conchal cartilage and use of retention sutures are keys to maintaining a wide open meatus.

POSTOPERATIVE CARE: EAR CANAL SURGERY

In most cases of ear canal surgery discussed above, canal packing with absorbable gelatin sponge (e.g. Gelfoam) is used. The patient is instructed to apply ototopical drops containing antibiotic and steroid daily. Topical antibiotics help prevent infection, and the steroids reduce postsurgical inflammation. Dry ear precautions should be maintained. Packing is gradually removed over 4 to 6 weeks postoperatively.

Depending on graft take and degree of postsurgical swelling, the tendency is toward slower removal of packing after repair of canal stenosis or atresia surgery to ensure sufficient stenting of the grafts circumferentially to limit restenosis during the healing phase. A custom plug may be created to help prevent restenosis. Close monitoring and aggressive treatment of any infection during the postoperative period are crucial to achieve optimal results.

REFERENCES

1. Kroon DF, Strasnick BS. Diseases of the auricle, external auditory canal, and tympanic membrane. In: Glasscock ME, Gulya AJ (Eds). Glasscock-Shambaugh's Surgery of the Ear, 5th edition. Hamilton, Ontario, Canada: BC Decker Inc; 2003. pp. 345-67.
2. Storper IS, Canalis RF, Lambert PR. Disease of the auricle and periauricular region. In: Canalis RF, Lambert PR (Eds). The Ear: Comprehensive Otology, 1st edition. Philadelphia, PA: Lippincott Williams and Wilkins; 2000. pp. 325-39.
3. Francis HW. Anatomy of the temporal bone, external ear, and middle ear. In: Flint PW, Haughey BH, Lund VJ, Niparko JK, Richardson MA, Robbins KR, Thomas JR (Eds). Cumming's Otolaryngology Head and Neck Surgery, 5th edition. Philadelphia, PA: Mosby Elsevier; 2010. pp. 1821-30.
4. Van Gilse PHG. Des observations ulterieures sur la genes des exostoses du conduit externe par l'irritations d'eau froide. Acta Otolaryngol (Stockh). 1938;26:343.
5. Wong BF, Cervantes W, Doyle KJ, et al. Prevalence of external auditory canal exostoses in surfers. Arch Otolaryngol Head Neck Surg. 1999;125:969-72.
6. Fisher EW, McManus TC. Surgery for external auditory canal exostoses and osteomata. J Laryngol Otol. 1994;108:106-10.
7. Morrison AW. Keratosis obturans. J Laryngol Otol. 1956;70: 317-21.
8. Corbridge RJ, Michaels L, Wright T. Epithelial migration in keratosis obturans. Am J Otolaryngol. 1996;17:411-4.
9. Piepergerdes JC, Kramer BM, Behnke EE. Keratosis obturans and external auditory canal cholesteatoma. Laryngoscope. 1980;90:383-90.
10. Shinnabe A, Hara M, Hasegawa M, et al. A comparison of patterns of disease extension in keratosis obturans and external auditory canal cholesteatoma. Otol Neurotol. 2013; 34(1):91-4.
11. Revadi G, Prepageran N, Raman R, et al. Epithelial migration on the external ear canal wall in normal and pathologic ears. Otol Neurotol. 2011;32(3):504-7.
12. Dubach P, Mantokoudis G, Caversaccio M. Ear canal cholesteatoma: meta-analysis of clinical characteristics with update on classification, staging and treatment. Curr Opin Otolaryngol Head Neck Surg. 2010;18(5):369-76.
13. Heeneman H. Surgical correction of the stenosed ear canal. J Otolaryngol. 1979;8:461-2.
14. El-Sayed Y. Acquired medial canal fibrosis. J Laryngol Otol. 1998;112:145-9.
15. Selesnick S, Nguyen TP, Eisenman DJ. Surgical treatment of acquired external auditory canal atresia. Am J Otol. 1998; 19:123-30.
16. McCary WS, Kryzer TC, Lambert PR. Application of split-thickness skin grafts for acquired diseases of the external auditory canal. Am J Otol. 1995;16:801-5.
17. Jahrsdoerfer RA. Surgery for congenital aural atresia. In: Glasscock ME, Gulya AJ (Eds). Glasscock-Shambaugh's Surgery of the Ear, 5th edition. Hamilton, Ontario, Canada: BC Decker Inc; 2003. pp. 389-99.
18. Cole RR, Jahrsdoerfer RA. Congenital aural atresia. Clin Plast Surg. 1990;19(2):367-71.
19. Spring PM, Gianoli GJ. Congenital aural atresia. J La State Med Soc. 1997;149(1):6-9.
20. Shih L, Crabtree JA. Long-term surgical results for congenital aural atresia. Laryngoscope. 1993;103(10):1097-102.
21. Service GJ, Roberson JB Jr. Current concepts in repair of aural atresia. Curr Opin Otolaryngol Head Neck Surg. 2010;18(6): 536-8.
22. Cressman WR, Pensak ML. Surgical aspects of congenital aural atresia. Otolaryngol Clin North Am. 1994;27(3):621-33.
23. Jahrsdoerfer RA, Lambert PR. Facial nerve injury in congenital aural atresia surgery. Am J Otol. 1998;19:283-7.
24. Jahrsdoerfer RA, Yeakley JW, Aguilar EA, et al. Grading system for the selection of patients with congenital aural atresia. AM J Otol. 1992;13:6-12.
25. Eze N, Jiang D, O'Connor AF. The atretic plate—a conduit for drill vibration to the inner ear? Acta Otolaryngol. 2014; 134(1):14-8.

CHAPTER

4 Otosclerosis and Stapedectomy

Seilesh C Babu, Emily Z Stucken

INTRODUCTION

Otosclerosis is a disorder of bone metabolism characterized by osteoclastic breakdown of otic capsule bone followed by its replacement with immature vascular, and eventually, dense sclerotic bone. Otosclerosis is inherited by autosomal dominant transmission with incomplete penetrance, and likely represents a complex genetic disease that requires a combination of genetic and environmental factors to become manifest.[1]

HISTORICAL PERSPECTIVE

The pathological process underlying the disease now known as otosclerosis was first described by Valsalva in 1735. This disease process was termed "otosclerosis" by Politzer in 1893.[2] Attempts at surgical correction of otosclerosis date back to 1876, when Kessel described a procedure designed to counteract stapes fixation through mobilization or removal of the stapes. In the 1900s, the treatment paradigm shifted to semicircular canal fistulization to improve hearing without altering the ossicular chain. In the early 1950s, stapes mobilization once again became the operation of choice to treat otosclerosis, and in 1954, Shambaugh introduced the operating microscope to stapes mobilizations. Shortly thereafter, Shea described a technique of stapedectomy that set the framework for most modern stapes operations: stapedectomy with the maintenance of an intact ossicular chain and a covered oval window.[2]

CONCEPTS IN SURGICAL TREATMENT

Since the original description by Shea in 1958, several major modifications of stapes surgery have been described. Both complete stapedectomy procedures and small-fenestration stapedotomy procedures are currently practiced. In a complete stapedectomy, the entire stapes footplate is removed and the oval window is covered with a tissue graft that supports a prosthesis. This is in contrast to the stapedotomy procedure in which a fenestration is created into an intact and fixed footplate to seat the prosthesis; this is then surrounded by fascia. Currently, stapedotomy procedures are favored by many and are performed more frequently. Though some studies have favored stapedotomy technique,[3,4] others have surmised that both techniques are effective in practiced hands.[5,6]

THE USE OF LASERS IN STAPES SURGERY

Lasers were introduced to stapes surgery in 1980 by Perkins.[7] The use of the laser in stapes surgery, and particularly in revision stapes surgery, facilitates a surgeon's ability to perform atraumatic tissue dissection. Operating with the laser, a surgeon is able to vaporize tissue while leaving underlying attachments undisturbed and thus reduce mechanical trauma to normal structures. The laser is also used by many surgeons to create a precise stapedotomy fenestration. The two main classes of lasers used in stapes surgery are visible spectrum lasers (Argon, 488 nm and KTP, 532 nm), and infrared spectrum lasers (CO_2, 10,600 nm). Visible spectrum lasers were first to be described in stapes surgery. The visible wavelength of the Argon and KTP lasers allows for simultaneous aiming and vaporizing, and these lasers are easily delivered through a fiberoptic cable. The chromophore for the Argon and KTP lasers is melanin, which has led to a concern that laser energy may pass unencumbered through the perilymphatic fluid and be absorbed by the underlying pigmented stria vascularis. This could theoretically lead to cellular damage and sensorineural hearing loss, a dreaded complication of stapedectomy surgery.[8] The CO_2 laser, conversely, is in the infrared spectrum and thus requires a Helium-Neon aiming beam that must be calibrated and checked before each use. Until recently, the CO_2 laser could only be delivered by a micromanipulator under direct line of sight; however, the introduction of the OmniGuide (OmniGuide, Inc, Cambridge, MA) system has allowed for delivery through a flexible laser fiber. The chromophore for the CO_2 laser is water; thus, laser energy is absorbed by the footplate bone and superficial perilymph, and heat is not transmitted to the underlying neurosensory portion of the cochleovestibular system.[8] While there is a theoretical risk with the use of visible spectrum lasers in stapedectomy, studies have not demonstrated an increased risk of sensorineural hearing loss in practice,[9] and both classes of laser are routinely used for stapedectomy surgery.

PATIENT SELECTION

The vast majority of patients affected by otosclerosis will exhibit a conductive or mixed hearing loss. A small percentage with cochlear otosclerosis may present with a purely sensorineural loss. Patients are most often diagnosed in young adulthood; those who present at a younger age should be considered to have congenital stapes fixation or other congenital ossicular abnormality. Fifty percent of patients will have a family history of otosclerosis.[10] Candidates for stapedectomy should exhibit at least a 15 dB air-bone gap on audiogram. The conductive loss usually presents in the low frequencies early on in the disease. As the disease progresses, a wider frequency range is affected and a greater air-bone gap is seen. Audiogram may also demonstrate a Carhart's notch—a depression in the bone conduction line most prominent at 2,000 Hz. Carhart's notch is attributed to the absence of normal ossicular vibration when a bone conduction device is placed on the mastoid, and usually improves with surgical correction of stapes fixation. Those patients who present with mixed hearing loss may achieve improved hearing aid use with closure of their air-bone gap. Patients who present with mainly sensorineural hearing loss may be difficult to diagnose. Discovery of the chronicity of hearing loss with inspection of prior audiograms as well as a family history of otosclerosis may provide clues to the diagnosis in this patient population.

Impedance testing is a valuable adjunct to audiological testing. Acoustic reflexes are generally absent to bilateral stimuli in patients affected by otosclerosis. This test can be used to distinguish patients with otosclerosis from patients with superior semicircular canal dehiscence who may demonstrate a similar conductive hearing loss in the presence of intact acoustic reflexes. Patients with superior semicircular canal dehiscence will also display characteristic findings on vestibular evoked myogenic potential (VEMP) testing and CT scans of the temporal bone that will clarify the diagnosis. Other etiologies of conductive hearing loss include tympanosclerosis, middle ear effusion, cholesteatoma, ossicular discontinuity, Paget's disease, and osteogenesis imperfecta; these should be evaluated for prior to consideration of stapedectomy.

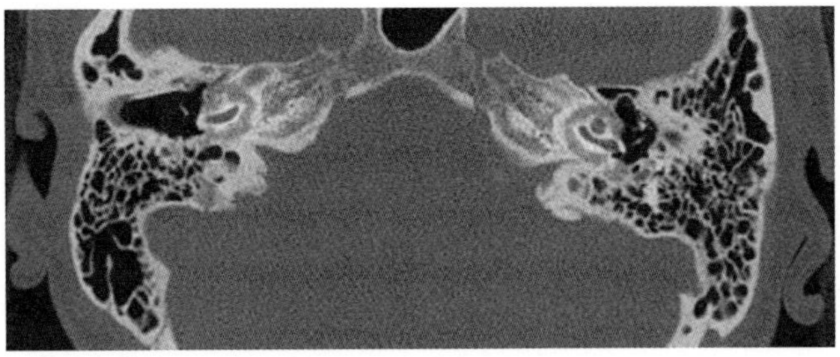

Fig. 4.1: Axial CT scan through the cochlea demonstrating the double ring sign, indicative of cochlear otosclerosis.

On examination, patients should have a relatively normal otoscopic examination without middle ear fluid, perforation of the tympanic membrane, retraction, cholesteatoma, or other evidence of chronic infections such as significant myringosclerosis. Evidence of chronic infection may lead the examiner to suspect an etiology of conductive hearing loss other than otosclerosis. An examination with a 512 Hz tuning fork should elicit a negative response to Rinne testing (bone conduction greater than air conduction), and a Weber test will lateralize to the side with the greater conductive loss.

Imaging is not necessary in majority of cases, but it may be useful if superior semicircular canal dehiscence, congenital hearing loss, or revision surgery is being considered. In the case of otosclerosis, a CT scan of the temporal bones is often normal. In some instances, a focus of lucency at the fissula ante fenestram may be identified. Advanced disease may be signified by sclerotic filling of the oval window niche, and the classic "double ring," or "halo" sign may been seen in cochlear otosclerosis (Fig. 4.1).

PREOPERATIVE COUNSELING AND INFORMED CONSENT

All patients with otosclerosis should be offered the options of observation and hearing amplification as alternatives to surgery. If the patient elects to pursue surgical correction, primary stapedectomy has a success rate of 90–95% of closure of the air-bone gap to within 10 dB.[11] Success rates with stapedectomy surgery are dependent on operator experience,[12] and so a surgeon should quote their personal success rate with the operation in addition to published data. Revision stapedectomy success rates are decidedly lower, though published success rates vary widely from 18% to 80%.[9] The patient should be informed of the risk of a dead ear, which in most series is 1% or less.[11] This risk rises up to 14% in revision procedures.[9] Significant sensorineural hearing loss may occur even after a routine, uncomplicated procedure. The patient should be informed of the possibility of postoperative taste disturbance that may be temporary or permanent. Facial nerve paralysis is extremely rare. The patient should understand the possibility of the need for future surgery, as up to 20% of cases may eventually require a revision surgery.[13]

PROSTHESIS SELECTION

Numerous prostheses are available for stapedectomy. The composition of different prostheses varies and includes titanium, platinum, Teflon, Nitinol, gold, and stainless steel. Consideration should be made of the use of nonferromagnetic implants so as to allow for MRI compatibility. Good results have been reported using an array of prostheses. Ultimately, the choice of prosthesis used should be made on the basis of surgeon preference.

SURGICAL TECHNIQUE: STAPEDOTOMY

Patient Positioning

The patient is placed in a supine position with the head turned away from the operative side. No pillows are used, and the patient's head may need to be lowered to optimize visualization of and access to the posterior mesotympanum.

Anesthesia

Stapedotomy can be performed under local anesthesia with intravenous sedation or under general anesthesia. Local anesthesia allows the surgeon to monitor for symptomatic perturbations of the inner ear that may cause dizziness. In this way, the surgeon may make real-time adjustments in surgical technique or prosthesis length and position. This technique also allows a surgeon to receive immediate feedback of hearing restoration. When local anesthesia with sedation is used at our institution, the anesthesiologist gives a bolus of Propofol in preparation for an injection of local anesthetic. A four-quadrant injection with 1% lidocaine with 1:100,000 epinephrine is performed. Sedation is allowed to wear off following the injection of local anesthetic.

Step 1

Preoperative antibiotics are administered. Intravenous dexamethasone may be administered preoperatively, unless contraindicated by a medical condition.

Step 2

The ear is sterilely prepped and draped.

Step 3

A four-quadrant injection of the ear canal skin is performed. Local anesthetic should be injected slowly and carefully; an adequate injection will be illustrated by blanching of the canal skin without creating a bleb. A hasty or inadequate injection will may lead to difficulty with hemostasis later in the procedure. The postauricular region is injected as well.

Step 4

Attention is turned to the postauricular region where a small piece of fascia (several millimeters) is harvested through an incision measuring approximately 5–6 mm. Hemostasis is achieved with bipolar electrocautery if needed, and the incision is closed with 5-0 fast-absorbing suture. The harvested fascia is divided into 1 mm or smaller fragments, set aside, and kept moist.

Step 5

The largest permissible size ear speculum is inserted into the ear canal and advanced with a twisting motion. The speculum is secured with a speculum holder to allow greater maneuverability of the surgeon's hands.

Step 6

A canal incision is made 6–8 mm lateral to the annulus.

Step 7

A tympanomeatal flap is elevated using a large round knife and a size 20 suction (Fig. 4.2). The middle ear is not entered until the annulus has been clearly identified. The annulus is elevated and the middle ear is entered with a fine dissector or Rosen needle. The annulus is elevated superiorly and inferiorly until middle ear exposure has been achieved from the facial nerve superiorly to the round window inferiorly. Care is taken not to disrupt the chorda tympani nerve when elevating the annulus and tympanic membrane. The elevated portion of the tympanic membrane is reflected anteriorly to provide visualization of the posterior mesotympanum (Fig. 4.3).

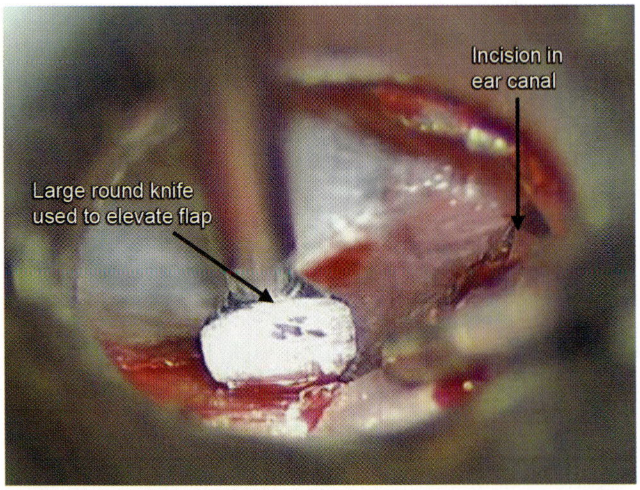

Fig. 4.2: A tympanomeatal flap is elevated in a left ear using a large round knife and size 20 suction.

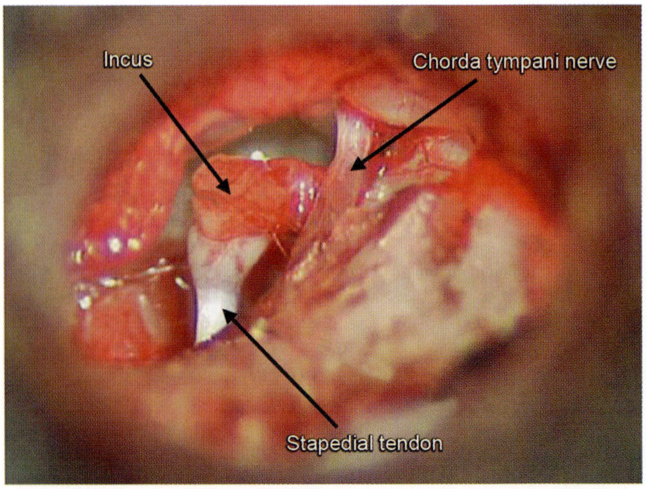

Fig. 4.3: Access to the posterior mesotympanum after elevation of the tympanomeatal flap. The chorda tympani nerve, incudostapedial joint, and stapedial tendon are visualized.

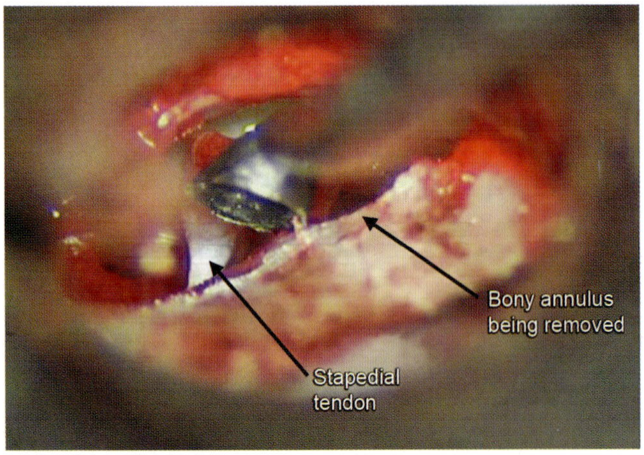

Fig. 4.4: The posterior-superior bony annulus is removed with a curette to improve access to the stapes footplate.

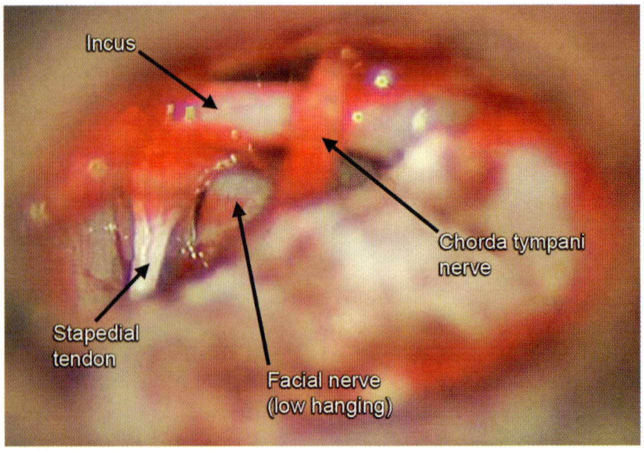

Fig. 4.5: Exposure of the posterior mesotympanum after removal of the posterior-superior bony annulus.

Step 8

Any overhanging posterior-superior bony annulus is removed to optimize visualization of the stapes footplate. This can be accomplished using any combination of a microdrill and a stapes curette. When using the curette, the sharp edge of the instrument is seated firmly against the obstructing bone, and the instrument is rotated to allow for bone removal. The curette should not be used in a linear fashion, and the trajectory of force should always be away from the facial nerve (Fig. 4.4).

Step 9

The chorda tympani nerve often obstructs a surgeon's view of the working field. The chorda tympani should be gently retracted anteriorly or posteriorly, depending on the patient's anatomy, in order to achieve proper visualization of the long process of the incus and the stapes.

Step 10

Adequate exposure requires the identification of the facial nerve superior to the stapes footplate, the stapedial tendon and pyramidal eminence posteriorly, the round window inferiorly, and the long process of the malleus anteriorly (Fig. 4.5).

Step 11

Once the surgeon begins work in the middle ear, the suction is changed to a size 22. The ossicular chain is

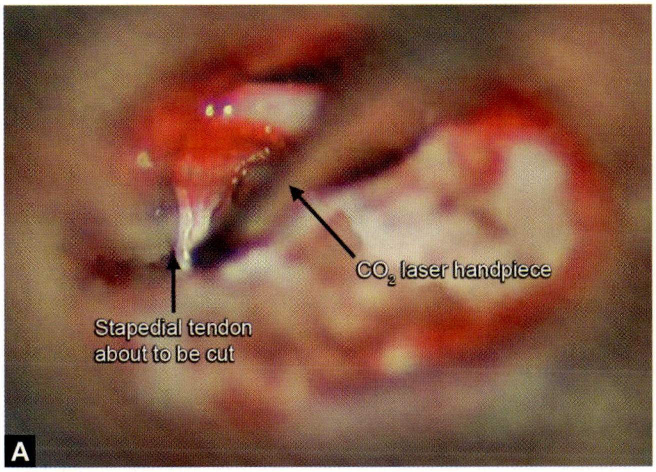

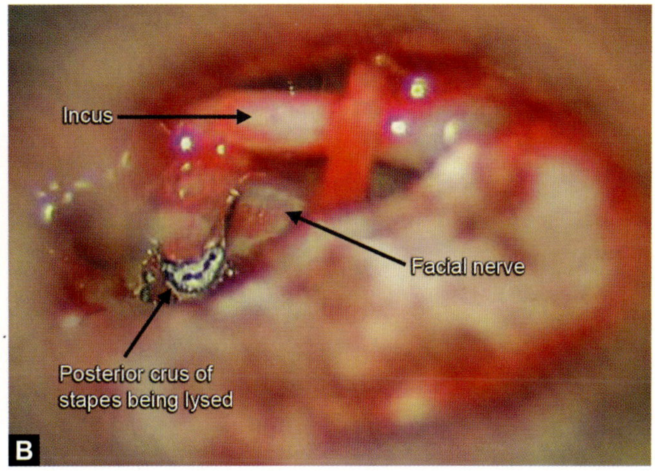

Figs. 4.6A and B: (A) The CO_2 laser is positioned to lyse the stapedial tendon. (B) The CO_2 laser is used to lyse the posterior crus of the stapes. This is performed as close to the promontory as possible to avoid interference of the residual posterior crus when placing the prosthesis.

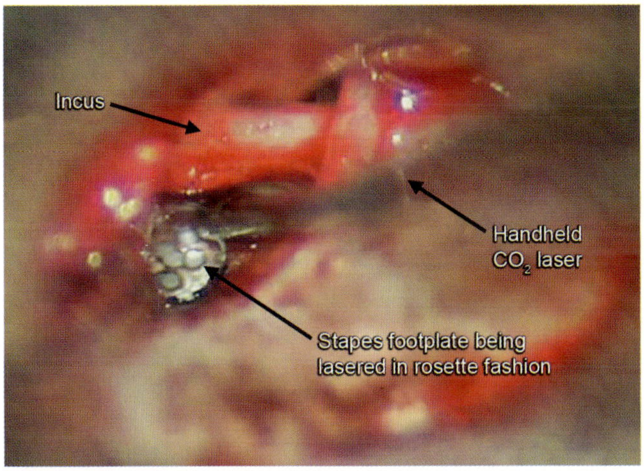

Fig. 4.7: The laser is applied to the footplate in a rosette pattern to create a 0.7 mm stapedotomy.

palpated with a curved needle to confirm the diagnosis of stapes fixation as well as to ascertain mobility of the lateral ossicular chain. Gentle palpation also allows the surgeon to precisely locate the position of the incudostapedial joint; the joint will become well defined as the mobile lenticular process of the incus moves with respect to the fixed stapes capitulum.

Step 12

The laser is applied to the mucosa overlying the incudostapedial joint.

Step 13

The incudostapedial joint is separated with a joint knife or small right-angle hook.

Step 14

The laser beam is then focused more sharply and used to lyse the stapedial tendon and the posterior crus of the stapes (Fig. 4.6A). This step is performed after separation of the incudostapedial joint in order to maintain stability of the superstructure during joint separation. The posterior crus is vaporized near its insertion into the stapes footplate; this location is chosen to prevent interference from the residual crura during prosthesis placement (Fig. 4.6B). If the anterior crus can be visualized, this is also lasered.

Step 15

The stapes suprastructure is downfractured using a small right-angle hook or a Rosen needle applied to the stapes capitulum with controlled swift pressure in an inferior direction (away from the facial nerve). The suprastructure is removed.

Step 16

The stapes footplate should now be well visualized. The laser is used at a 0.2 mm spot size in a rosette pattern to create a stapedotomy in the posterior midportion of the stapes footplate measuring approximately 0.7 mm (Fig. 4.7). Once the footplate has been penetrated, a rasp is used to remove the bone over this area. Care should be taken not to laser the perilymph once the bone has been vaporized or removed (Fig. 4.8). Once a stapedotomy has been created, the suction should never be used directly over the stapedotomy. If the perilymphatic fluid is inadvertently suctioned, the stapedotomy should immediately be bathed in saline.

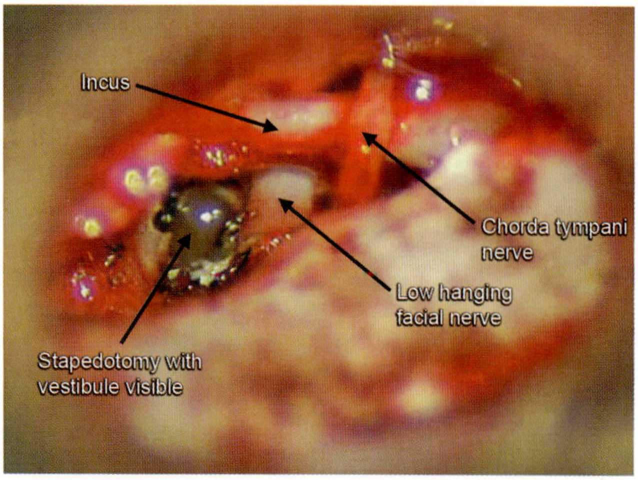

Fig. 4.8: A stapedotomy has been created in the posterior third of the stapes footplate. Note the position of the facial nerve just above the oval window.

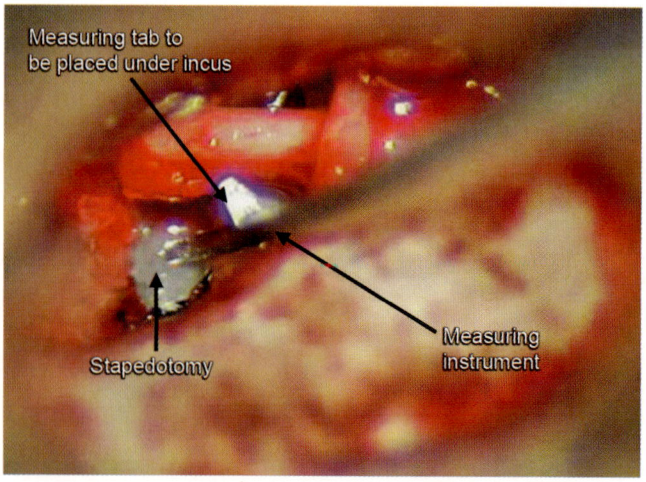

Fig. 4.9: A measuring stick is used to measure the distance from the undersurface of the incus to the vestibule.

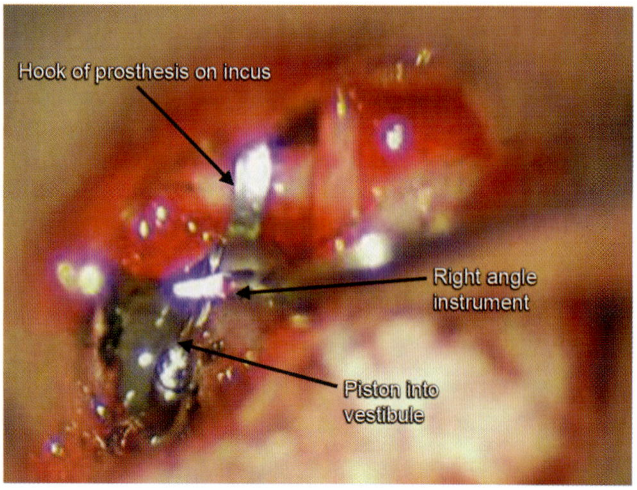

Fig. 4.10: The prosthesis is positioned so that the loop lies over the long process of the incus and the piston lies in the stapedotomy.

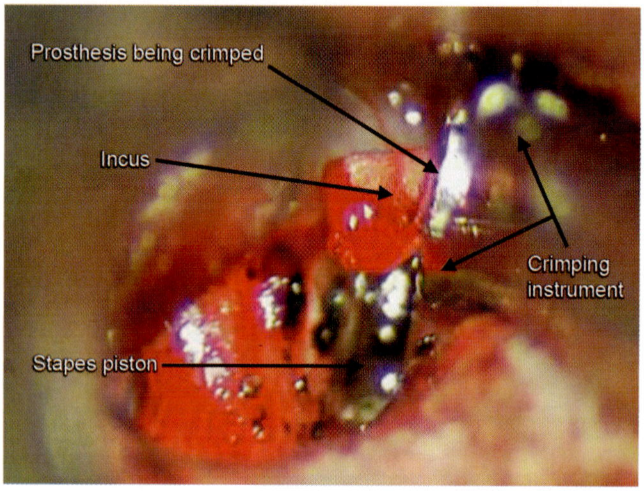

Fig. 4.11: The prosthesis is crimped onto the incus.

Step 17

A measuring instrument is used to measure the distance from the undersurface of the long process of the incus to the stapes footplate (Fig. 4.9).

Step 18

A proper sized prosthesis is selected. A prosthesis 4.25 mm in length and 0.5 mm in diameter will be appropriate for the majority of patients, though occasionally a different length must be used.

Step 19

The prosthesis is loaded on a positive-locking forceps, and gently and precisely placed such that the loop lies over the long process of the incus and the piston lies in the stapedotomy (Fig. 4.10).

Step 20

The hook of the prosthesis is crimped to the long process of the incus (Fig. 4.11). The final position of the prosthesis is demonstrated in Figure 4.12.

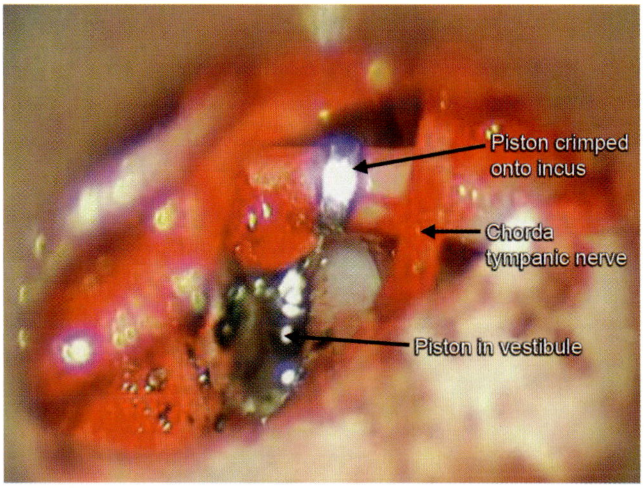

Fig. 4.12: Final position of the stapes prosthesis in the vestibule. Proper position and mobility are confirmed with gentle palpation of the malleus.

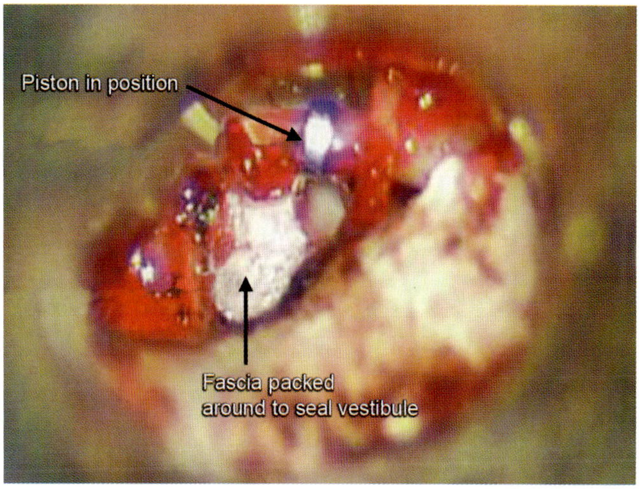

Fig. 4.13: Fascia fragments are placed around the prosthesis piston.

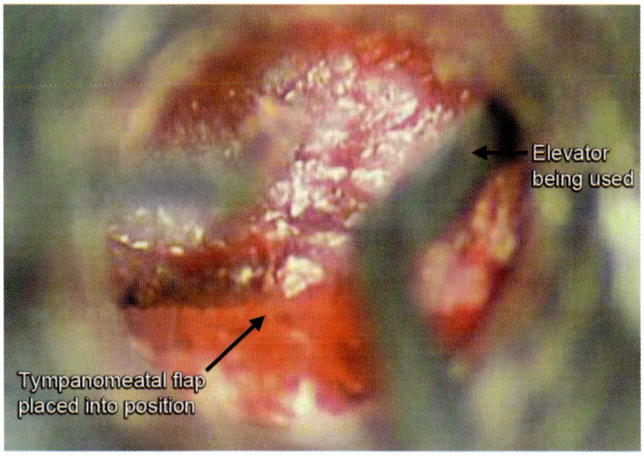

Fig. 4.14: The tympanomeatal flap is replaced.

Step 21

Fascia fragments are applied around the prosthesis to seal off the perilymph space (Fig. 4.13).

Step 22

Placement is confirmed with gentle palpation of the malleus, which should transmit motion to both the incus and the prosthesis.

Step 23

The tympanomeatal flap is replaced (Fig. 4.14). The patient is asked to repeat whispered words as a test of hearing if performed under sedation.

Step 24

Gelfoam soaked in saline or antibiotic solution is placed over the tympanomeatal flap and tympanic membrane. Care is taken not to pack the canal tightly.

INTRAOPERATIVE CONSIDERATIONS

Obliterated Footplate

An obliterated footplate exists when the otosclerotic process has advanced such that the margins of the stapes footplate cannot be defined. When an obliterated footplate is encountered, it should be thinned with a microdrill using a small diamond burr until the footplate is blue lined. Adequate irrigation should be used to assure that bone dust is cleared and that heat is not transferred to the inner ear compartment. At this point, a laser stapedotomy can be performed as described above.

Overhanging Facial Nerve

The tympanic segment of the facial nerve may be inferiorly positioned such that it partially or totally obscures the stapes footplate and oval window niche. If there is a question of whether a stapedotomy can safely be performed due to the position of the facial nerve, the procedure should be aborted. An experienced surgeon may elect to proceed if the surgeon is able to safely work around or gently displace the nerve. This can be performed by using a size 26 suction to carefully elevate the nerve off of the stapes footplate and maintain the nerve in a safe position while creating a stapedotomy at the inferior portion of the footplate. If the resting position of the facial nerve makes contact with the prosthesis, this potentially may cause dysfunction of the nerve and should be monitored closely postoperatively.

Floating Footplate

A floating footplate results when the footplate is destabilized from the annular ligament, and thus is "floating" in the oval window niche. A mobilized footplate may be depressed into the inner ear with manipulation, thus it should be approached with caution by only an experienced surgeon. A 1 mm space may be drilled into the promontory at the edge of the oval window. Working through this port, a small right-angle hook is inserted and rotated to elevate the footplate out of the oval window niche. Once the footplate has been adequately displaced, it may be grasped and removed.

Persistent Stapedial Artery

The stapedial artery forms in utero as a branch off of the internal carotid artery; in the normal sequence of development, this artery regresses before birth. In rare instances, however, the artery may fail to degenerate and may course over the stapes footplate between the anterior and posterior crura. This anomaly should be approached with caution as accidental disruption of the vessel can lead to substantial bleeding. Bipolar electrocautery should be used to coagulate the vessel on both sides of the footplate. Often, the artery will be positioned over the anterior aspect of the footplate, and a stapedotomy can safely be performed posterior to the vessel.

Perilymphatic Gusher

A perilymphatic gusher occurs when there is a significant connection between the subarachnoid space and perilymphatic space, and the pressure differential between the intracranial space and the middle ear space allows for rapid efflux of cerebrospinal fluid (CSF) through the inner ear into the middle ear at the time of stapedectomy. This often occurs in the presence of a widened cochlear aqueduct or internal auditory canal, and is more prevalent in cases of congenital stapes fixation. CSF should be allowed to drain until the pressure gradient has lowered. At this point, the stapedotomy should be packed with a fascia graft, which is held in place with the stapes prosthesis. Additional Gelfoam packing should be placed around the stapedotomy to prevent recurrent or persistent egress of CSF. The patient should be monitored postoperatively for persistent CSF leak. The need for lumbar drain placement to decrease CSF pressure is rare.

Imaging may demonstrate a widened cochlear aqueduct or fundus of the internal auditory canal, heralding a warning to the surgeon preoperatively. Cases of perilymph gusher have been reported, however, in the absence of radiologic abnormality.[14] A sensorineural component to the hearing loss preoperatively may be another harbinger of a gusher. A high index of suspicion should be maintained when considering stapedectomy for cases of congenital stapes fixation, as the occurrence of perilymphatic gusher increases the risk of postoperative sensorineural hearing loss.[15]

Narrow Oval Window Niche

A narrow oval window niche may preclude adequate exposure for stapedotomy fenestration and prosthesis placement. If the bony promontory encroaches on the oval window niche, 1 mm of the promontory bone on the inferior aspect of the oval window may be lasered or drilled to improve access.

POSTOPERATIVE CARE

Most stapedectomy surgery is performed as an outpatient procedure, though patients are given the opportunity to stay overnight if they live at a distance or have other concerns. Patients are instructed to avoid heavy lifting or nose blowing, and to sneeze with their mouth open for 3 weeks. Patients may fly after 3 weeks. They are seen in the office 10–14 days after surgery to check the ear and remove any remaining packing, and a postoperative audiogram is routinely obtained at 3 months.

COMPLICATIONS OF STAPEDECTOMY SURGERY

Patients may complain of postoperative dizziness, tinnitus, or hearing loss. The most common etiology of postoperative dizziness after stapes surgery is serous labyrinthitis. Patients will present with vertigo that responds well to a short course of steroids. Other etiologies of postoperative dizziness including a perilymphatic fistula, overly long prosthesis, or reparative granuloma. Perilymphatic fistula presents with fluctuating or progressive hearing loss with tinnitus, and often vertigo. Examination will reveal a positive fistula test. Treatment is re-exploration with placement of a tissue seal around the oval window. The incidence of reparative granuloma has decreased such that it is now a rare complication. This complication should be considered in the case of persistent dizziness after stapedectomy. A reparative granuloma may lead to sensorineural hearing loss if left untreated. Packing should be removed from the ear; a reddish hue may be visualized along the undersurface of the tympanomeatal flap and the lenticular process of incus. If reparative granuloma is suspected, the patient should be urgently returned to the operating room, the prosthesis removed, and the granuloma cleared with the laser. A tissue seal should be placed over the oval window, and the region should be left to heal. Revision surgery may be considered after 6 months, or the patient may elect hearing amplification through nonsurgical means.

REFERENCES

1. Schrauwen I, Van Camp G. The etiology of otosclerosis: a combination of genes and environment. Laryngoscope. 2010;120:1195-202.
2. Glasscock ME 3rd, Storper IS, Haynes DS, et al. Twenty-five years of experience with stapedectomy. Laryngoscope. 1995;105:899-904.
3. Cremers W, Beusen J, Huygen P. Hearing gain after stapedotomy, partial platinectomy, or total stapedectomy for otosclerosis. Ann Otol Rhinol Laryngol. 1991;100:959-61.
4. Kursten R, Schneider B, Zrunek M. Long-term results after stapedectomy versus stapedotomy. Am J Otol. 1994;15:804-6.
5. House HP, Hansen MR, Al Dakhail AA, et al. Stapedectomy versus stapedotomy: comparison of results with long-term follow-up. Laryngoscope. 2002;112:2046-50.
6. Esquivel CR, Mamikoglu B, Wiet RJ. Long-term results of small fenestra stapedectomy compared with large fenestra technique. Laryngoscope. 2002;112:1338-41.
7. Perkins R. Laser stapedotomy for otosclerosis. Laryngoscope. 1980;90:228-40.
8. Lesinski SG, Palmer A. Lasers for otosclerosis: CO2 vs. Argon and KTP-532. Laryngoscope. 1989;99 (Suppl 46):1-8.
9. Stucken EZ, Brown KD, Selesnick SH. The use of KTP laser in revision stapedectomy. Otol Neurotol. 2012;33:1297-9.
10. Donnell GN, Alfi OS. Medical genetics for the otorhinolaryngologist. Laryngoscope. 1980;90:40-6.
11. Vincent R, Sperling NM, Oates J, et al. Surgical findings and long-term hearing results in 3,050 stapedotomies for primary otosclerosis: a prospective study with the otology-neurotology database. Otol Neurotol. 2006;27:S25-47.
12. Yung MW, Oates J, Vowler SL. The learning curve in stapes surgery and its implication to training. Laryngoscope. 2006;116:67-71.
13. Ozuer MZ, Olgun L, Gultekin G. Revision stapes surgery. Otolaryngol Head Neck Surg. 2012;146:109-13.
14. Krouchi L, Callonnec F, Bouchetemple P, et al. Preoperative computed tomography scan may fail to predict perilymphatic gusher. Ann Otol Rhinol Laryngol. 2013;122:374-7.
15. Dornhoffer JL, Helms J, Hoehmann DH. Stapedectomy for congenital fixation of the stapes. Am J Otol. 1995;16:382-6.

CHAPTER 5

Stapes Mobilization

Robert T Sataloff

Most otologists stopped performing stapes mobilization years ago because of its high failure rate. I have continued to perform stapes mobilization electively (following a comprehensive consent discussion with my patients) throughout my practice, having learned the procedure from my father, Joseph Sataloff, who performed approximately 10,000 stapes operations; many of them were mobilizations. This decision is not because of a disagreement with any of the data that were utilized by the otologists who advocated abandoning stapes mobilization in favor of stapedectomy. Rather, it is based on a different stratification of priorities, which resulted in a judgment in favor of stapes mobilization, based upon the same data.

In 1979, Brookler published an article reviewing 120,132 stapedectomy cases.[1] He identified sensorineural hearing loss reported in 0.97% (approximately 1%) of cases. It was not possible to separate a "dead" ear from less severe sensorineural hearing loss in all of these cases. Most active otologists agree that the incidence is at least 1–2% commonly and probably higher in less experienced hands. I have reviewed many of the published articles on stapes mobilization,[2-16] totaling 10,811 cases. They revealed a 0.036% incidence of sensorineural hearing loss and 0.064% incidence of a "dead" ear. This results in a total sensorineural hearing loss incidence of approximately 0.1% among stapes mobilization patients, a tenfold decrease in comparison with stapedectomy.

The reported long-term success rate of stapes mobilizations gleaned from these articles was about 55%. This number has remained accepted for decades, perhaps because no one has tried to improve it. However, if we were to initiate research to advance the techniques and outcomes of stapes mobilization surgery, it is conceivable that better outcomes might prove possible. Nevertheless, this chapter assumes a "failure" rate of about 50%.

There is something intrinsically unappealing about a procedure with a failure rate that approaches 50%; but we still must ask whether it is worth paying the price necessary to achieve a success rate closer to 98% by performing stapedectomy instead of stapes mobilization. At the beginning of my career, I decided that it was not; and that judgment has not changed.

If we accept as our guiding principle Primum non nocere (First do no harm), then perhaps stapes mobilization has a place in otologic surgery. If we have a patient with bilateral 70 dB conductive hearing loss, have a stapes mobilization fail and have to proceed with stapedectomy, little is lost other than a few minutes in the operating room. However, if we perform a stapedectomy on that patient and end up with a 70 dB hearing loss in one ear and a "dead ear" on the other side, we have not done the patient a service. Hence, I would submit that anything that we can do to decrease the incidence of severe or profound sensorineural hearing loss should be considered seriously.

My personal experience has been similar to that in the literature. I care for patients for whom I performed stapes mobilization 30 years ago, and patients operated upon by my father 50 years ago, who still have normal conductive hearing, and who achieved it with minimal risk of sensorineural hearing loss. Of course, I also care for others who are returned to the operating room to undergo stapedectomy within a few months following stapes mobilization. Our stapedectomy results in patients who have undergone stapes mobilization do not differ from results in patients who have never undergone stapes surgery, and the procedure has been particularly trouble-free since the advent of laser stapedotomy which virtually eliminates the problem of "floating footplate".

Stapes mobilization and stapedectomy are both excellent operations. Their risks and benefits differ and

Adapted in part from Sataloff RT. Stapes mobilization revisited: Primum non nocere. ENT J. 2007;86(3):126-29, with permission.

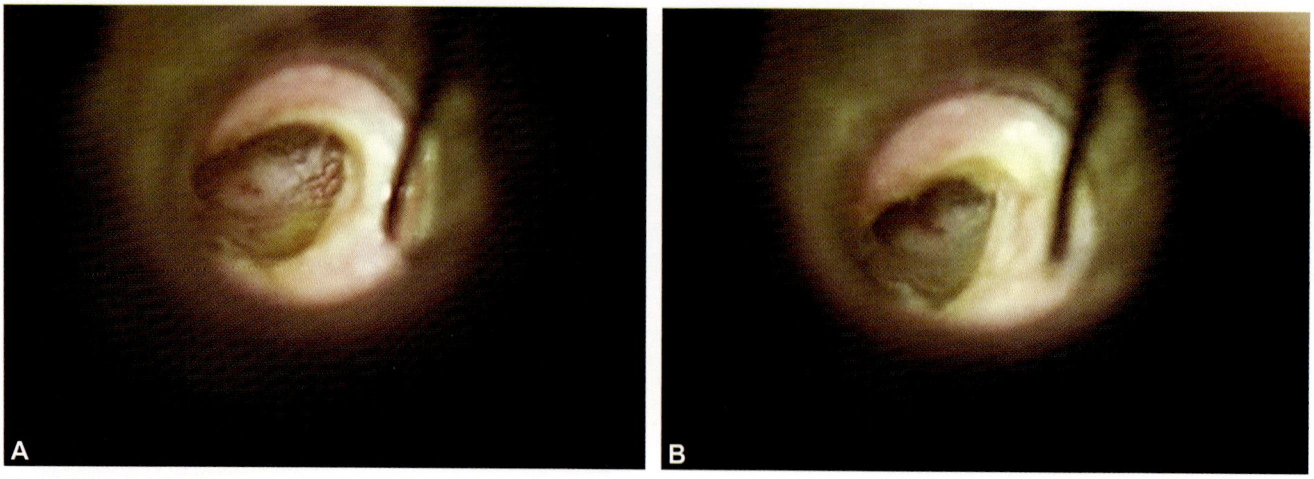

Figs. 5.1A and B: (A) Xylocaine with epinephrine is injected into the posterior-superior quadrant. (B) Dissection of the anesthetic results in blanching and elevation of the external auditory canal skin.

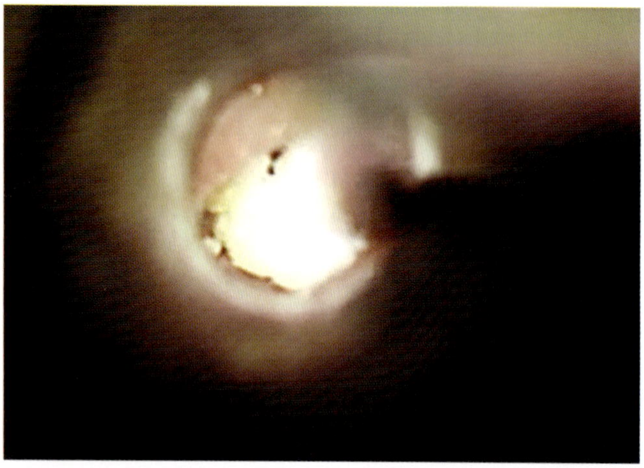

Fig. 5.2: A cotton ball is used to compress the external auditory canal skin after injection.

are worthy of reconsideration. The judgment of the field of otology to select stapedectomy in order to eliminate the high failure rate associated with stapes mobilization is certainly understandable. However, even if half of the patients who undergo stapes mobilization fail and require stapedectomy, the successful half has achieved good hearing with a 0.1% risk instead of a 1% risk of irreversible sensorineural impairment. Furthermore, if half return for secondary stapedectomy, that would mean that only half of our otosclerosis patients are subjected to the 1% (or greater) risk of sensorineural hearing loss associated with stapedectomy, and that would cut the overall risk in our surgical otosclerosis patients nearly in half. It appears worth considering any procedure that decreases the incidence of one of our worst complications by tenfold in half of our patients, and by half in the stapes surgical population as a whole. We also may want to reprioritize our criteria for success. From my perspective, a good hearing result that required two trips to the operating room seems like a success; a dead ear surely does not.

SURGICAL TECHNIQUES

Step 1

This author performs stapes mobilization and stapedectomy under local anesthesia with sedation. The table is placed into about 20° of Trendelenburg, and the neck is extended. If the position is correct, when the surgeon is sitting comfortably with the microscope line of sight perpendicular to the floor, the surgeon should be looking directly at the region of the oval window, without having to angle the microscope or his/her body into an awkward position. The largest speculum that provides adequate visualization should be used. The ear is anesthetized by injecting xylocaine with epinephrine. The first injection is placed in the posterior-superior quadrant of the external auditory canal (Fig. 5.1A). During injection, blanching of the epithelium can be seen (Fig. 5.1B). If the blanching extends far enough anteriorly and inferiorly (below the tympanomastoid suture), this single injection is often sufficient. After injection, a small cotton ball on a heavy alligator is used to compress the xylocaine within the epithelium (Fig. 5.2). This helps distribute the injected liquid, and flattening the epithelium makes it easier to incise the skin and elevate the tympanomeatal flap.

Step 2

An incision is made in the posterior aspect of the external auditory canal (Fig. 5.3A). The horizontal incision should

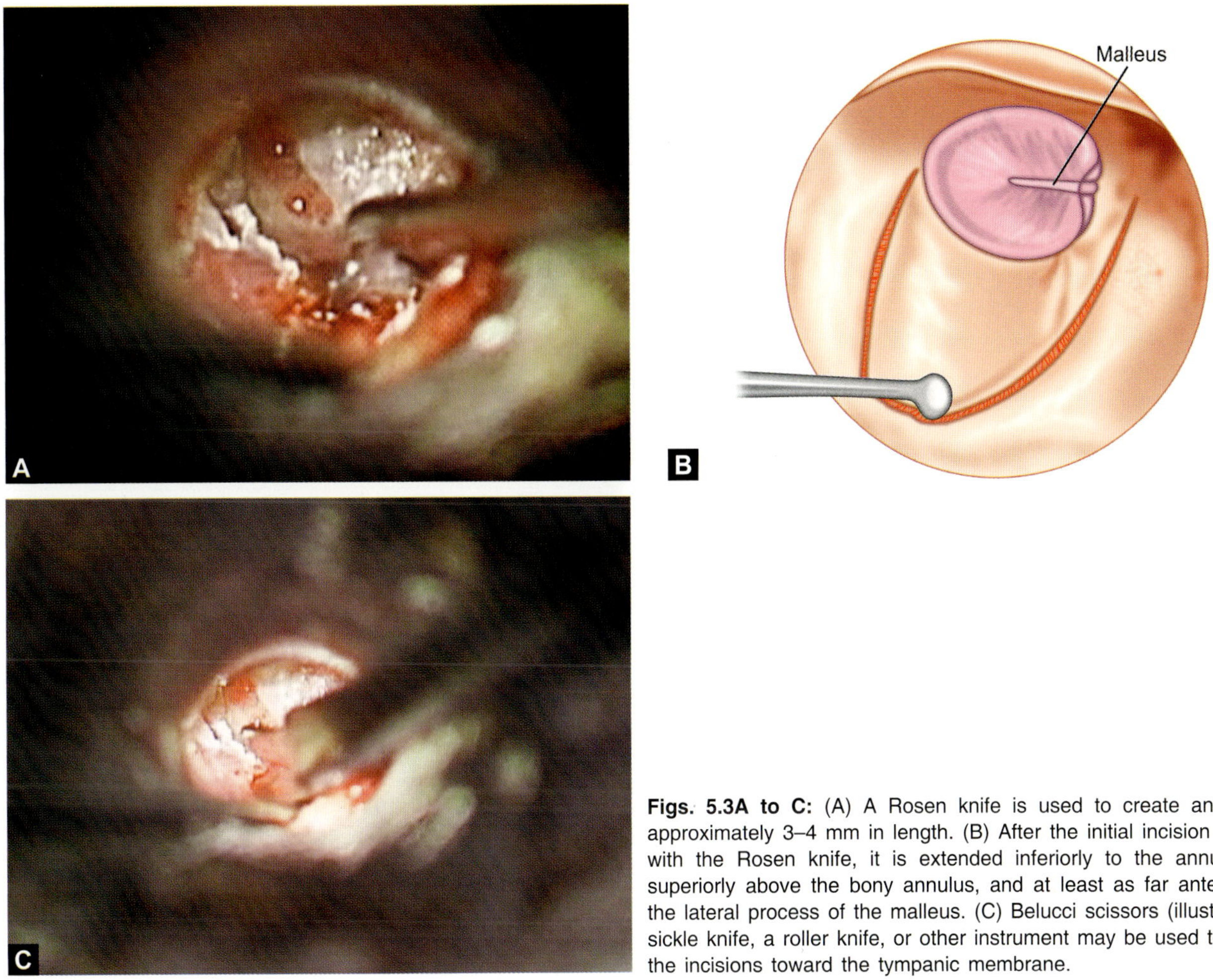

Figs. 5.3A to C: (A) A Rosen knife is used to create an incision approximately 3–4 mm in length. (B) After the initial incision is made with the Rosen knife, it is extended inferiorly to the annulus and superiorly above the bony annulus, and at least as far anteriorly as the lateral process of the malleus. (C) Belucci scissors (illustrated), a sickle knife, a roller knife, or other instrument may be used to extend the incisions toward the tympanic membrane.

be relatively small (usually 3–4 mm). The edges of the incision are carried toward the annulus inferiorly (going low enough to permit visualization of the round window region), and superiorly to a level approximately even with the lateral process of the malleus and 2 mm superior to the bony edge of the external auditory canal (Fig. 5.3B). The position of this incision allows easy anterior extension if malleus fixation is encountered. If a superior incision ends at the bony edge rather than above it, anterior extension may result in perforation. The trapezoidal design of the flap minimizes the amount of tissue in the surgeon's way (there is much more tissue on the flap with a larger horizontal incision and rectangular-shaped flap) which is especially important with small ear canals. The author prefers to make the horizontal incision with a Rosen knife and the longitudinal incisions with Belucci scissors (Fig. 5.3C). The inferior tine is placed firmly against bone. Alternatively, the incisions can be made with a roller knife, sickle knife or other instrument. However, some of these instruments (especially the sickle knife) may tear the flap if they are unexpectedly dull. Such problems are prevented by using the scissors.

Step 3

The tympanomeatal flap is elevated, scrapping the Rosen knife firmly against the bone of the external auditory canal (Fig. 5.4A). Lifting the knife away from bone (prying the flap up) may tear the flap. The tympanomeatal flap should be elevated throughout its entirely breadth (Fig. 5.4B), not in narrow tunnels. The Rosen knife should be allowed to gently drop over the medial edge of the bony annulus, taking care not to let it extend too far into the middle ear where it might traumatize important structures such as the ossicles. It is often safest to enter the middle ear low, in the posterior-inferior quadrant. Many surgeons switch instruments at this point, using a Sheehy annulus elevator or curved pick (Rosen needle).

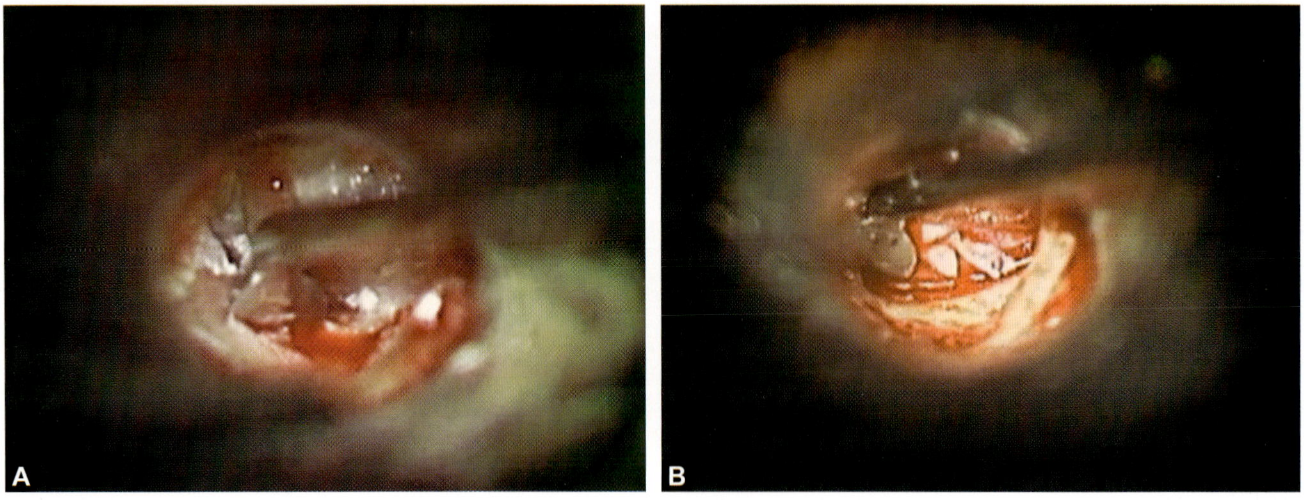

Figs. 5.4A and B: (A) The Rosen knife is pressed against bone, and the flap is pushed medially in order to elevate it. (B) Elevation should proceed over the whole breadth of the flap as illustrated, not in narrow tunnels.

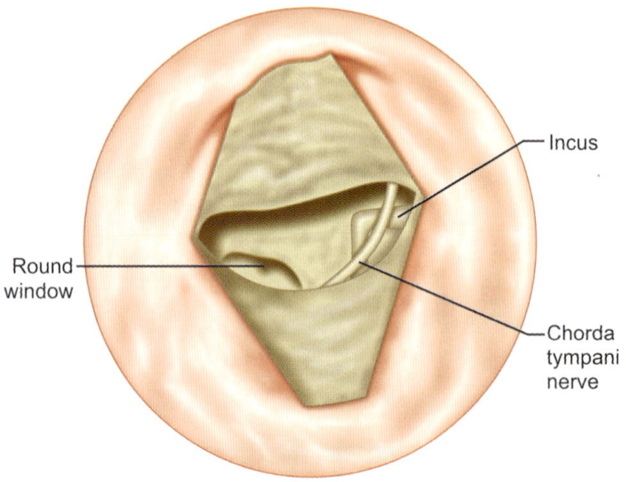

Fig. 5.5: When the tympanomeatal flap is elevated, the incus, stapes superstructure, chordatympani nerve, and round window niche should be visible.

This author prefers to simply pull the Rosen knife posteriorly, placing it firmly against the bony annulus. It can then be swept superiorly, serving as an annulus elevator, while taking care not to injure the chorda tympani nerve.

Step 4

Either the Rosen knife or a curved pick can be used to lift the flap anteriorly. If the superior incision is sufficiently anterior as described above, the flap folds easily at the level of the malleus and does not impede visualization of the area of the stapes (Fig. 5.5).

Step 5

The malleus is palpated to confirm malleus and incus mobility. The stapes is palpated through the distal aspect of the incus. If visualization is not adequate, bone can be curetted posteriorly. However, if the head and neck position is optimal, this is not necessary in most cases. The chorda tympani nerve should be preserved whenever possible, but if substantial stretching is required, division of the nerve may be preferable.

Step 6

There are several techniques for stapes mobilization, but the technique used by the author most of the time utilizes a curved pick. It is placed against the distal aspect of the incus directly over the stapes capitulum (Fig. 5.6). If the pick is placed too far proximally or distally on the incus, it will fracture. Firm pressure is applied to the pick through an imaginary plumb line that goes directly to the center of the footplate and perfectly parallel to the crura. When necessary, slightly extra pressure can be applied anteriorly toward the fissula ante fenestra. However, if the pressure is not perfectly parallel with the crura, crural fracture is common. Mobilization requires more force than most people expect. Typically, the stapes mobilizes suddenly with a snap. The pressure is created by squeezing the thumb and forefinger together, with very little motion toward the vestibule. This helps prevent sudden, excessive medial displacement of the stapes footplate into the vestibule. Most of the time, mobilization can be accomplished easily without seeing perilymph.

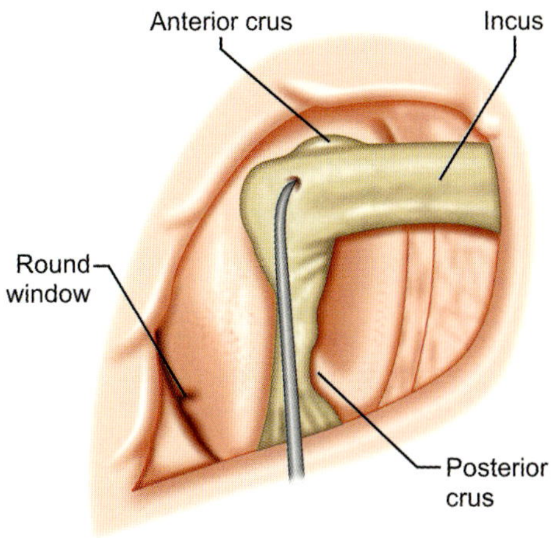

Fig. 5.6: Using a curved pick (Rosen needle), pressure is applied through the incus, with the pick placed directly over the center of the stapes capitulum. Force is directed through an imaginary plumb line that runs to the center of the footplate.

Step 7

If stapes mobilization cannot be accomplished, stapedectomy is performed. If stapes mobilization has been accomplished, good footplate mobility should be confirmed by palpating the malleus and watching the center of the footplate, or by observing a round window reflex. It is also useful sometimes to palpate the center of the footplate with a 24 gauge suction (rather than a sharp pick) to confirm stapes footplate mobility (as opposed to crural fracture with a fixed footplate).

Step 8

The tympanomeatal flap is replaced. Hearing is tested with whispered voice and a tuning fork. If good results are confirmed, the ear is packed. The author uses a wick, acetic acid drops, and a cotton ball in the meatus.

REFERENCES

1. Brookler KH. Otosclerosis Surgery: Reassessment of its value in 1978. Laryngoscope. 1979;89:725-9.
2. Bellucci RJ. Survey of stapes surgery: 5 year study. Arch Otolaryngol. 1969;89:408-11.
3. Derlacki EL, Shambaugh GE, Harrison WH. The Evolution of a Stapes Mobilization Technique. Laryngoscope. 1957;67: 420-47.
4. Goodhill V, Holcomb AL. A study of 500 stapes mobilizations. Laryngoscope. 1957;67:615-42.
5. Harrison WH, Shambaugh GE, Derlacki EL, et al. Perilymph fistula in stapes surgery. Laryngoscope. 1967;77:836-49.
6. Holmgren L. Mobilization and stapediolysis. Primary and long-term results. Acta Otolaryngol. 1960;158:316-27.
7. House HP. Trends in mobilization surgery. Laryngoscope. 1959;69:1805-107.
8. Kinney CE. Statistical analysis of the stapes mobilization procedure. Laryngoscope. 1956;66:1339-45.
9. Kos CM, Shapley JL, Iles PB. Results of 939 stapes mobilization operations. Ann Otol. 1960;69:206-21.
10. Kraus RN, Elliott LL, Moore EW. Stapes mobilization. Experience in the U.S.A.F. U.S.A.F. School of Aerospace Med. 1961;88:1-11.
11. Lewis DK. Some unsolved problems of stapes mobilization. Ann Otol. 1960;69:222-35.
12. Meurman Y, Meurman O. Stapes mobilization in otosclerosis. Arch Otolaryngo. 1955;62:164-72.
13. Myers D, Ronis BJ. Improvement of hearing in otosclerosis by means of stapes mobilization operation. Arch Otolaryngo. 1956;64(4):370-23.
14. Rosen S. Results of mobilization of fixed stapedial foot plate in otosclerosis deafness. JAMA. 1956;161:595-9.
15. Sataloff J, Menduke H. Mobilization of the stapes in older patients with otosclerosis. J Amer Ger Soc. 1960;8:277-83.
16. Scheer AA. Observations of 500 cases of transtympenio mobilization of the stapes. Arch Otol. 1957;65(3):245-54.

CHAPTER

6

Tympanoplasty and Ossiculoplasty

Eric L Slattery, Dennis I Bojrab

INTRODUCTION

Tympanoplasty is a procedure that (1) produces a mobile tympanic membrane, (2) allows for an aerated middle ear cleft, and (3) conducts sound successfully into the fluid-filled inner ear. Its application within otology is wide, including cholesteatoma resection, tympanic perforation repair, and ossicular chain evaluation and modification.

HISTORICAL PERSPECTIVE

In 1640 Banzer attempted the first recorded tympanoplasty by stretching a portion of pig bladder over a perforated tympanic membrane, which allowed for temporary improvement of hearing.[1] Other early attempts included Toynbee in 1853[2] placing a rubber disk attached to silver wire onto a perforation and Blake in 1877[3] placing a paper patch over a perforation. Tympanoplasty as a concept is credited to Berthold, who in 1878 de-epithelialized a tympanic membrane with plaster, and placed a skin graft over it.[4]

Modern tympanoplasty began in the 1950s as reported by Wullstein[5] and Zollner,[6] and later House and Sheehy[7] and Plester.[8] Skin grafts were initially employed, and later abandoned after high failure rates. Despite the low success rates in these early procedures, the management of chronic middle ear disease was radically changed. The 1960s laid the foundation for many current techniques. Austin and Shea[9] along with Tabb[10] described use of autologous vein in what today would be considered an underlay or medial technique for repair of perforations. Storrs described fascia grafting for the first time in the early 1960s.[11] His description was a type of overlay or lateral technique, which with some modification, became the main methodology at the House Ear Clinic during the ensuing decades. Glasscock in 1973 reported on a large series of underlay and overlay fascia graft techniques.[12] The transcanal approach for tympanoplasty was described by Austin.[13] Contributions by many others have helped shape tympanoplasty into its current state, with new techniques continuing to be described.[14-17]

CONCEPTS IN SURGICAL TREATMENT

Tympanoplasty is utilized in many pathologies of the middle ear. These include tympanic membrane perforations, adhesive otitis media, chronic suppurative otitis media, tympanosclerosis, ossicular fixation, retraction pockets, cholesteatoma, glomus tympanicum, and conductive hearing loss.

Due to the wide applications of tympanoplasty for different middle ear conditions, variations in the size of middle ear cleft and different size of perforations, many techniques have been described. Two dominant methodologies for drum grafting have evolved. The first is the overlay or lateral (here forward described as overlay) technique, which places the graft lateral to the tympanic annulus. The second is the underlay or medial (here forward described as underlay) technique, which places the graft medial to the annulus. Both are described. Another technique, the over-under graft, which is a modification of medial grafting, will also be discussed. Ossiculoplasty refers specifically to work performed on the ossicular chain to restore conductive hearing function and is discussed as well. Often tympanoplasty is performed with mastoidectomy techniques in order to remove disease. Mastoidectomy can aid in access of the epitympanum through a posterior atticotomy or the middle ear through a posterior tympanotomy (facial recess). Mastoidectomy techniques are varied and are described within the chapter on Mastoidectomy.

CLASSIFICATION OF TECHNIQUES

Wullstein provided an early classification of tympanoplasty;[18] however, this classification's applicability to current procedures is limited. Instead most techniques can be described by (1) approach to the tympanic membrane/middle ear, (2) choice of grafting material (if used), (3) how the graft is placed in reference to the native tympanic membrane, a nd (4) ossiculoplasty type (if performed) (Table 6.1).

PATIENT SELECTION

Common clinical presentations include (1) stable and dry perforation of the tympanic membrane, (2) chronic suppurative otitis media, (3) deep retraction pockets or cholesteatoma, and (4) conductive hearing loss. Most cases are elective as medical alternatives often exist and should be discussed with the patient. In the case of a dry perforation, methods of keeping the ear dry are important and, if meaningful hearing loss exists, use of a hearing aid may be offered. The use of a hearing aid may allow ear canal moisture to occur, causing ear infections; therefore, hearing aids should be used with caution. Initial attempts to control draining ears without signs of cholesteatoma usually include frequent office aural debridement and antibiotic drops with or without oral antibiotics for several weeks before deciding on surgical intervention.Often ear drops with the presence of a steroid can help decrease inflammation. In cases refractory to treatment, gram stain and culture may aid therapy. Many of these situations will have a narrow middle ear cleft with some mucosalization of the surrounding perforation edges on a malleus that is adherent to the promontory, necessitating surgical repair. In patients with cholesteatoma, some small pockets can be managed with routine debridement in the office; however, many need removal by surgery. Rarely complications from infections such as facial nerve palsy, subperiosteal abscess, meningitis, brain abscess, and otitic hydrocephalus can occur. In cases presenting only with conductive hearing loss, awareness of the status of the ossicles on examination or old operative notes if possible should be sought, and rare inner ear "third mobile window" entities such as superior canal dehiscence excluded.

Otomicroscopic evaluation is invaluable and is important for any treatment plan. The presence of infection can be confirmed with purulent discharge. Polyps or mucosalization of the drum or external auditory canal (EAC) may occur. The size and location of perforations within the tympanic membrane can be assessed, as larger perforations and those centered over the round window can cause increased conductive hearing loss. Classification of the perforation as central or marginal should be done, with any squamous debris tracking through the perforation noted. The middle ear mucosa can be evaluated for inflammation, infection, or cholesteatoma. Tympanosclerosis of the tympanic membrane and/or the middle ear can be seen.

All patients should have audiometric testing that includes pure tone (air and bone conduction) and speech audiometry at the minimum. This information can help in the preoperative counseling if there is a greater likelihood for ossiculoplasty or not. Risk factors such as a labyrinthine or cochlear fistula can be assessed in cases of sensorineural hearing loss. Tuning fork testing should be performed to confirm audiometric testing. CT scan may be of benefit, especially in cases that have signs or symptoms of complications of otitis media including facial paresis, vertigo/imbalance, or cerebrospinal fluid leak.

Factors that may predispose to poor healing include ongoing Eustachian tube function, infection, diseased middle ear mucosa, allergies, reflux, or smoking. Eustachian tube function is often correlated with the age of the patient. Younger patients with chronic suppurative otitis media fail more often. Delaying surgery on patients until 5–8 years of age is generally felt to be prudent, although there is no strict age threshold and the condition of the contralateral ear should be noted. Despite this, there is no set testing of the Eustachian tube that can be performed ahead of surgery to ensure success, but judgment comes from experience. In fact Sheehy is attributed with stating, "Sometimes the best test... is a tympanoplasty."[19]

Table 6.1: Classification of tympanoplasty

Approach	*Graft material*	*Graft placement*	*Ossiculoplasty*
Post- (or retro-) auricular	Fascia	Underlay	Autograft
Transcanal	Perichondrium	Overlay	Alloplastic prosthesis
Endaural	Cartilage	Over-under	Partial vs. total
	Periosteum		
	Fat		
	Homograft (e.g. AlloDerm)		

Many treatment decisions are made intraoperatively. The grafting technique (overlay, underlay, or over-under) chosen may be influenced by narrowness of the middle ear, location of the needed repair, presence of cholesteatoma, and the need for ossicular repair. Staging ossicular chain reconstruction is made at the time of surgery and is influenced by previously failed tympanoplasty, recurrent cholesteatoma, or marked middle ear inflammatory disease.

Most tympanic repairs are performed using fascia or perichondrium, although cartilage grafting is increasing in popularity at some centers. Potential situations in which cartilage grafting may be of benefit include repair of scutal defects, repair or posterior retraction pockets, previously failed tympanoplasty, and total tympanic membrane perforations.

When considering ossiculoplasty, the middle ear should be free of infection, marked inflammation, or cholesteatoma. The tympanic membrane should not be markedly retracted. Ossiculoplasty can be performed at the time of the initial surgery or at future staged surgery. Understanding acoustic mechanics is necessary for the surgeon who wishes to perform successful ossiculoplasty. Merchant et al. provide an in-depth description of middle ear mechanics.[19] In general, the function of the middle ear is to act as a sound transducer from the low impedance air to the high impedance fluid-filled inner ear. The acoustic transformer consists of the tympanic membrane, the ossicular chain, and hydraulic lever. The tympanic membrane is designed so that the manubrium of the malleus receives the greatest energy. The ossicles, with the malleus being longer than the incus, afford a 1.3 fold sound increase. Finally, the surface area of the tympanic membrane to the oval window is approximately 20.8 to 1 and accounts for the majority of the hydraulic lever effect. Other phenomena that help in the transmission of sound include the optimal frequency resonance of the pinna, ear canal, and ossicles.

The choice of type of ossiculoplasty depends on the status of the ossicles and their availability for use in reconstruction. Autograph ossiculoplasty with the incus or head of the malleus is preferred in many centers. Autograft fixation (in the case of cortical bone or ossicles) or warping (when cartilage is used) is a concern. Alloplastic prostheses are an alternative. Over 300 prostheses have been designed with many different materials. Table 6.2 shows a sample of the many alloplastic prostheses available. In general, smaller and lighter prostheses function better. Extrusion rates vary, with all alloplasts extruding at higher rates than autografts. Alloplasts also have higher costs than autografts, but the costs become comparable when considering the additional OR time and disposable drill bits needed to sculpt autografts.

PREOPERATIVE COUNSELING AND INFORMED CONSENT

Alternatives to surgery should be discussed with the patient. Proper preoperative counseling of realistic expectations aids in patient satisfaction. We address the ear situation and list the problems, e.g. perforation, chronic suppurative otitis media, or hearing loss. Then we explain that success may be seen in repair of the perforation, cessation of the ear infection or improvement of hearing. We explain that hearing loss may need to be addressed at a later surgery or with hearing aid technology.

Complications that can occur with tympanoplasty include reperforation of the tympanic membrane, chorda tympani nerve injury (temporary or permanent), recurrence of cholesteatoma, transient imbalance, and continued conductive hearing loss. Rarely sensorineural hearing loss and facial nerve injury can also occur. Often providing the patient this information redundantly (e.g. speaking about risks, benefits, and alternatives in the

Table 6.2: Commonly used prostheses for middle ear reconstruction

	Prosthesis	*Type*	*Material*	*Weight*
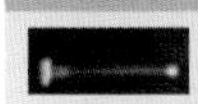	Bojrab HA + Ti	Total	HA/Titanium	10 mg
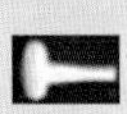	Torp	Total	Dense HA	47 mg
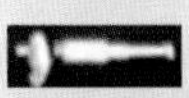	Torp	Total	Dense HA/Flex HA	43 mg
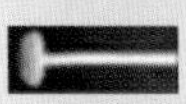	Top	Total	Polycel	4 mg
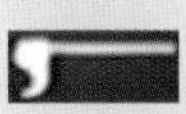	Incus-stapes	Total	HA/Hapex	28 mg
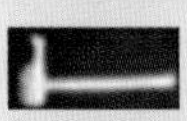	Incus-stapes	Total	HA/Plasti-Pore	16 mg
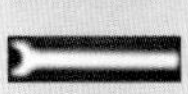	Strut	Total	Dense HA	16 mg
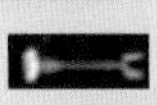	Bojrab HA + Ti	Partial	HA/Titanium	8 mg
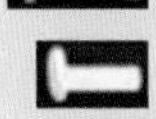	Porp	Partial	Dense HA	44 mg
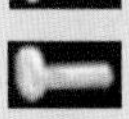	Porp	Partial	Dense HA/Flex HA	39 mg
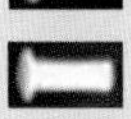	Pop	Partial	Polycel	6 mg
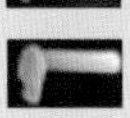	Porp	Partial	HA/Hapex	28 mg
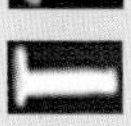	Porp	Partial	HA/Plasti-Pore	17 mg
	Strut	Partial	Dense HA	21 mg

office, providing written material, access to electronic media, and finally repeating on the day of surgery) helps to convey the information to the patient and his or her family.

SURGICAL TECHNIQUES

Myringoplasty

Myringoplasty is defined as a procedure to repair the tympanic membrane without elevating a tympanomeatal flap. The procedure is typically done transcanal. Small perforations without concomitant infection, cholesteatoma, other disease of the middle ear, or ossicular abnormalities/unexpectedly large conductive hearing loss are candidates for myringoplasty (Fig. 6.1).

Step 1: Basic techniques include de-epithelializing the edges of the perforation and placement of a paper patch, small fat graft harvested from the medial side of the lobule, or fascia graft (Figs. 6.2 and 6.3).

Step 2: A modified technique of myringoplasty utilizes the CO_2 laser and is used in tympanic membranes with deep retraction pockets (atelectasis). Defocusing the beam allows for the laser not to penetrate the tympanic membrane. The resulting heat and coagulative effect tightens the atelectatic drum (Fig. 6.4).[20]

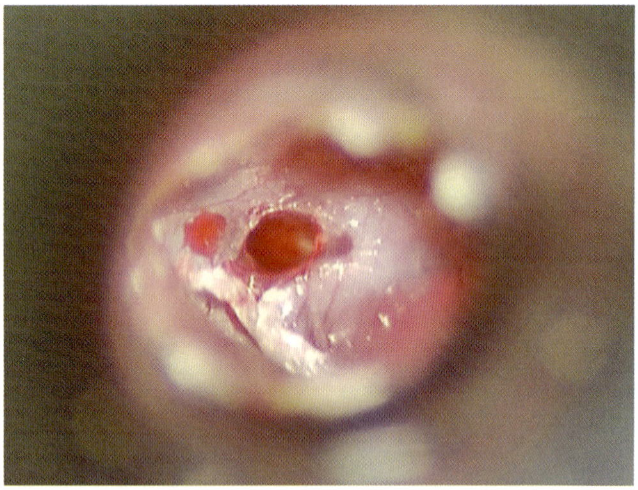

Fig. 6.1: Transcanal view of a perforated tympanic membrane following tube removal.

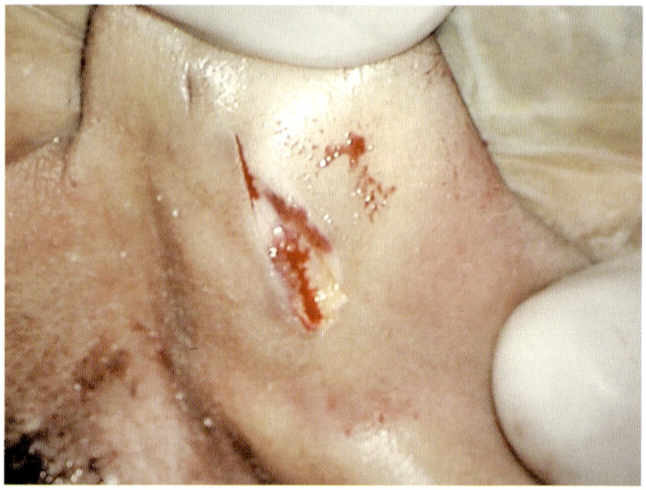

Fig. 6.2: Incision of the medial side of lobule for fat harvesting.

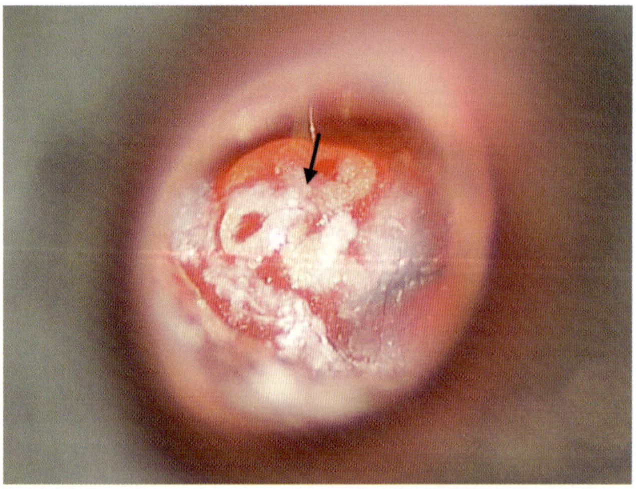

Fig. 6.3: Placement of a fat graft through a perforation after de-epithelialization of the perforation. Arrow is on the fat graft.

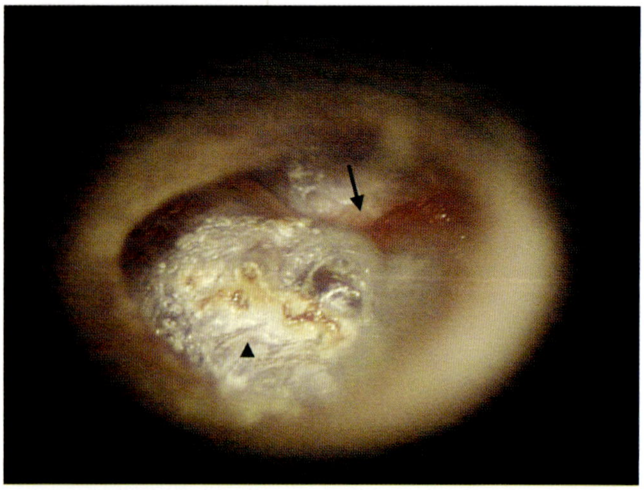

Fig. 6.4: View of the tympanic membrane following a myringoplasty of a posterior atrophic and an atelectatic tympanic membrane. Long arrow denotes the umbo, arrowhead on the lasered tympanic membrane.

Step 3: A small tympanostomy tube (0.76 mm diameter) may be placed to help with ventilation during healing of the tympanic membrane following laser myringoplasty.

Transcanal Approach Setup

If a transcanal approach is decided, the procedure can be done easily under either general or local anesthesia with intravenous sedation.

Step 1: An appropriately sized ear speculum is placed and under binocular microscopy (working distance is typically 250–300 mm) and the ear is cleaned of debris. A speculum holder, if desired, is placed.

Step 2: Visualization of the posterior canal wall, tympanic membrane, malleus (if present), and perforation(s) are then confirmed, and the decision to proceed transcanal, endaural, or postauricular is decided at this step (Fig. 6.5). If the transcanal approach is pursued, the canal skin is injected in quadrants with 1% lidocaine with 1:100,000 epinephrine just medial to the bony-cartilaginous junction. Approximately 1 cc of solution is injected at this step. Slow injection within the correct plane helps to prevent blebs, allows for blanching of the canal skin to the tympanic membrane, and provides hemostasis.

Step 3: Canal cuts are then performed using the round, roller, sickle, or Beaver knife depending on surgeon preference (Fig. 6.6). Many flaps have been described. Usually a long tympanomeatal flap of 5–7 mm is designed that allows the flap to be displaced anteriorly.

Step 4: The skin is then elevated using a dissecting elevator. Occasionally, microscissors may be needed to cut the thicker skin of the superior canal. The annulus is then identified and lifted from the tympanic sulcus. If the case is done under local anesthesia, frequent use of 1% lidocaine-soaked Gelfoam applied during elevation decreases discomfort, especially at the annulus.

Step 5: The middle ear is then entered (Fig. 6.7).

Postauricular Approach Setup

Step 1: Canal cuts may be made first via the transcanal approach (Fig. 6.8) or from the postauricular approach. Many skin flap incisions have been designed. Most are laterally based, such as the vascular strip incision, which allows the pinna and the skin flap to be pulled from the bony canal and retracted forward to visualize the middle ear. Three canal incisions are made to create the vascular strip: incisions at 12 and 6 o'clock from the annulus to the cartilaginous canal and a medial cut with a 72 Beaver blade just lateral to the annulus. Alternatively incisions along the tympanosquamous and tympanomastoid sutures with a connecting incision 5–7 mm from the annulus can be made. Following these transcanal cuts, the speculum is removed and the postauricular incision is made with a #15 blade through the skin between 5 mm and 10 mm from the postauricular sulcus (Fig. 6.9). The incision is typically carried down to near the mastoid tip and carried up over the superior attachment of the pinna (Fig. 6.10). The dissection can then be continued with either electrocautery or with a knife. With lateral retraction of the ear, tissue planes can be more readily identified. The temporalis fascia, which covers the temporalis muscle, is identified in the superior portion of the

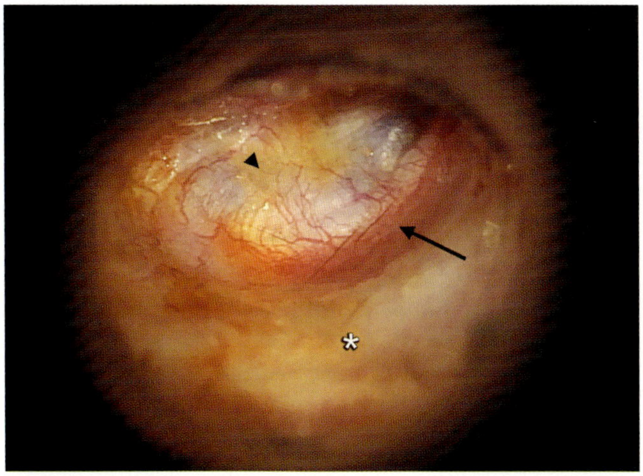

Fig. 6.5: Transcanal view. Posterior canal wall is seen with transition to the annulus and tympanic membrane. Arrowhead is on the tympanic membrane, arrow shows annulus, and asterisk denotes the posterior canal wall.

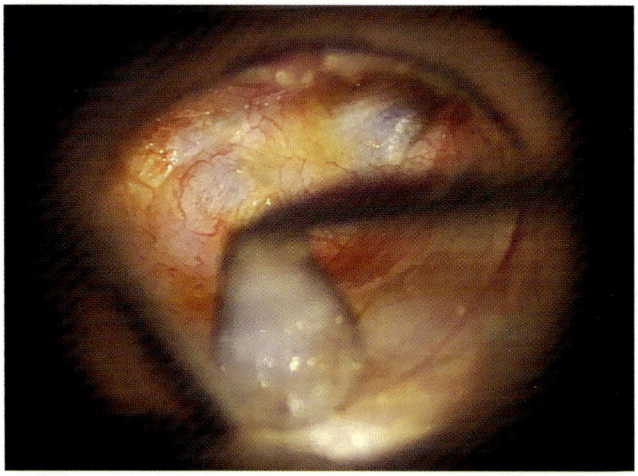

Fig. 6.6: A transcanal incision. An incision for the tympanomeatal flap made approximately 5 mm from the annulus.

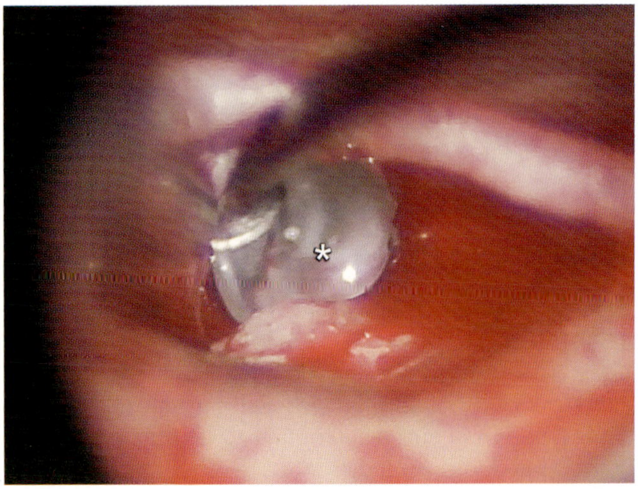

Fig. 6.7: Entering middle ear via a transcanal approach. The tympanomeatal flap is lifted anteriorly and the mucosa of the middle ear is seen beyond the instrument. An asterisk shows an opened middle ear cleft.

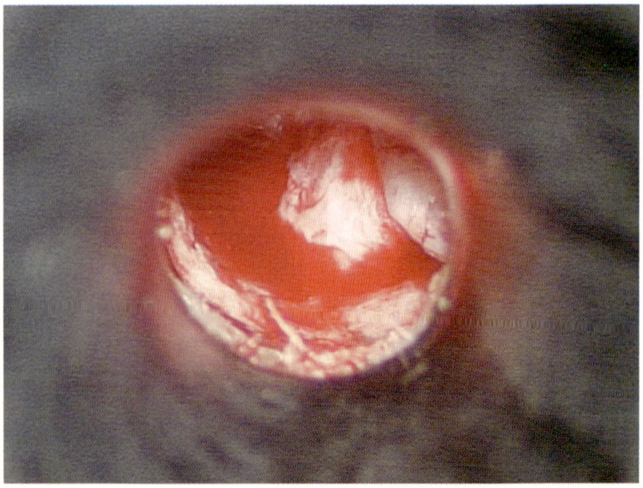

Fig. 6.8: A transcanal incision prior to a postauricular incision.

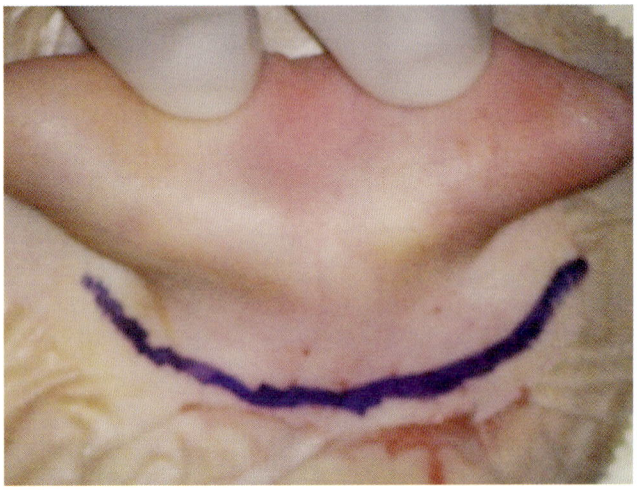

Fig. 6.9: Plan of a postauricular incision, which is placed approximately 5–10 mm posterior to the auricular sulcus.

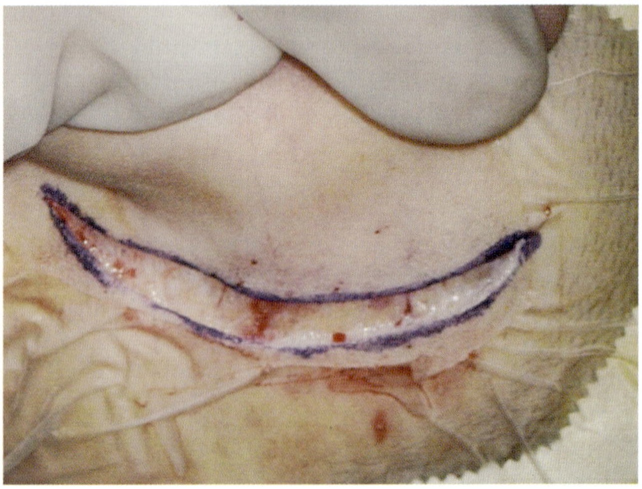

Fig. 6.10: An incision through skin of the postauricular area.

incision. Once this avascular plane is identified, the dissection is then carried at the same plane inferiorly toward the mastoid tip, through the postauricular muscle. This dissection should be carried toward the root of the zygoma and up to, but not through, the skin of the ear canal.

Step 2: A self-retaining retractor is placed and then the musculoperiosteal incision is performed from the root of the zygoma along the linea temporalis over the ear canal and back toward the mastoid (Fig. 6.11). A perpendicular limb is then dropped from this incision in either a "T" or "7" configuration (Fig. 6.12). Using a periosteal elevator, the musculoperiosteal flap is then elevated anteriorly toward the canal.

Step 3: Once at the canal, the dissection is carried out under the microscope and the flap is raised first off the spine of Henle, then away from the posterior ear canal with a smaller (e.g. Freer or Shambaugh) elevator. The skin is elevated medially in the ear canal until the canal cuts are identified. The skin of the vascular strip is the retracted forward, allowing visualization of the tympanic membrane (Fig. 6.13). Alternatively, no transcanal cuts are made, and the incisions of the vascular strip are made after elevating the skin from the canal from behind (Figs. 6.14 to 6.17).

Step 4: Following the postauricular exposure, the middle ear is entered by lifting the tympanomeatal flap.

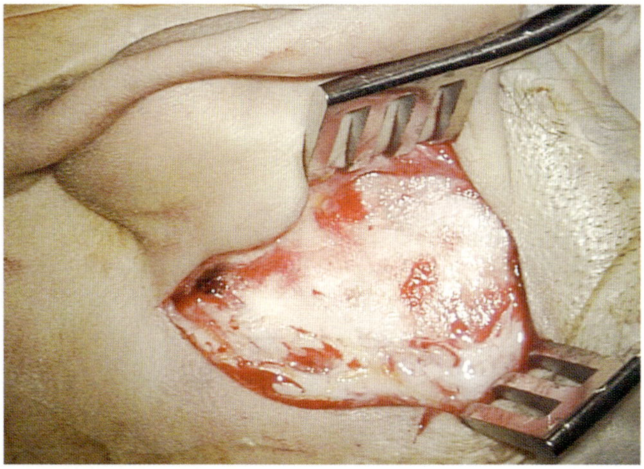

Fig. 6.11: The location of the temporalis fascia. The avascular plane immediately superficial to the temporalis fascia is identified.

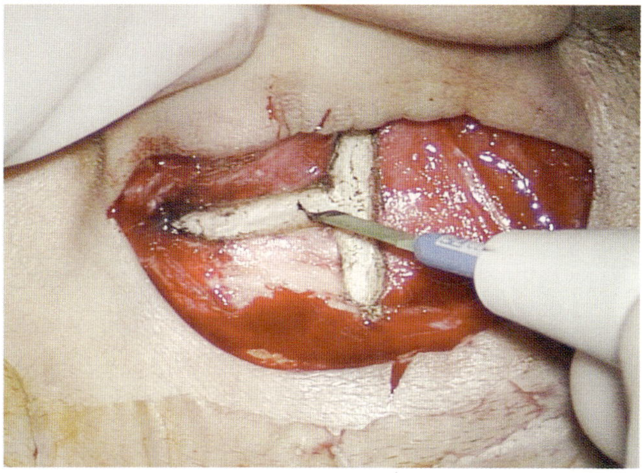

Fig. 6.12: A musculoperiosteal incision, which is place along the linea temporalis and carried down to mastoid tip. The incision is made to the mastoid cortical bone.

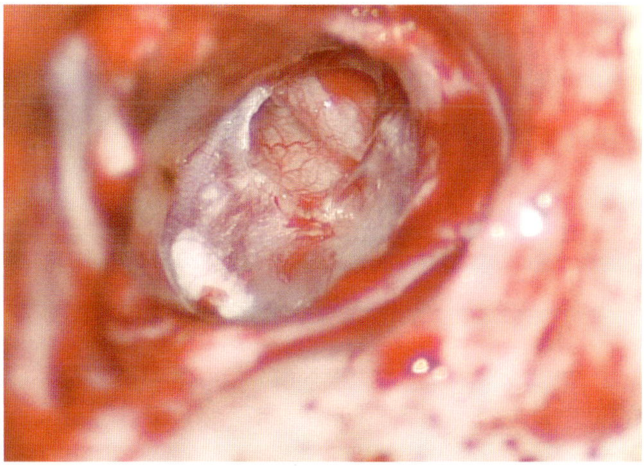

Fig. 6.13: Standard postauricular exposure. The tympanic membrane with a perforation is visualized after retraction of the vascular strip.

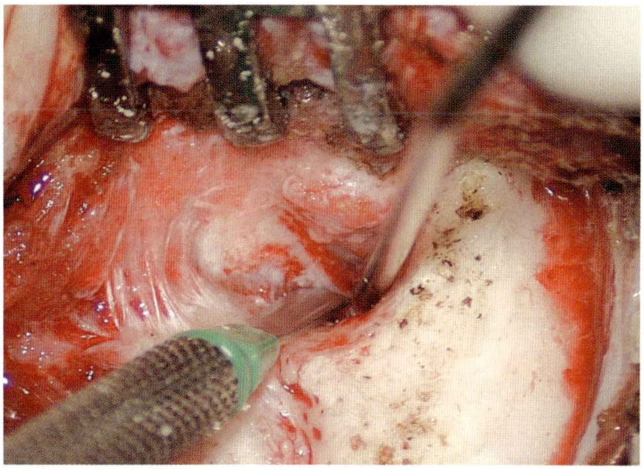

Fig. 6.14: The vascular strip incision made from a postauricular exposure. A Beaver 6400 blade is used.

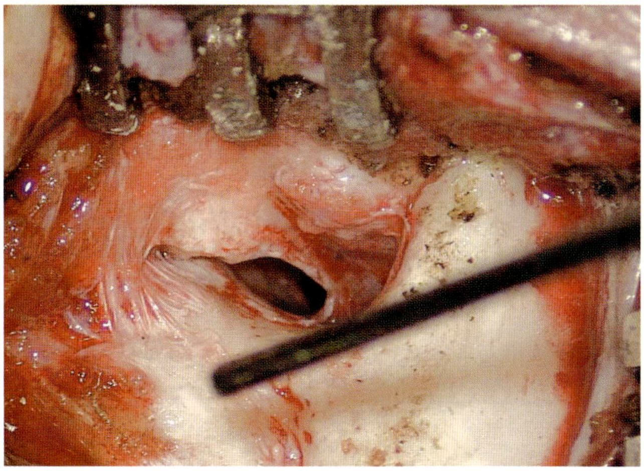

Fig. 6.15: An incision is made along the tympanomastoid suture.

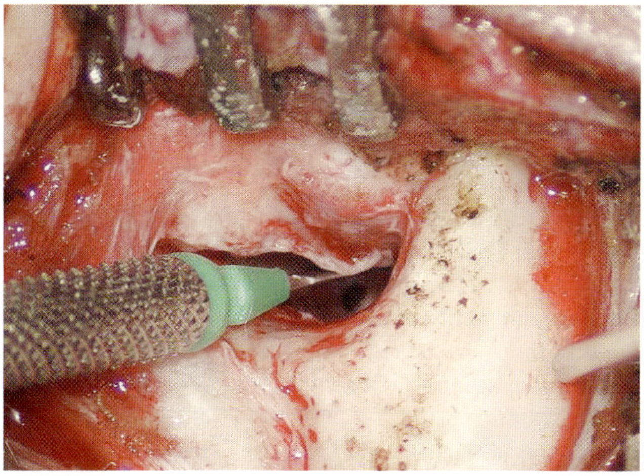

Fig. 6.16: An incision from the medial tympanomastoid suture to the tympanosquamous suture is demonstrated.

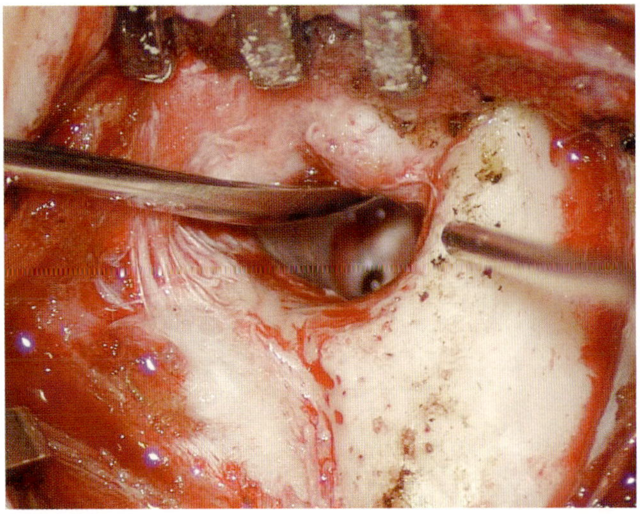

Fig. 6.17: View after completion of the tympanosquamous incision.

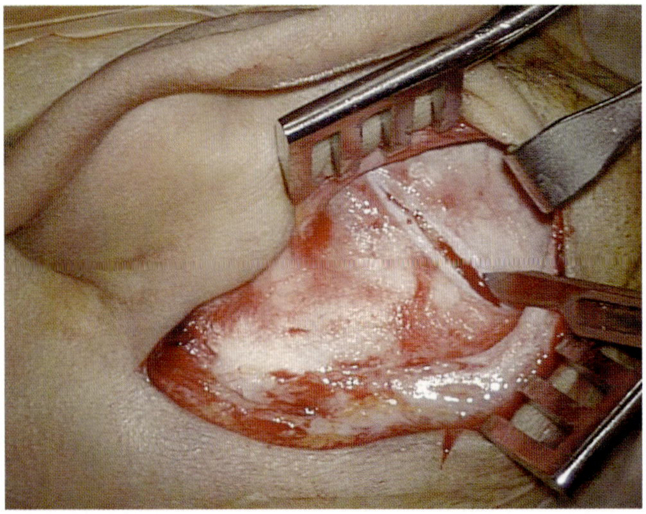

Fig. 6.18: Incising the temporalis fascia. An initial incision is made with a #15 blade for harvesting the temporalis fascia.

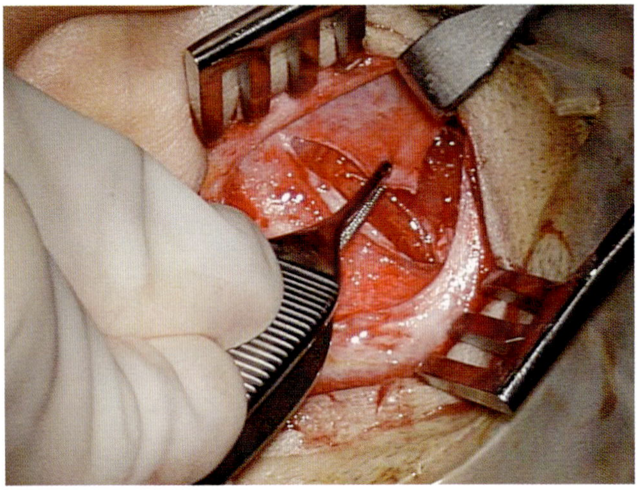

Fig. 6.19: Harvesting temporalis fascia.

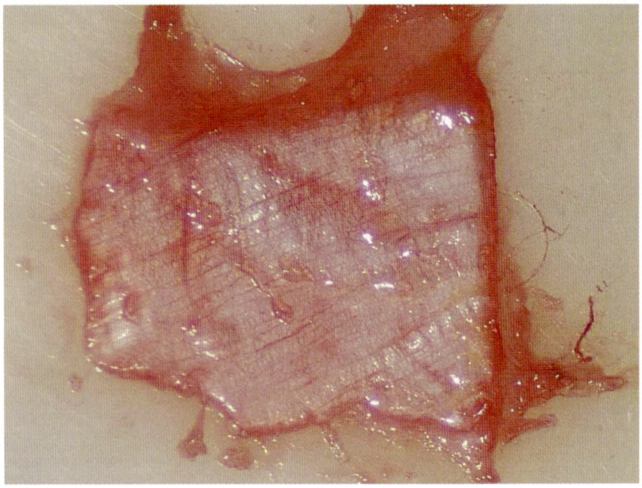

Fig. 6.20: Shaping of the graft can happen after drying the fascia.

Step 5: At the end of the case, the incision is closed with deep dermal 3-0 Vicryl sutures, and skin reapproximated with an absorbable suture or tissue adhesive.

Harvesting Temporalis Fascia

Temporalis fascia is a common grafting material used in modern tympanoplasty. The fascia is readily available through a postauricular incision:
Step 1: Incision of the fascia takes place with a #15 blade and continued either with a knife or with scissors (Figs. 6.18 and 6.19).
Step 2: The underlying muscle is trimmed from the graft. For a near total perforation a 10 × 20 mm graft should be sufficient.
Step 3: The graft is then dried for use (Fig. 6.20). Trimming of the graft occurs after drying.

Harvesting Tragal Cartilage

If cartilage is sought then the tragal cartilage is often used.
Step 1: An incision is made medial to the lateral edge of the tragus in the ear canal. The incision is carried through the tragal cartilage, leaving a small lateral "cap" for cosmesis (Fig. 6.21).
Step 2: A single-prong hook is placed to allow exposure and the cartilage is then dissected free from its surrounding soft tissue with scissors and removed (Fig. 6.22).
Step 3: Often perichondrium on at least one side of the graft is desirable (Fig. 6.23). After removal of the

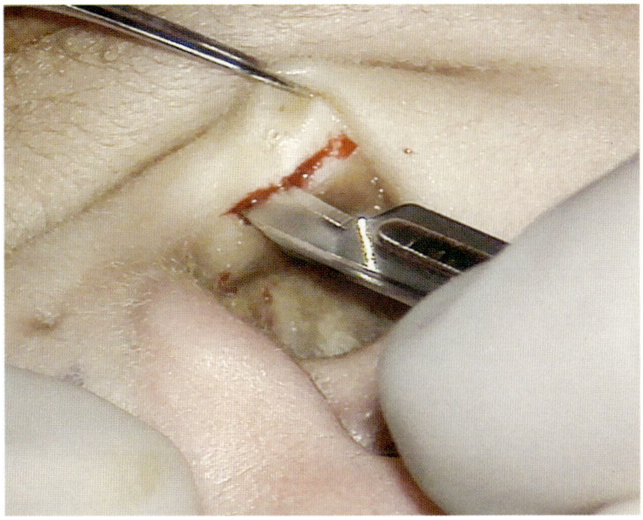

Fig. 6.21: Tragal cartilage graft initial incision. The lateral most cartilage is maintained for cosmesis.

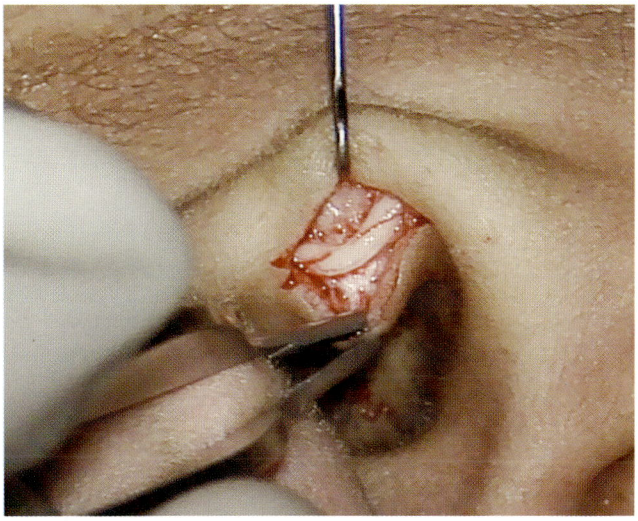

Fig. 6.22: Identification of tragal cartilage.

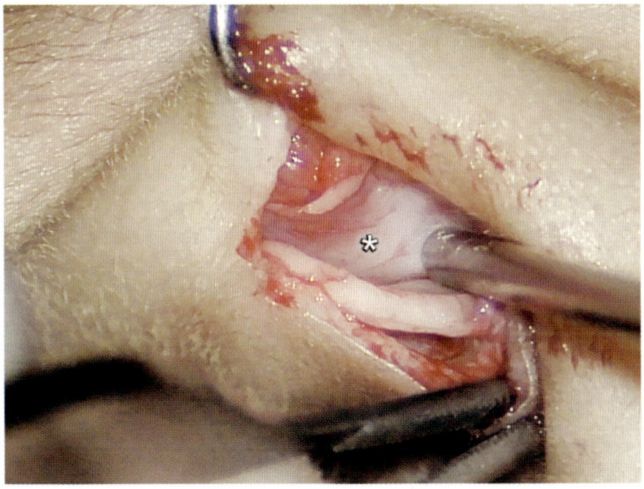

Fig. 6.23: Release of the anterior perichondrium from the cartilage graft (asterisk denotes anterior perichondrium being lifted from tragal cartilage).

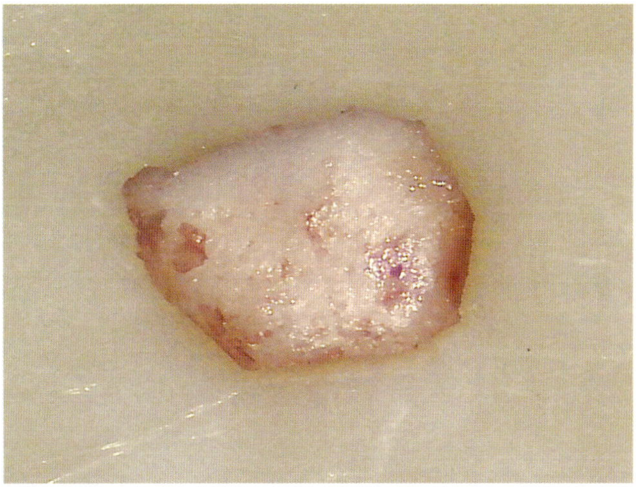

Fig. 6.24: Tragal cartilage graft.

cartilage, it can be further shaped as needed (Fig. 6.24). Alternatively exposure of the cartilage with resection of only the perichondrium can be performed if cartilage is not needed.

Step 4: The incision can be closed using interrupted fast absorbing suture.

Harvesting Conchal Cartilage

Another source of cartilage and/or perichondrium is from conchal cartilage. This can be accessed through a pre-existing postauricular incision or by a smaller incision made directly on the posterior pinna in transcanal cases.

Step 1: The overlying soft tissue is dissected away sharply until the cartilage is located (Fig. 6.25).

Step 2: It is then incised and freed from the surrounding tissue for use sharply using either a knife or scissors. Care must be ensured not to enter the lateral skin, which would then cause a through-and-through defect in the pinna.

Entering the Middle Ear

Step 1: Once the skin flap is raised to the sulcus of the annulus, the white cord-like structure of the fibrous annulus (which is the beginning of the fibrous portion

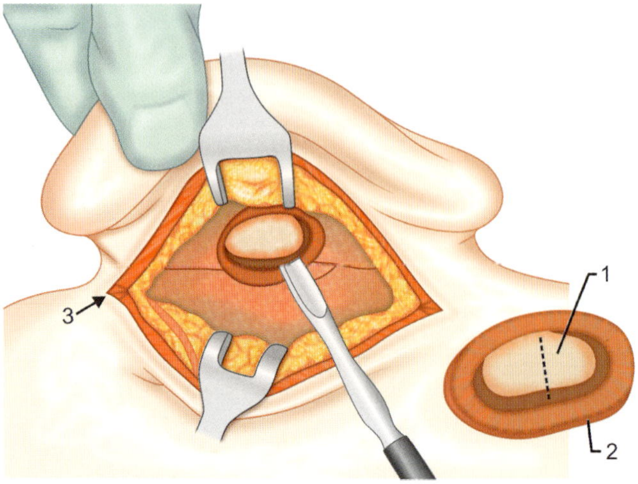

Fig. 6.25: Harvesting conchal cartilage. Sharp dissection is used to release the soft tissue.

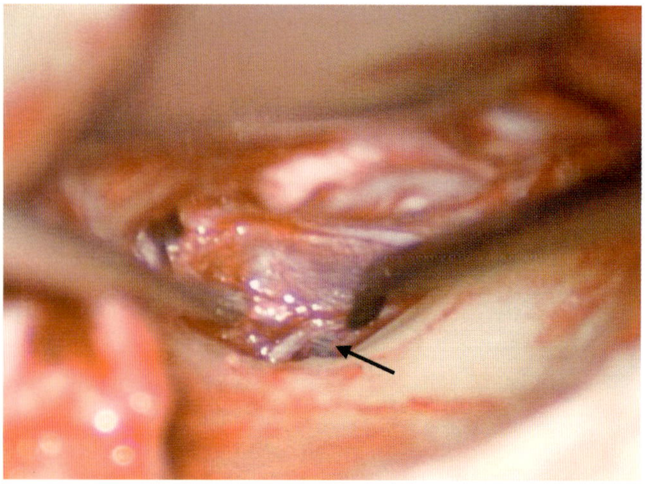

Fig. 6.26: Identification of the fibrous annulus. The instrument points to the annulus, which has been lifted from the tympanic sulcus. The arrow points to the middle ear mucosa medial to annulus.

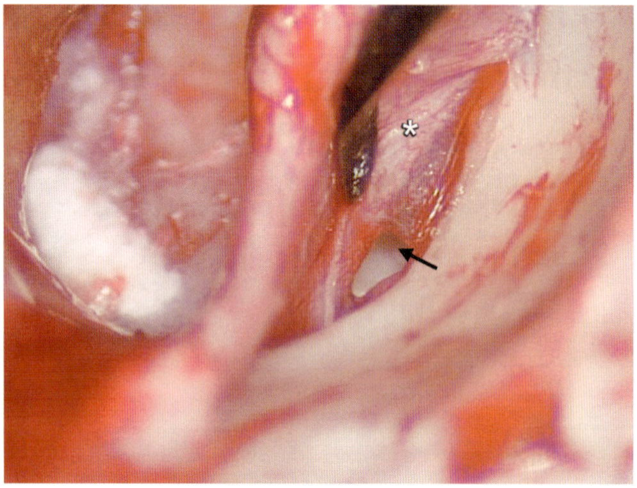

Fig. 6.27: Entrance into the middle ear. A small opening into middle ear mucosa is made immediately medial to the annulus. The arrow points to opened middle ear space through mucosa. An asterisk is on fibrous annulus.

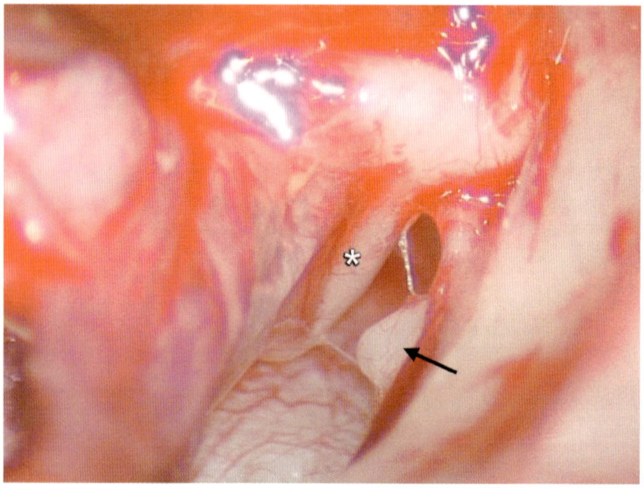

Fig. 6.28: Exposure of middle ear. The tympanomeatal flap has been lifted and the malleus (asterisk) and lenticular process of incus (arrow) seen.

of the tympanic membrane) is then elevated from the sulcus with a small elevating instrument (Fig. 6.26).

Step 2: The thin web-like mucosa (often bluish in healthy ears, red and thick in diseased ears) is then entered bluntly with a dissecting instrument (Fig. 6.27).

Step 3: The fibrous annulus is raised inferiorly and superiorly from its bony sulcus. The fibrous annulus starts as a structure lateral to the bony sulcus and then continues to have a close association in the bony sulcus.

Step 4: The chorda tympani nerve, which lies medial to the annulus, exits the tympanic bone often superiorly, but its location can be variable in individuals. This is especially true in revision cases. Often a fine needle is needed to remove the chorda tympani nerve from the surrounding tissue.

Step 5: The superior dissection should be carried to the malleus (Fig. 6.28).

Inspection of the Middle Ear for Disease and Evaluation/Palpation of the Ossicles

Step 1: After entering and gaining wide exposure to the middle ear, the mucosa should be assessed. Middle ear

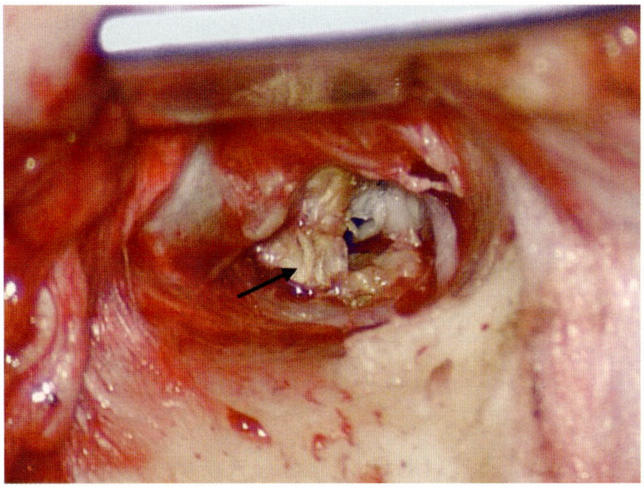

Fig. 6.29: Cholesteatoma. Middle ear with cholesteatoma (arrow) after postauricular exposure.

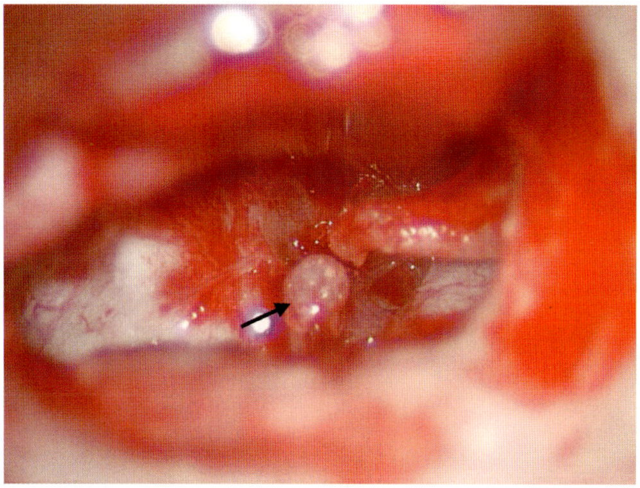

Fig. 6.30: Incus erosion. The capitulum of stapes (arrow) is not connected to the incus.

disease should be noted. Cholesteatoma (Fig. 6.29), which often is seen prior to entering the middle ear, can track posteriorly into the sinus tympani, superiorly into epitympanum and aditus, or inferiorly to the hypotympanum. Removal of diseased tissue should then ensue.

Step 2: The ossicular chain should be examined. Erosion or discontinuity should be assessed (Fig. 6.30). The incudostapedial joint should be scrutinized. Sometimes a fibrous union is seen, which transmits sound inefficiently. A myringoincudostapedio- or myringostapediopexy may exist, and the drum may need to be lifted from these structures.

Step 3: Palpation of the ossicles, regardless if they are connected or not, should be performed. First applying gentle lateral pressure to the malleus, followed by palpation of the long process of the incus, the stapes superstructure and finally the footplate. Sometimes fixation can seem to be associated with all the ossicles and disarticulation of the incudostapedial joint with repeat palpation can help ascertain the location of fixation.

Step 4: At this point if the bony anatomy of the ear canal inhibits visualization a canalplasty can be performed.

The Underlay Technique

The underlay grafting technique consists of placement of the graft medial to the annulus.

Step 1: All perforations should be assessed for skin tracking medially and along the undersurface of the tympanic membrane prior to grafting. These diseased portions should be resected. Tympanosclerosis of the drum abutting the perforation should be excised. If the tympanosclerosis is very thick in the remaining portion of the drum, it should be resected. If the tympanosclerosis is thin, then this is left in place as it adds stability to the reconstruction.

Step 2: The edges of the perforation should be de-epithelialized with a right angle pick.

Step 3: The tympanic membrane is lifted anteriorly, and the middle ear is packed with moist Gelfoam to act as support for the graft.

Step 4: The graft is then trimmed and placed with suction and fine instruments.

Step 5: Following placement, the tympanic membrane is placed back on top of the graft (Fig. 6.31). No gaps between the graft and the native drum should be present.

Step 6: The skin of the tympanic membrane and canal should be unrolled to prevent an iatrogenic cholesteatoma with the vascular strip meticulously placed over the graft and canal. The ear canal is then packed with Gelfoam soaked in antibiotic solution or an ear canal sponge pack.

The Over-Under Modification of the Underlay Technique

Situations in which the underlay grafting often fails include when a perforation abuts or is anterior to the malleus, and with narrow middle ear clefts (Figs. 6.32A and B). One technique that greatly increases the versatility of the underlay technique is the over-under procedure. This procedure also allows for easier prosthesis placement under the malleus without the interference of the grafting material.

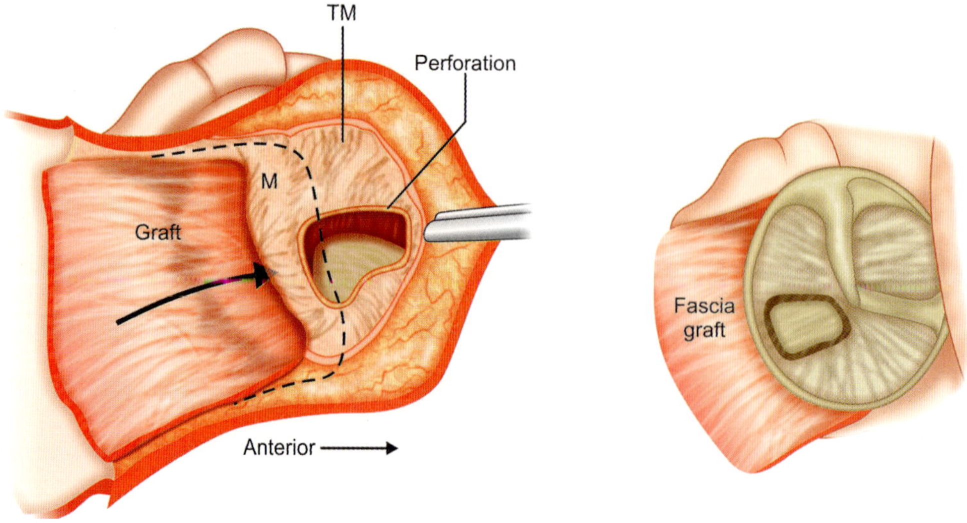

Fig. 6.31: Underlay technique. The fascia graft is placed medial to the malleus and annulus.

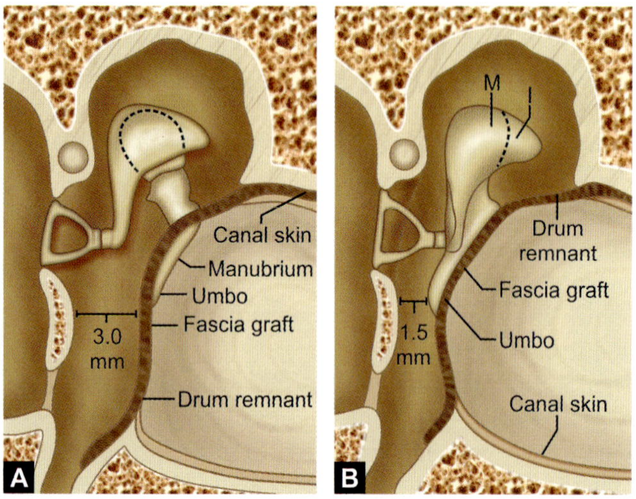

Figs. 6.32A and B: Configurations of the middle ear cleft. (A) Favorable middle ear cleft with space for graft placement. (B) Unfavorable middle ear cleft with narrow space for graft placement.

Step 1: Similar to the underlay technique, the edges of the perforation should be de-epithelialized and any skin folded under the perforation removed.

Step 2: Unlike the traditional underlay technique, the drum is lifted from the malleus sharply with a fine needle with care—especially if the ossicular chain is intact. The fibrous attachment at the umbo can be sharply divided with microscissors or with the aid of the laser (Figs. 6.33A and B). The laser may allow for less manipulation of the ossicular chain.

Step 3: Once this is done the graft can then be placed lateral to the malleus but still medial to the annulus (Fig. 6.34). The malleus then becomes an asset in helping maintain the graft as opposed to a hinderance. This technique also allows for placement of a prosthesis under the malleus without interference from the fascia graft, as it lies lateral to the manubrium.

Step 4: When the middle ear cleft is narrow, laying the inferior graft lateral to the bony tympanic sulcus helps minimize graft failure. Usually, this involves back elevation of the anterior and inferior canal wall skin.

The Overlay Technique

The overlay technique involves placement of the graft lateral to the annulus.

Step 1: Exposure of the tympanic membrane is by the postauricular approach, allowing for necessary visualization anteriorly.

Step 2: The skin circumferentially is removed from the canal and taken off the fibrous layer of the tympanic membrane as one piece (Fig. 6.35). Usually, a curved needle is needed to free the skin layer from the fibrous layer at the anterior annulus. This free graft is removed and set on the back table (Fig. 6.36). Care is needed to remove all squamous epithelium as retained skin will form an iatrogenic cholesteatoma.

Step 3: Following exposure of the tympanic membrane canalplasty is performed. Drilling the anterior canal wall allows for a better angle at the anterior sulcus to prevent blunting.

Step 4: The graft is then placed on the fibrous layer (Figs. 6.37A and B) and up the anterior canal wall. Approximately, half the graft is placed on the canal and half on the drum (Fig. 6.38). Generally, the graft is cut in a manner to hook it under the umbo/manubrium of the malleus to prevent lateralization.

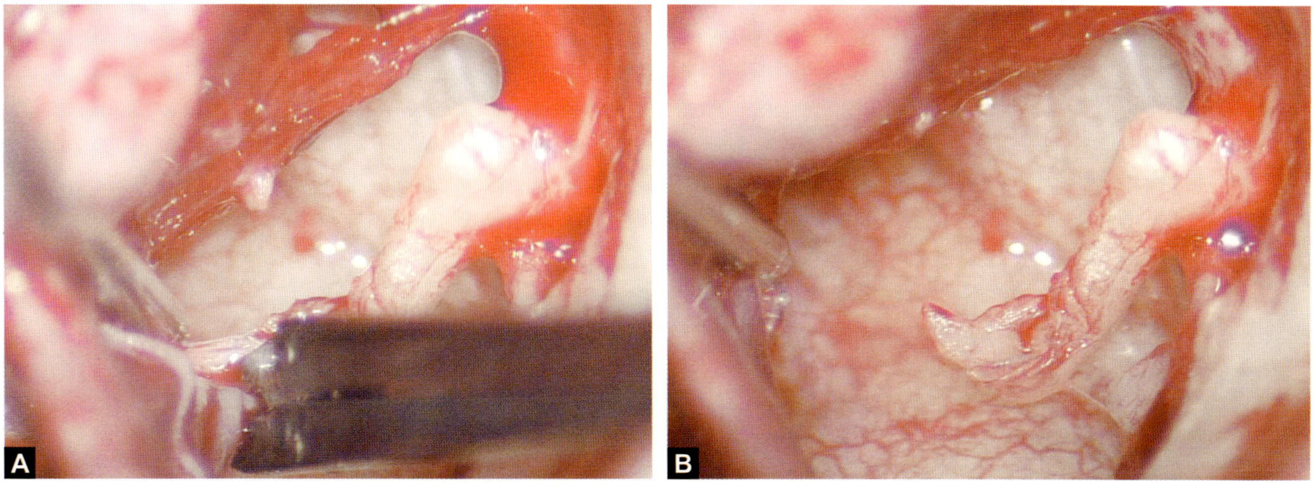

Figs. 6.33A and B: Lifting the tympanic membrane from the malleus. (A) The last fibrous attachments of the tympanic membrane to the umbo are released with microscissors. (B) Malleus completely free from the tympanic membrane.

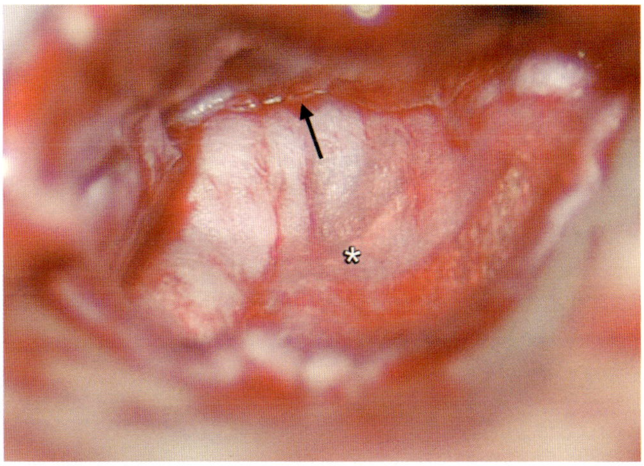

Fig. 6.34: Placement of a graft in the over-under technique. The graft (asterisk) is placed under the annulus anteriorly, and over the malleus. The remnant of the drum (arrow) is seen anteriorly.

Step 5: Packing is placed to reinforce the anterior sulcus to create a sharp angle in order to reduce blunting. Packing is then placed in the rest of the ear canal.

Drilling of the External Ear Canal (Canalplasty)

In all tympanoplasty procedures, the anatomy of the bony canal can prohibit visualization. Bony canalplasty can enlarge the canal in these cases.

Step 1: In general, drilling starts at the spine of Henle at the lateral canal. Care must be used not to enter the mastoid air cells, which could result in a fistula. If air cells are entered, bone wax can be applied to seal the opening.

Step 2: Once the spine is removed the tympanomastoid and tympanosquamous suture lines are assessed. Further drilling of these structures then proceeds if needed (Fig. 6.39).

Step 3: As one works medially, often a small (4–5 mm) aluminum foil disk (protector) is fashioned and placed to keep from drilling on the flap, canal skin, or ossicles (Fig. 6.40).

Step 4: Anterior drilling, if needed, is then accomplished. Care must be taken not to open the glenoid fossa. It is of note that most exposure for successful canalplasty surgery is with careful dissection and removal of the superior portion of the bony canal and tympanosquamous suture line, then extending anteriorly when needed.

Meatoplasty

Soft tissue meatoplasty may be needed in cases for narrowed ear canals. This may occur either with or without bony canalplasty. Most often meatoplasty is performed in cases of canal-wall-down mastoidectomy. There are many techniques that have been described. Important is the release of conchal cartilage that provides a "spring" effect for the meatus to resume its original shape. Only after accomplishing this release is the meatus allowed to relax.

Step 1: Following a bony canalplasty or canal-wall-down mastoidectomy, a nasal speculum is placed in the ear.

Step 2: Extension of the superior incision along the tympanosquamous suture is carried out laterally with a small 6400 Beaver blade toward the meatus.

Step 3: A second incision from the tympanomastoid suture toward the meatus is performed.

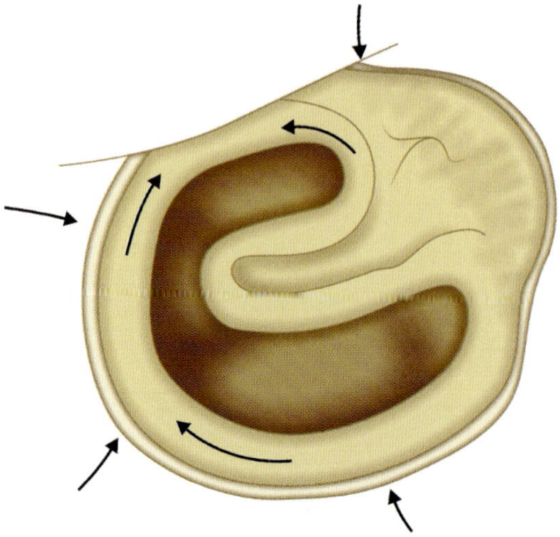

Fig. 6.35: Removal of skin from the tympanic membrane as seen in the overlay technique.

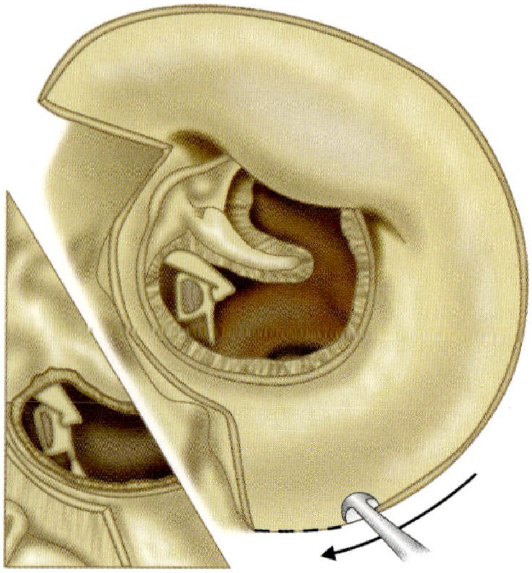

Fig. 6.36: Removal of the surrounding canal skin is performed prior to the overlay graft placement.

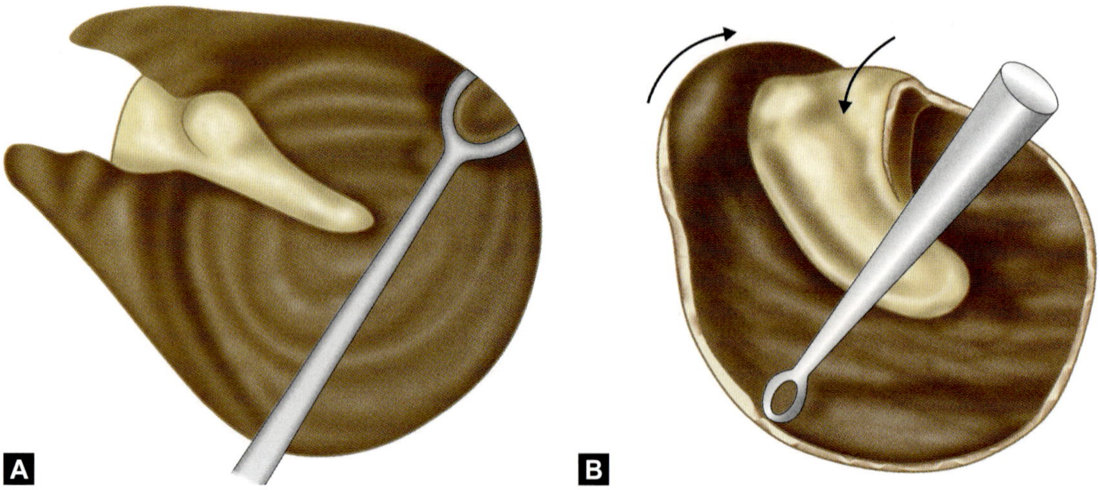

Figs. 6.37A and B: Placement of fascia in the overlay technique. The graft is tucked under the malleus and over the fibrous remnant of the tympanic membrane.

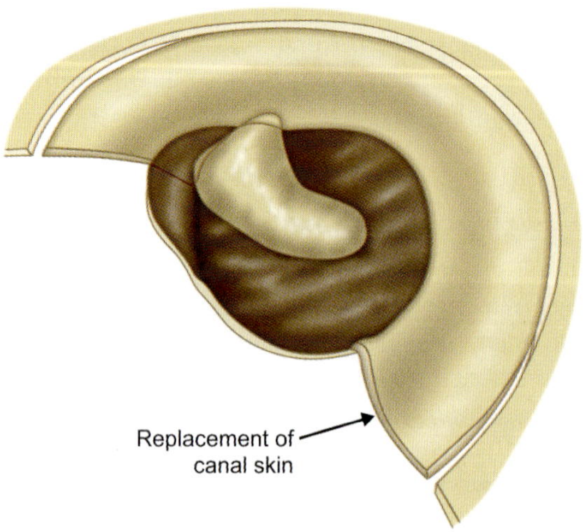

Fig. 6.38: Replacement of the canal skin following fascia placement.

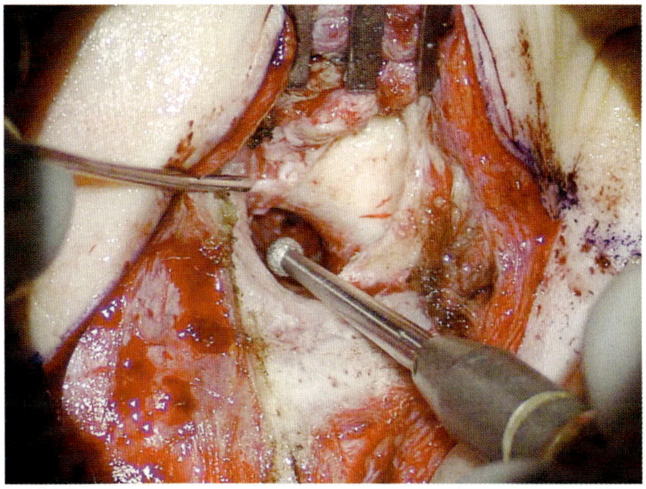

Fig. 6.39: Drilling of the bony canal.

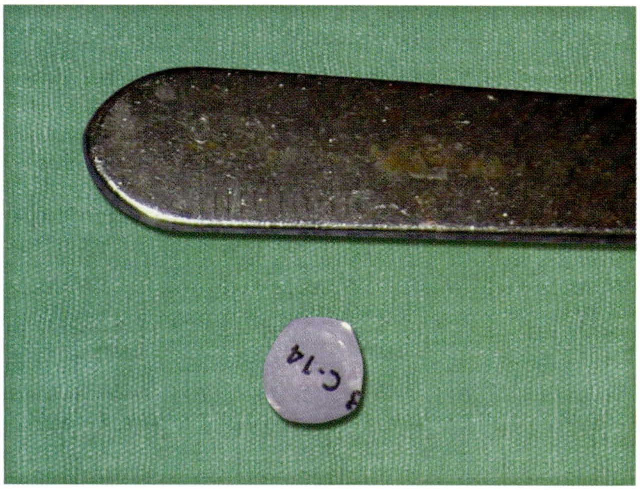

Fig. 6.40: Creation of an aluminum disk used to protect the skin during drilling.

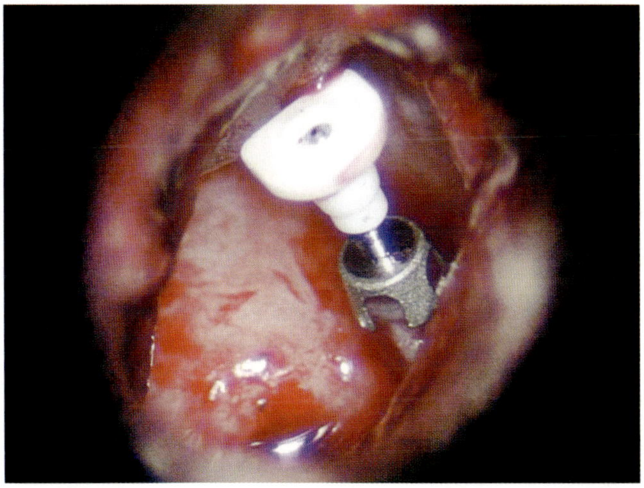

Fig. 6.41: Placement of a partial ossicular replacement prosthesis (PORP). The prosthesis attaches from the malleus to the capitulum of the stapes.

Step 4: From the postauricular incision the vascular strip is then thinned with scissors.

Step 5: Then either through the meatus or postauricularly the conchal cartilage of the posterior meatus is resected from the flap. This allows the vascular strip to then conform to the bony canal.

Step 6: The meatus is then packed with strips of Gelfoam soaked in antibiotic solution with or without an ear Merocel ear pack. In general, no suturing of the meatus is necessary with this technique, which can lead to rotation of the pinna; however, absorbable retaining sutures can be placed at the edge of the cartilage resection and positioned posteriorly to enlarge the canal.

Ossiculoplasty

If ossiculoplasty is needed, the decision to perform an ossiculoplasty is made intraoperatively.

Step 1: Assessment of all the ossicles, their movement and structural integrity is carried out. In general, maintaining the integrity of the ossicles is desired. Incus erosion is the most common problem encountered (Fig. 6.30). Minor erosion of the incus can be repaired with hydroxyapatite cement. Hearing results may not be as good as expected due to stiffness of the incus and malleus, and long-term hearing results from large series do not exist for this technique. A larger erosion may call for bypass of the incus. If the stapes is mobile and structurally sound, a partial ossicular replacement prosthesis (PORP) extending from the malleus to the capitulum is a solution (Fig. 6.41). If the superstructure of the stapes is partially or totally missing or has poor integrity, and the footplate is intact and mobile, placement of a total ossicular replacement prosthesis (TORP) from the malleus or drum to the footplate may be needed (Figs. 6.42A and B). The placement of a TORP with a shoe that inserts over the footplate can add stability in some cases (Fig. 6.43). Some prostheses are universal—meaning that they can act as a PORP or TORP by cutting the prosthesis. Such prostheses maybe hollow and taper distally, and thus by leaving it longer it can act as a columella to the footplate (Fig. 6.44), but cut shorter it can adapt to the capitulum as a PORP (Fig. 6.45).

Step 2: If the malleus is present, attempting to use it for stabilization is helpful. If possible, maintaining the malleus head with its anterior malleolar ligament and the

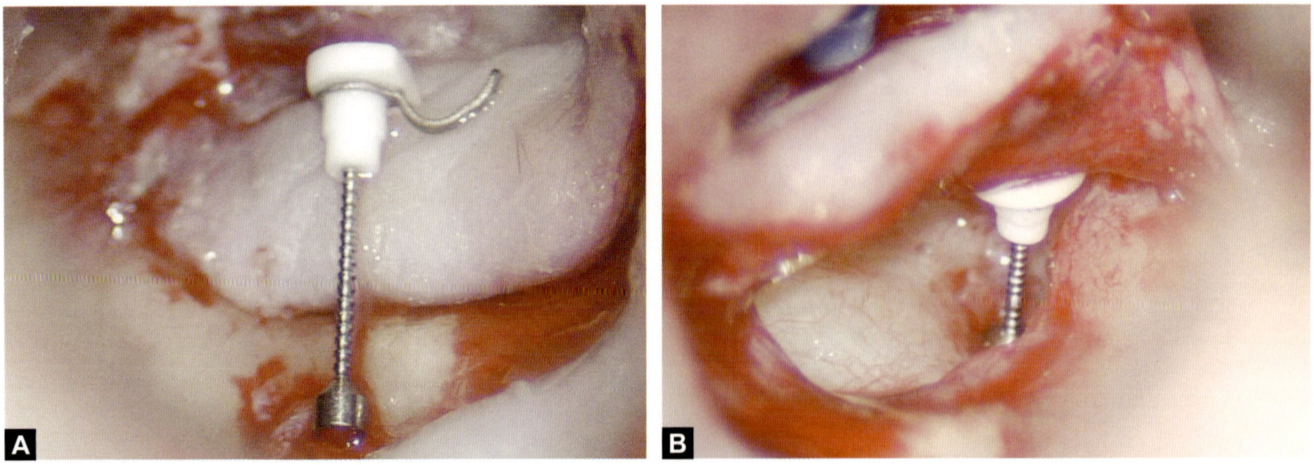

Figs. 6.42A and B: Total ossicular replacement prosthesis (TORP) ossiculoplasty. (A) TORP without oval window shoe prior to placement. (B) Arrangement of a TORP from the malleus to the oval window.

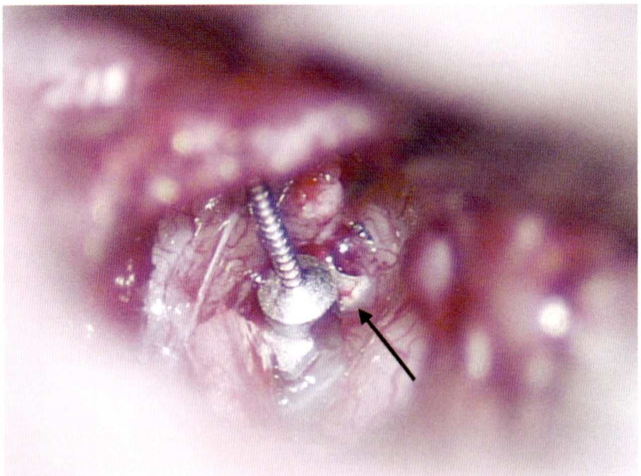

Fig. 6.43: A total ossicular replacement prosthesis (TORP) with shoe. The anterior phalange of the shoe is shown with the arrow.

tensor tympani also help with stabilization. However in ears with a narrow middle ear cleft, release of the tensor tendon allows lateralization of the malleus resulting in increased size of the middle ear cleft.

Step 3: Autografts such as the incus or malleus head, cortical bone, or cartilage can be shaped for placement (Fig. 6.46). Sculpting of the ossicle requires fixation with an ossicle holder and use of a 1 mm drill bit at lower speeds (10,000 to 40,000 rpm). Rarely is extrusion seen with autologous materials.

Step 4: A large variety of prostheses comprised of biocompatible materials exist, with many contemporary prosthesis made of titanium, hydroxyapatite, plastic, or composite. Many are adjustable and often these prostheses come with sizers that help predict the correct length. While performing ossiculoplasty minimizing footplate movement and medial force on the footplate is crucial. Use of a small-caliber suction in one hand and a fine instrument in the other allows for guidance of the graft or prosthesis into place.

Step 5: One should make sure that the autograft or prosthesis is secure after placement without ready displacement. It should also clear the posterior canal wall, which could impede its movement should fusion occur. Small pieces of Gelfoam soaked in saline are placed around the prosthesis to help support it. In some situations, a small-bore tympanostomy tube may be placed to limit tympanic membrane movement during the healing phase.

Ossicular Fixation and Incus Bypass

Ossicular fixation can be seen with otosclerosis (*see* chapter on Stapedectomy) or in tympanosclerosis, which is a sequela of chronic otitis media. Fixation can also be congenital. Fixed ossicles can be approached in two ways: (1) incus bypass and (2) exploration of the epitympanum and freeing of the impinging structure on the ossicle(s). Fixed ossicles may be of the lateral chain (malleus and/or incus) or stapes. Lateral chain fixation is handled by mobilization of the chain manually with additional section of the tensor tympani tendon. The preferred method is for removal of the incus and PORP reconstruction. Otherwise an epitympanum exploration and freeing of the impinging structures on the ossicles can be undertaken.

Step 1: A fine instrument such as a curved needle is used to palpate the ossicles. The head of the malleus and body of the incus are common sites for fixation. The incudostapedial joint is separated with posterior to anterior force using a joint knife or right angle knife.

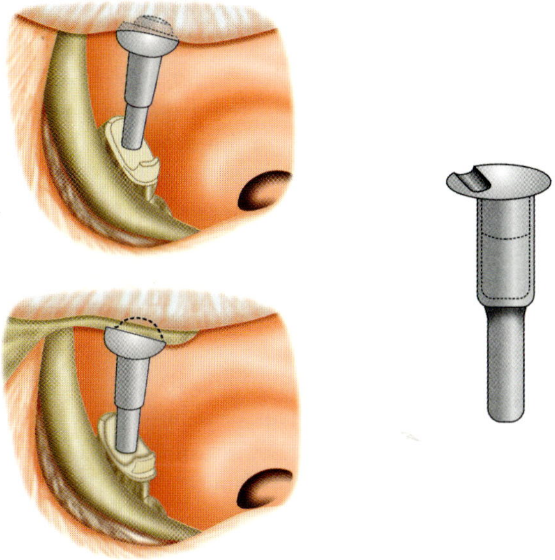

Fig. 6.44: Example of a universal prosthesis used as a total ossicular replacement prosthesis (TORP).

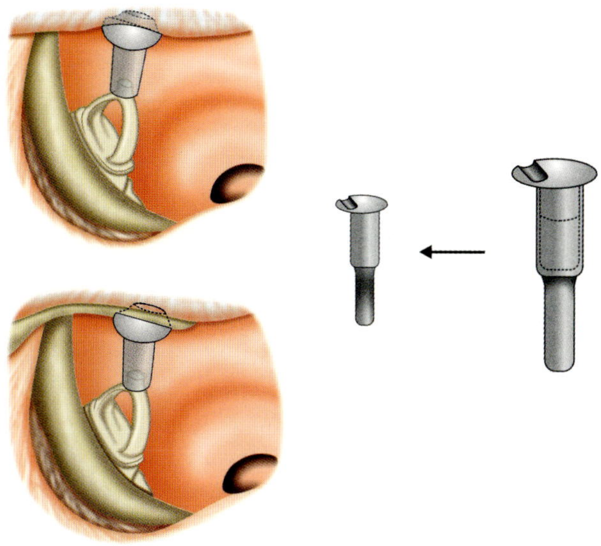

Fig. 6.45: Example of a universal prosthesis used as a partial ossicular replacement prosthesis (PORP).

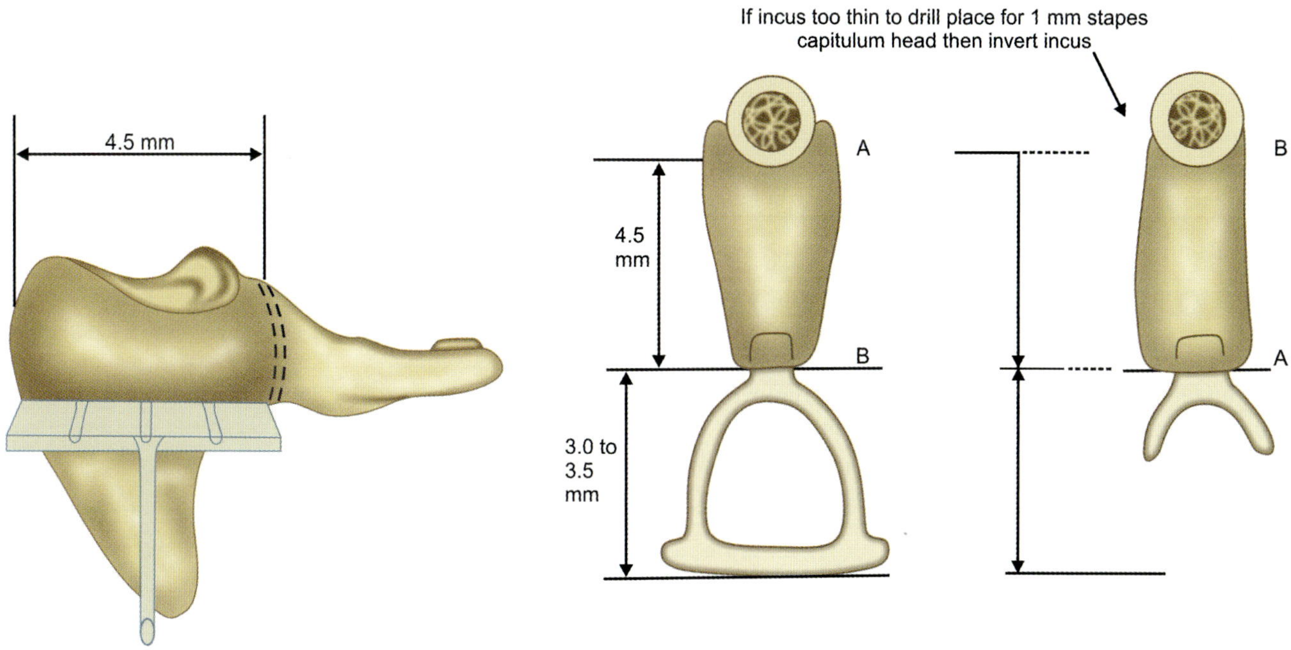

Fig. 6.46: An incus interposition graft from the malleus to the stapes capitulum.

Step 2: If any question exists that the footplate is fixed, the stapes should be repalpated after disarticulation. If the stapes is mobile, the incus is separated from the malleus with a right angle pick and the incus is then delivered into the middle ear. Palpation of the malleus is repeated. *Step 3*: If the malleus is mobile, then a PORP ossiculoplasty can be placed.

Step 4: If the malleus is still fixed, the head should be removed using a malleus nipper at the neck above the tensor tympani insertion. If the malleus is still fixed, the tensor tympani should be severed.

Ossicular fixation can also be dealt with by posterior atticotomy via a mastoidectomy or transcanal atticotomy (*see* chapter on Mastoidectomy).

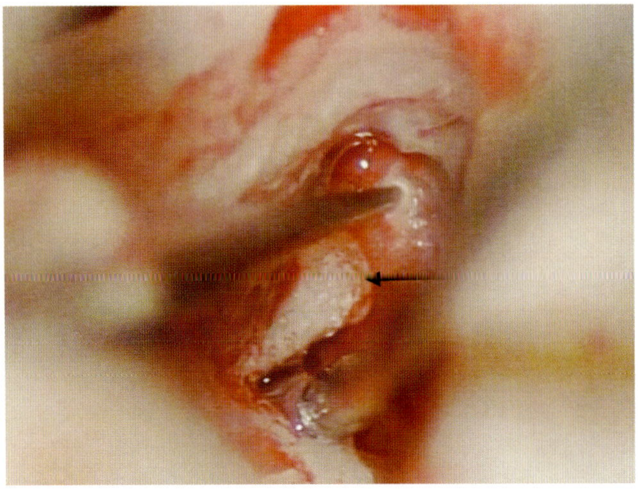

Fig. 6.47: Malleus fixation. Drilling of a fixation point superior to the head of the malleus (arrow) through a posterior atticotomy via a mastoidectomy approach. The short process of the incus is shown with an arrow.

Step 1: Assessment of fixation of ossicles is performed as above.

Step 2: Exposure of the epitympanum is achieved with cutting burs (care is taken not to drill on the ossicles) by a cortical mastoidectomy. Any fixation points within the epitympanum that are identified are removed with a drill or hand-held instruments (Fig. 6.47). Many times a piece of thin Silastic is placed between the ossicular heads and the epitympanum to prevent bony regrowth.

POSTOPERATIVE CARE

Most cases are performed as outpatient surgery. Any dressing placed at the time of surgery can be removed the next day. Usually, the patients have packing in their ear canal. They are instructed to use antibiotic drops until the return visit, which is 1–2 weeks postoperatively. Patients are to sneeze with their mouth open and avoid blowing their nose for 2 weeks. Packing is removed at the first visit down to the level of the graft and incisions are inspected. Patients can fly one month after surgery assuming good healing is noted at their postoperative visit. Patients are instructed to keep water out of the ear canal until healing is complete. Postoperative audiograms are obtained after 2 months or when healing is complete.

COMPLICATIONS

In general, complications of tympanoplasty include reperforation, ear infection, loss of hearing (total loss less than 1%), tinnitus, dizziness, taste disturbance, facial nerve injury, bleeding, and general anesthetic risk.[21] These issues should be discussed with the patient preoperatively. Complications specific to the underlay technique include graft medialization, possible skin tracking into the middle ear or recurrence of the perforation. A rare complication unique to the over-under technique is lateralization of the drum from the malleus. Complications of the overlay technique include anterior canal wall blunting, lateralization of the graft, and cholesteatoma formation if skin is left under the fascia graft. In general, overlay techniques have a higher take rate but cause more scarring of the drum itself. In ossiculoplasty, migration or slippage of the prosthesis from its intended place can occur. Many newer prosthesis have means of lateral stabilization with either a grooved hydroxyapatite head or a titanium extension that fits under the malleus for stabilization. Medial stabilization of the prosthesis is offered by using a partial prosthesis that fits over the capitulum then over part of the crura. Fixation of autografts can occur especially to the posterior canal wall. Alloplastic prostheses have a higher extrusion rate than autografts. In cases of cholesteatoma recurrence can be as high as 20–30%, and a second look procedure is generally recommended.[22]

REFERENCES

1. Banzer M. Disputatio de Audiotone Laesa. Wittenbergae: Johannis Rohrerei; 1651.
2. Toynbee J. On the Use of an Artificial Membrane Tympani in Cases of Deafness Dependent Upon Perforations or Destruction of the Natural Organ. London: J Churchill & Sons; 1853.
3. Blake CJ. Transactions of the First Congress of the International Otological Society. New York: D Appleton & Company; 1887.
4. Berthold E. Über myringoplastik. Wier Med Bull. 1878;1:627.
5. Wullstein H. The restoration of the function of the middle ear, in chronic otitis media. Ann Otol Rhinol Laryngol. 1956; 65:1021-41.
6. Zollner F. The principles of plastic surgery of the sound-conducting apparatus. J Laryngol Otol. 1955;69:637-52.
7. House WF, Sheehy JL. Myringoplasty. Use of ear canal skin compared with other techniques. Arch Otolaryngol. 1961; 73:407-15.
8. Plester D. Myringoplasty methods. Arch Otolaryngol. 1963; 78:310-16.
9. Austin DF, Shea JJ, Jr. A new system of tympanoplasty using vein graft. Laryngoscope. 1961;71:596-611.
10. Tabb HG. Closure of perforations of the tympanic membrane by vein grafts. A preliminary report of twenty cases. Laryngoscope. 1960;70:271-86.
11. Storrs LA. Temporalis muscle fascia and denatured fat grafts in middle-ear surgery. Laryngoscope. 1963;73:699-701.

12. Glasscock ME, 3rd. Tympanic membrane grafting with fascia: overlay vs. undersurface technique. Laryngoscope. 1973;83:754-70.
13. Austin DF. Transcanal tympanoplasty. Otolaryngol Clin North Am. 1972;5:127-43.
14. Dornhoffer J. Cartilage tympanoplasty: indications, techniques, and outcomes in a 1,000-patient series. Laryngoscope. 2003;113:1844-56.
15. McFeely WJ, Jr, Bojrab DI, Kartush JM. Tympanic membrane perforation repair using AlloDerm. Otolaryngol Head Neck Surg. 2000;123:17-21.
16. Kartush JM, Michaelides EM, Becvarovski Z, et al. Over-under tympanoplasty. Laryngoscope. 2002;112:802-7.
17. Gerber MJ, Mason JC, Lambert PR. Hearing results after primary cartilage tympanoplasty. Laryngoscope. 2000;110:1994-9.
18. Wullstein H. Theory and practice of tympanoplasty. Trans Am Laryngol Rhinol Otol Soc. 1956:548-65; discussion, 65-7.
19. Merchant SN, Ravicz ME, Puria S, et al. Analysis of middle ear mechanics and application to diseased and reconstructed ears. Am J Otol. 1997;18:139-54.
20. Ostrowski VB, Bojrab DI. Minimally invasive laser contraction myringoplasty for tympanic membrane atelectasis. Otolaryngol Head Neck Surg. 2003;128:711-8.
21. Fayad JN, Sheehy JL. Tympanoplasty-outer surface grafting technique. In: Brackmann D, Shelton C, Arriaga M (Eds). Otologic Surgery. Philadelphia, PA: Saunders; 2010.
22. Sheehy JL, Brackmann DE, Graham MD. Cholesteatoma surgery: residual and recurrent disease. A review of 1,024 cases. Ann Otol Rhinol Laryngol. 1977;86:451-62.

CHAPTER

7

Mastoidectomy

Eleanor Y Chan

INTRODUCTION

Although the advent of antibiotics has led to a dramatic reduction of complicated ear infections, mastoid surgery remains a bread and butter procedure for otolaryngologists in the management of chronic otitis media and cholesteatoma. Mastoidectomy is also the surgeon's gateway to structures deep within the temporal bone and beyond, providing access to the facial nerve, the jugular bulb, the labyrinth, the internal auditory canal, the petrous apex, as well as the middle and posterior fossae.

HISTORY OF MASTOIDECTOMY

Coalescent mastoiditis with osteothrombophlebitic extension arising from acute suppurative otitis media were not uncommon in the preantibiotic era.[1] Mastoid trephination was first described by Petit in 1774,[2] where a surgically created fistula was established to drain an infected mastoid. However, neurovascular complications abounded before aseptic technique was practiced, leading to abandonment of the procedure until it was repopularized by Schwartze who described the simple mastoidectomy in 1873.[3] Over the next century, the art and precision of mastoidectomy were refined with the introduction of the operating microscope and advances in microsurgical instrumentation. Technical variations designed to address the spectrum of disease encountered have led to the current classification of mastoidectomy types.

NOMENCLATURE OF MASTOIDECTOMY

Simple Mastoidectomy

Mastoid cortex is removed. The degree of mastoid air cell exenteration may be limited and is usually guided by the extent of disease. This may be performed for drainage of a subperiosteal abscess secondary to coalescent mastoiditis.

Intact Canal Wall Mastoidectomy

Cortical mastoidectomy is performed with maintenance of the normal anatomical division between the external auditory canal and the mastoid cavity. The posterior canal wall is usually preserved, but if removed, it is reconstructed with autologous or alloplastic material. Facial recess is classically included. Intact canal wall (ICW) mastoidectomy is often combined with transcanal exploration of the tympanic membrane and middle ear.

Canal Wall Down Mastoidectomy

The mastoid cavity is exteriorized to the external auditory meatus by complete removal of mastoid air cells including the superior and posterior portions of the canal wall. The lateral cortical edges are saucerized. Meatoplasty is required. Concomitant tympanoplasty is often performed with preservation or grafting of the tympanic membrane. The mucosal-lined middle ear space is maintained. Ossicular chain can be reconstructed to restore hearing.

Bondy Procedure or Modified Radical Mastoidectomy

Pars tensa is normal with intact ossicular chain. The healthy middle ear is left undisturbed. Tympanic membrane is not elevated. Mastoid disease is limited to the epitympanum and remains lateral to the malleus head and body of incus. Atticoantrostomy is performed by removing the scutum with adjacent superior and posterior canal wall regions to allow drainage of the attic to the aditus ad antrum. Cholesteatoma matrix lateral to the ossicular heads can be maintained as lining for the limited epitympanic cavity.

There is often confusion of terminology as some surgeons refer to the canal wall down (CWD) mastoidectomy as modified radical mastoidectomy (MRM). MRM is classically defined by the Bondy procedure,[4,5] and is especially useful in cases of middle-ear sparing cholesteatoma with good hearing.

Atticotomy

Limited attic cholesteatoma confined to the central epitympanic area is amenable to atticotomy. Extension of disease medial to the ossicles often requires removal of the incus and head of the malleus. Canalplasty with drilling of the scutum as well as removal of the superior and anterior tympanic bone are performed to allow complete visualization and excision of the cholesteatoma. Canal wall defects are reconstructed using cartilage, bone pâté, perichondrial, and temporalis grafting as needed. If there is posterior extension of disease into the mastoid, conversion to a formal CWD mastoidectomy may be required.

Radical Mastoidectomy

The lateral ossicular chain (malleus and incus) is removed. Stapes is preserved. If the stapes suprastructure is diseased and requires removal, then the footplate is maintained. Ossicular reconstruction is forfeited. Eustachian tube is packed and obliterated. Tympanic membrane is left open without grafting to allow epithelialization. Middle ear and mastoid form a common cavity and are both exteriorized.

Mastoid Obliteration

Mastoid is obliterated to reduce the size of the cavity after CWD procedures. Local tissue flaps (pedicled muscle), free grafts using autologous materials (e.g. bone pâté, bone chips, fat, cartilage, and fascia) or nonbiologic materials (e.g. hydroxyapatite crystals and calcium phosphate ceramic granules, bioactive glass) are employed. Any epithelium or keratin disease must be completely removed. Concerns of burying disease and lack of proven superiority compared to other forms of mastoidectomy have rendered obliteration a less popular technique.

INDICATIONS FOR MASTOIDECTOMY

Mastoidectomy is performed to eradicate cholesteatoma and chronic otitis media, and treat suppurative complications of ear infection. Choice of mastoidectomy technique is based on preoperative assessment with clinical examination and imaging as well as intraoperative findings. In the patient with an only-hearing ear, or where compliance with follow-up is questionable, a CWD mastoidectomy is preferred given the lower risk of recurrent or residual disease. Similarly, when a patient has multiple medical comorbidities and an inherently high anesthetic risk, a CWD surgery may eliminate the need for revision or second-look procedures. Anatomic variables may favor CWD mastoidectomy; a low-lying tegmen mastoideum with an anteriorly displaced sigmoid sinus may severely restrict the ability to create an effective ICW mastoid cavity. If cholesteatoma and infection have caused horizontal semicircular canal fistula or destruction of the posterior bony canal wall, a CWD mastoidectomy is warranted to achieve a safe, disease-free ear. Ultimately, intraoperative evaluation should dictate the extent of surgery, balancing a conservative approach with anatomical preservation but emphasizing the need to achieve complete disease elimination.[6–9]

Mastoidectomy is the prelude to various transtemporal skull base exposures used for tumor resection, facial nerve decompression, encephalocele repair, and control of cerebrospinal fluid leak. Access through the facial recess provides the channel for cochlear implantation and aids in the treatment of challenging middle ear disease. Exposure of the labyrinth via mastoidectomy allows semicircular canal occlusion and labyrinthectomy to be performed. Mastoidectomy is a versatile operation that can be tailored to the specific requirements of each case.

PREOPERATIVE COUNSELING AND INFORMED CONSENT

Counseling of patients should be individualized, and the rationale and goals for mastoidectomy discussed thoroughly before surgery is undertaken. Successful mastoidectomy is dependent upon the interplay of numerous elements including the precipitating ear pathology, the extent of middle ear and mastoid involvement, patient factors, genetic predispositions, as well as the surgeon's experience with the procedure. Success rate, as defined by the achievement of a safe dry ear, ranges in the literature from 80% to 98%.[9,10] The incidence of revision surgery is not insignificant, and must be conveyed as part of the informed consent process.[9]

Potential complications of mastoidectomy should be reviewed with the patient. Structures that are at risk for injury during mastoidectomy include the tegmen, semicircular canals, facial nerve, sigmoid sinus, and jugular bulb. Iatrogenic dehiscence of the tegmen should be promptly recognized and repaired. Extra caution must be taken if dura is exposed, as violation with cerebrospinal fluid leak introduces contamination into the intracranial compartment. Bleeding from the sigmoid and jugular bulb must be controlled and meticulous hemostasis

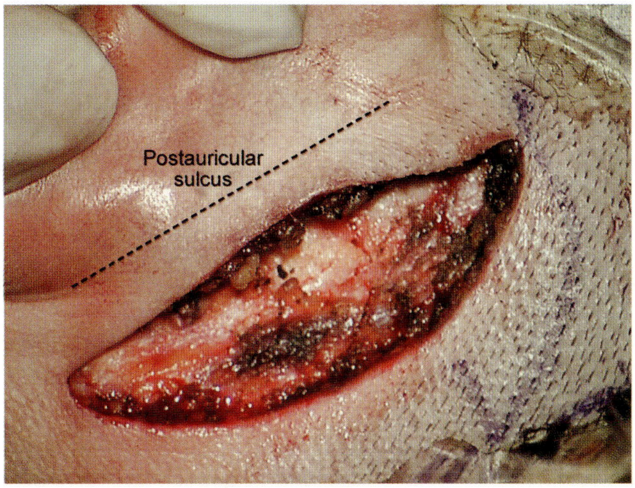

Fig. 7.1: Postauricular incision (left ear).

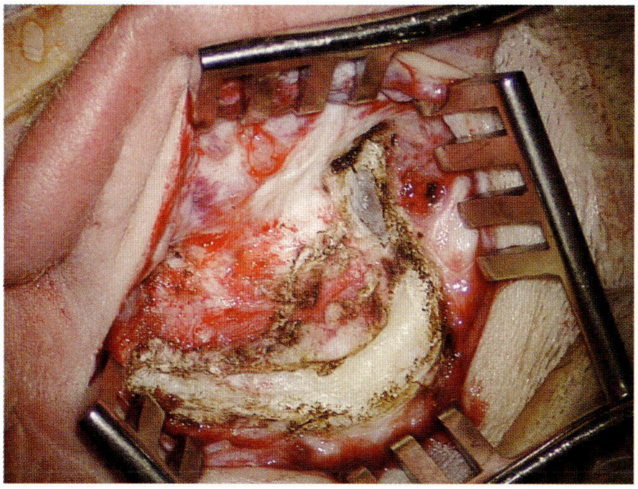

Fig. 7.2: Musculoperiosteal flap (left ear). Cuts are made in the musculoperiosteal layer to develop an anteriorly-based flap.

maintained throughout surgery. Permanent sensorineural hearing loss may result from inadvertent entry into the semicircular canals. Facial nerve injury is the most feared complication, occurring in 2–8% of cases.[11] Revision mastoidectomy, operating in severely diseased ears, as well as natural or acquired dehiscences along the fallopian canal all lead to increased risk of potential facial nerve trauma.

Creation of a postauricular incision results in a period of anesthesia affecting the pinna and periauricular region that usually takes weeks to months to normalize. The pinna tends to protrude laterally in the immediate postoperative phase, but this is rarely a cause for permanent cosmetic concern as long as meticulous wound closure in layers is adhered to. Although the majority of incisions heal without any untoward sequelae, persistent postauricular dysesthesia, otalgia, or keloid formation may be encountered in the occasional patient. These seemingly minor details should be clearly communicated, as the symptoms can be rather distressing to some patients.

SURGICAL TECHNIQUE

Surgical Steps: ICW Mastoidectomy

Step 1

A C-shaped incision is made about 5–10 mm behind the postauricular sulcus using a #15 scalpel (Fig. 7.1). The postauricular sulcus is generally avoided for incision placement due to difficulty with hygiene and tendency for debris to accumulate within the crease.

Step 2

Incision is carried through the subcutaneous tissues staying lateral to the temporalis fascia and musculoperiosteal layer.

Step 3

A T-shaped incision is made with the Bovie electrocautery along the temporal line, with a vertical limb perpendicular to it down toward the mastoid tip. The temporal line approximates the level of the middle fossa dura, but the true tegmen level may vary. In revision mastoidectomy, the vertical limb is placed behind the previously drilled mastoid cavity creating a semilunar musculoperiosteal flap (Fig. 7.2).

Step 4

Musculoperiosteal flaps are elevated using a Lempert to expose the mastoid cortex (Fig. 7.3). Weitlaner retractors are placed for exposure.

Step 5

Mastoidectomy is begun by outlining a triangular area of drilling defined by the temporal line, the posterior bony canal wall, and a line connecting the two (Fig. 7.4).

Step 6

As the mastoid cortex is removed, the tegmen mastoideum and sigmoid sinus are identified, and the posterior bony canal wall is thinned (Fig. 7.5).

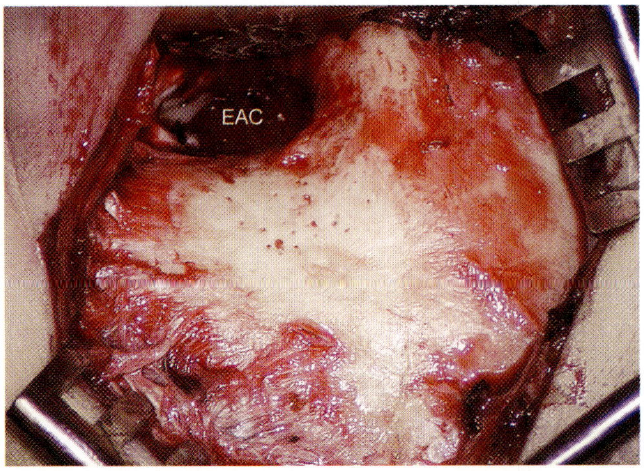

Fig. 7.3: Mastoid cortex in preparation for drilling (left ear). In this example, canal incisions have already been made to expose the ear canal proper (EAC) from the postauricular mastoid view.

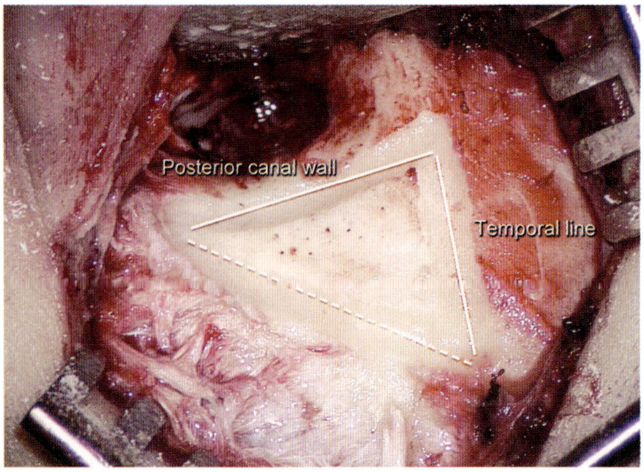

Fig. 7.4: Boundaries of mastoidectomy (left ear). Drilling area is defined by the temporal line superiorly and the posterior bony canal wall anteriorly.

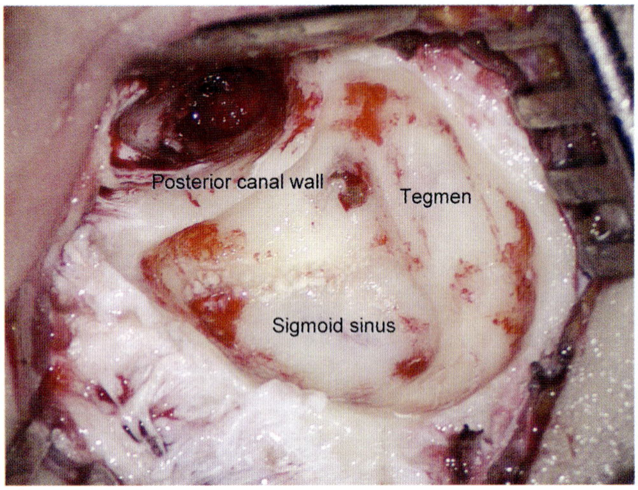

Fig. 7.5: Superficial mastoidectomy (left ear).

Step 7

The sigmoid sinus is followed superiorly to the sinodural angle and inferiorly toward the jugular bulb. A layer of bone should be kept over the sigmoid for protection in most routine mastoid procedures unless decompression is necessary.

Step 8

Saucerization of the mastoid cavity is achieved by drilling away the lateral cortical margins. The tegmen is followed medially into the antrum, the location of which is approximated laterally by the cribriform area just posterior to the suprameatal spine of Henle.

Step 9

Once all mastoid air cells lateral to Koerner's (petrosquamous) septum are removed, the antrum should be visible. The size of the antrum is variable based on the degree of pneumatization of the temporal bone.

Step 10

The dome of the horizontal semicircular canal can be seen at the floor of the antrum (Fig. 7.6), and serves as a key landmark in mastoid surgery.

Step 11

Further exposure of the antrum is attained by drilling anteriorly toward the zygomatic root, removing the bone lateral to the antrum and superiorly toward the tegmen and roof of the bony external auditory canal.

Step 12

The short process of the incus is identified at the aditus ad antrum (Fig. 7.7). With constant suction and irrigation, a "water reflex" usually lends to early visualization of the incus reflection prior to seeing the actual incus itself.

Step 13

Dissection can be extended toward the anterior epitympanum or supratubal recess if necessary to eradicate disease. Removal of the incus and malleus head greatly facilitates this exposure. The bone between the tegmen tympani and superior canal wall is removed with a small diamond.

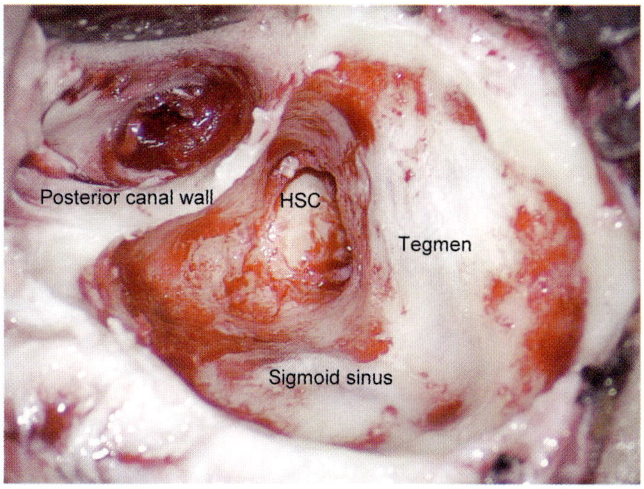

Fig. 7.6: Key landmarks of a simple mastoidectomy (left ear). Middle fossa tegmen (superior). Posterior bony external auditory canal wall (anterior). Sigmoid sinus (posterior). Horizontal semicircular canal (HSC) is noted at antrum.

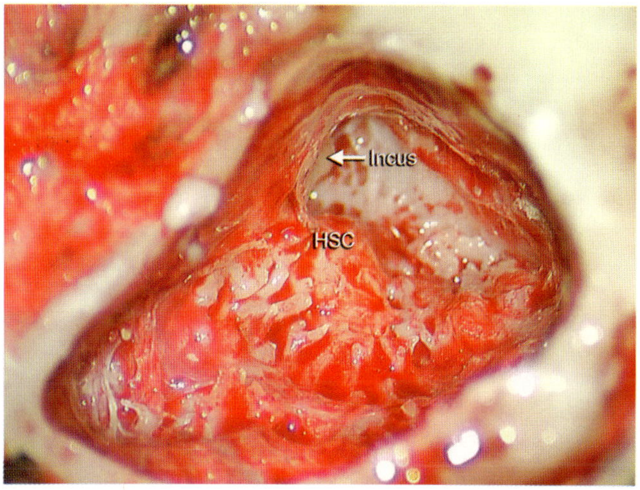

Fig. 7.7: Close-up of antrum demonstrating horizontal semicircular canal and incus (left ear).

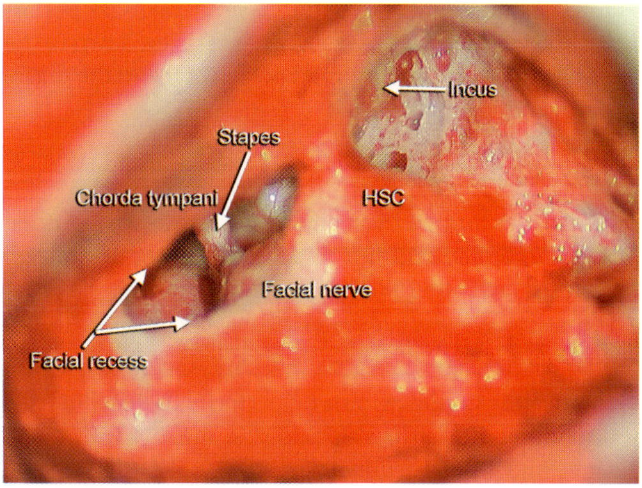

Fig. 7.8: Facial recess (left ear). Boundaries of the facial recess are formed by the fossa incudis (superior), chorda tympani (anterior/lateral), and facial nerve (posterior/medial).

Step 14

The facial nerve should be positively identified using several landmarks:

- The second genu of the facial nerve is located just anterior and medial to the dome of the horizontal semicircular canal.
- The mastoid segment of the facial nerve courses slightly anteriorly and laterally, as it descends from the second genu toward the stylomastoid foramen.
- The digastric ridge at the mastoid tip serves as a pointer for the facial nerve situated just anterior to it.

When drilling, bur strokes should be executed parallel to the course of the facial nerve to minimize chances of injury.

Step 15

The facial recess is opened. It is located just inferior and medial to the fossa incudis. The boundaries of the facial recess are formed by the fossa incudis superiorly, the chorda tympani anterolaterally, and the facial nerve posteromedially (Fig. 7.8).

Step 16

The size of the facial recess is dependent on the degree of pneumatization, but usually measures approximately 2 mm. Middle ear structures visualized through the recess include the promontory, round window niche, incudo-stapedial joint, malleus handle, and medial surface of tympanic membrane.

Step 17

An extended facial recess approach can be performed if needed by sacrificing the chorda tympani nerve, in which case the tympanic membrane annulus then forms the lateral boundary of dissection.

Surgical Steps: CWD Mastoidectomy

The CWD mastoidectomy aims to exteriorize the mastoid cavity to allow direct drainage and ventilation via the

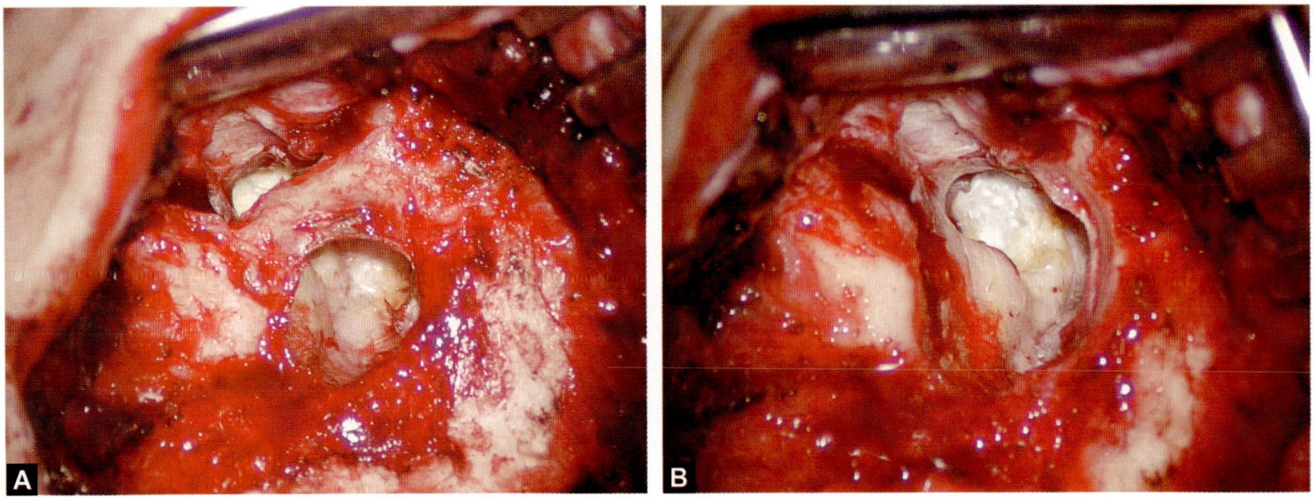

Figs. 7.9A and B: (A) Posterior canal wall just prior to canal wall down (CWD) mastoidectomy (left ear). (B) CWD mastoid cavity (left ear). Posterior bony canal wall is lowered completely to the facial ridge. Smooth transition from epitympanum into mastoid.

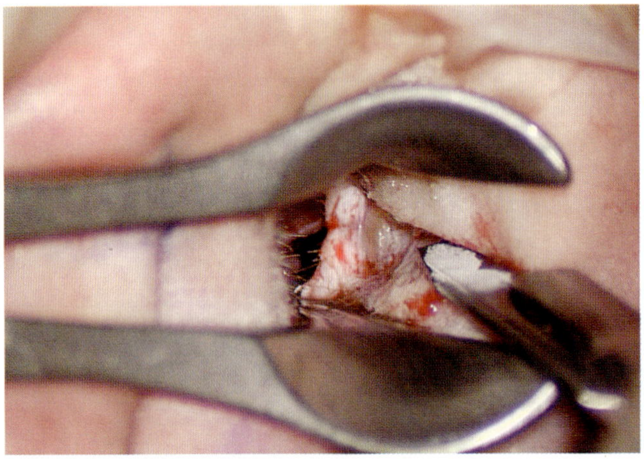

Fig. 7.10: Superior cut (12 o'clock) made at meatus (left ear).

external auditory meatus. The initial steps are carried out in a similar fashion as for ICW surgery (*see* Steps 1–13 of ICW Mastoidectomy).[12,13]

Step 1

Using the anatomical landmarks for the facial nerve (*see* Step 14 of ICW mastoidectomy), the posterior bony canal wall is lowered completely down to the level of the facial ridge (Fig. 7.9A).

Step 2

The superior canal wall (anterior buttress) is completely removed to achieve a smooth transition from epitympanum to mastoid cavity proper. Wide unobstructed view of the entire cavity is achieved without any bony overhangs (Fig. 7.9B).

Step 3

Extensive saucerization of the mastoid cavity is performed. The lateral edges of the cavity are taken down to the tegmen superiorly, the sigmoid posteriorly and the digastric ridge inferiorly.

Step 4

Irregularities formed by the mastoid air cells are polished with a large diamond bur to achieve a smooth uniform surface to facilitate future office maintenance.

Step 5

Generous meatoplasty must be performed. Relaxing cuts are made at 12 and 6 o'clock of the meatus with a #15 scalpel and brought out laterally. Visualization can be aided with use of a nasal speculum (Fig. 7.10).

Step 6

A rim of conchal cartilage with underlying soft tissues are resected to relax the constriction at the meatus (Fig. 7.11). Cartilage is usually the limiting factor in meatus restriction. Resection of subcutaneous tissues alone is inadequate to achieve a wide meatus.

Step 7

Retention sutures are applied to the cut edge of the conchal cartilage and secured posteriorly to the musculoperiosteal layer (Fig. 7.12A). Placement of three stitches along the superior, middle, and inferior aspects of the meatus works well to stent it open (Fig. 7.12B). Beware

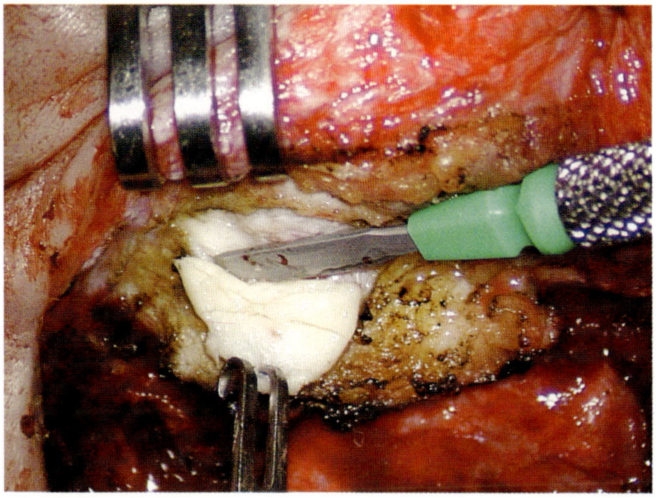

Fig. 7.11: Resection of conchal cartilage at meatus (left ear).

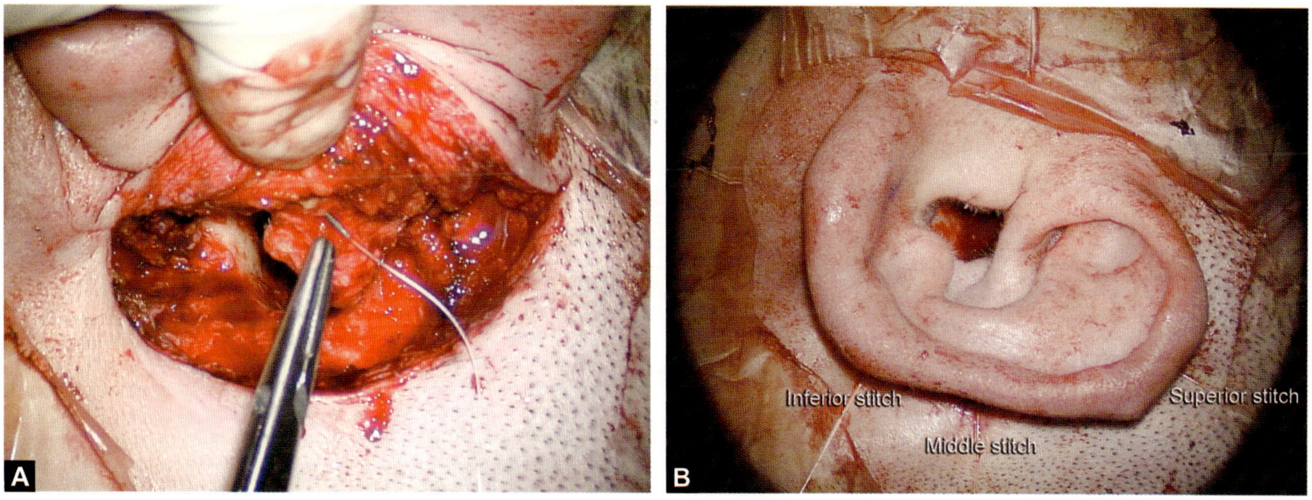

Figs. 7.12A and B: (A) Placement of retention sutures for meatoplasty (left ear). Suture is applied to the rim of conchal cartilage exposed after resecting the appropriate amount. (B) Strategic positioning of retention sutures to achieve wide meatoplasty (left ear).

of "ear cupping" with excessive tightening of the stitches. This can be avoided by modifying placement of the cartilage stitches.

Step 8

The vascular strip is laid back down into the mastoid to line the posterior cavity. Eventual healing and re-epithelialization of any bone-exposed areas is expected to occur. Alternatively, healing may be accelerated by lining such bare areas with split thickness skin graft or Alloderm (Fig. 7.13).

Step 9

A polyvinyl alcohol sponge pack (e.g. Merocel and Ambrus) is placed at the meatus and left for 1-2 weeks. Packing does not obviate the need for properly applied sutures, which provides the main force to keep the meatus stented open.

Surgical Steps: Atticotomy

Atticotomy is usually performed in conjunction with tympanoplasty, termed "tympanoatticotomy", to allow proper access and management of limited epitympanic disease (Fig. 7.14).

The complex anatomy of the epitympanic diaphragm, composed of the anterior, lateral and posterior malleal ligaments, the posterior incudal ligament, the tensor fold, and the lateral incudomalleal fold, along with the malleus and incus, determines the pathways of ventilation and connections to the mesotympanum and mastoid air

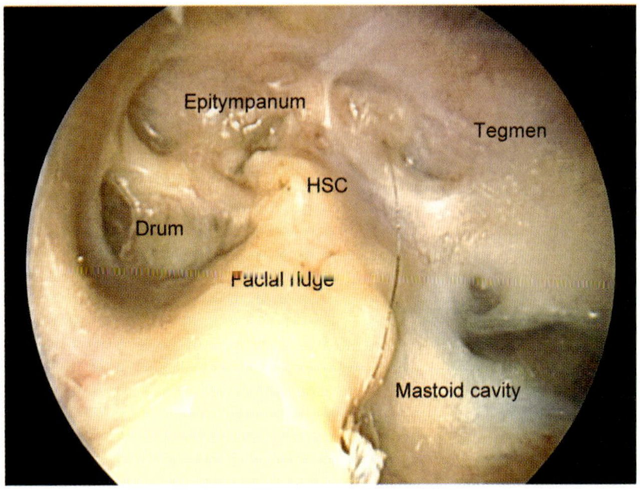

Fig. 7.13: Healed canal wall down mastoid cavity (left ear).

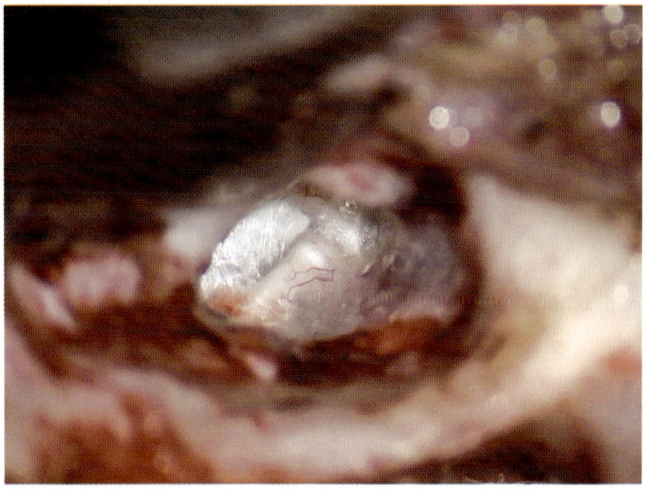

Fig. 7.14: Retraction cholesteatoma of central epitympanic region (left ear).

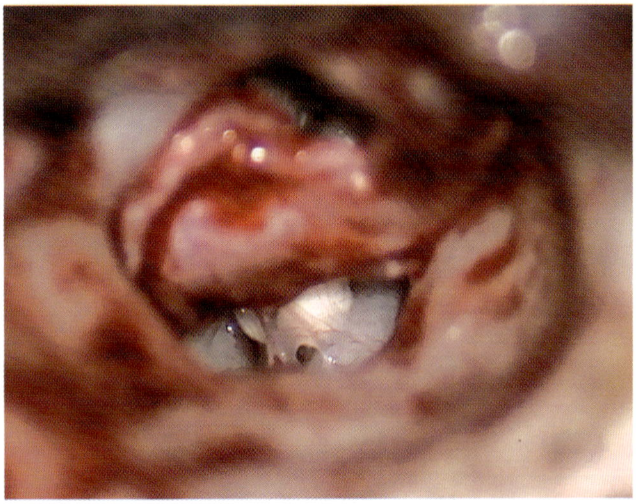

Fig. 7.15: Elevation of tympanomeatal flap (left ear). In this revision case, the previously inserted incus strut is visualized. A blanket of mucosal disease extends superiorly into the area of the attic cholesteatoma.

space. Understanding the routes of epitympanic pneumatization aids in proper disease eradication.[14]

Step 1

Canal incisions are made and a tympanomeatal flap is elevated as per usual for tympanoplasty (Fig. 7.15).

Step 2

Epitympanic exposure is facilitated by drilling of scutum, followed by removal of bone along the superior canal wall (Fig. 7.16).

Step 3

Complete removal of attic cholesteatoma and mucosal disease with exposure of anterior and posterior epitympanic compartments (Fig. 7.17).

Step 4

Cartilage reconstruction of scutum and superior canal wall defects (Fig. 7.18).

Step 5

Tympanomeatal flap is draped over cartilage graft and replaced back into original position (Fig. 7.19).

TECHNICAL DETAILS AND INTRAOPERATIVE CONSIDERATIONS

Mastoidectomy is performed using a high-speed drill system under constant irrigation with suction. The burs required for mastoid surgery range from 6.0 mm to 7.0 mm down to 0.5–1.0 mm, and comprise of cutting or diamond tips. Cutting or fluted burs are generally used to remove gross bone and allow dissection to progress quickly, whereas diamond burs are used for bone polishing and are employed around delicate structures.

In general, employing the largest bur possible for any given location allows for safe and effective drilling. Burs that are too small have the tendency to "punch holes" with greater risk of injuring important structures. A broad plane of dissection should be maintained while drilling to allow clear visualization of the entire mastoid.

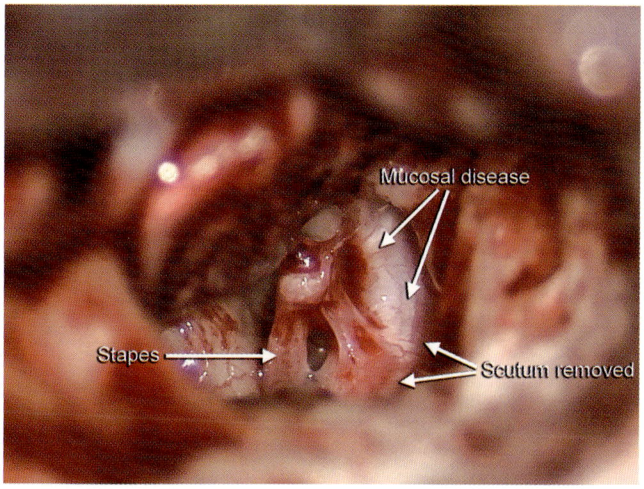

Fig. 7.16: Extending view of superior mesotympanum toward attic (left ear).

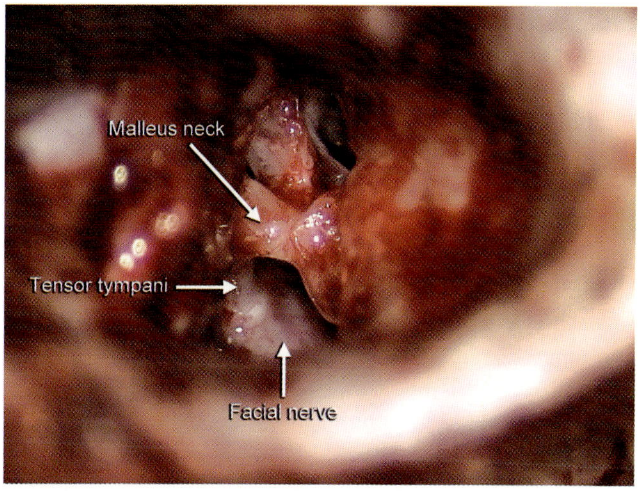

Fig. 7.17: Atticotomy (left ear). Malleus (neck, partial head) is visualized following complete resection of attic cholesteatoma. Tensor tympani and tympanic segment of facial nerve are noted.

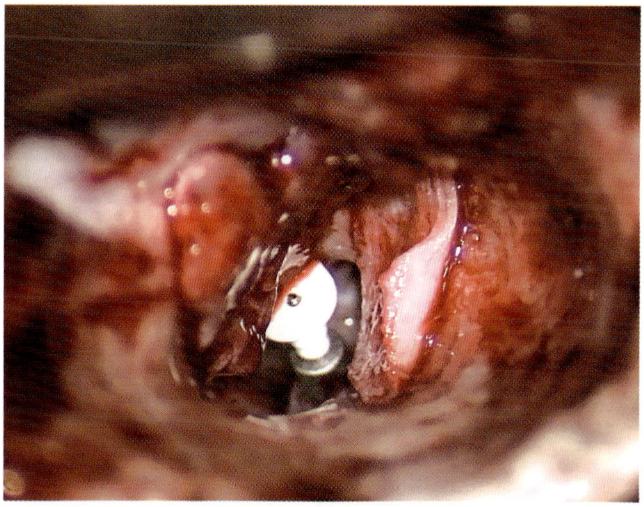

Fig. 7.18: Canal wall reconstruction using cartilage graft (left ear). A partial ossicular replacement prosthesis is placed between malleus and stapes.

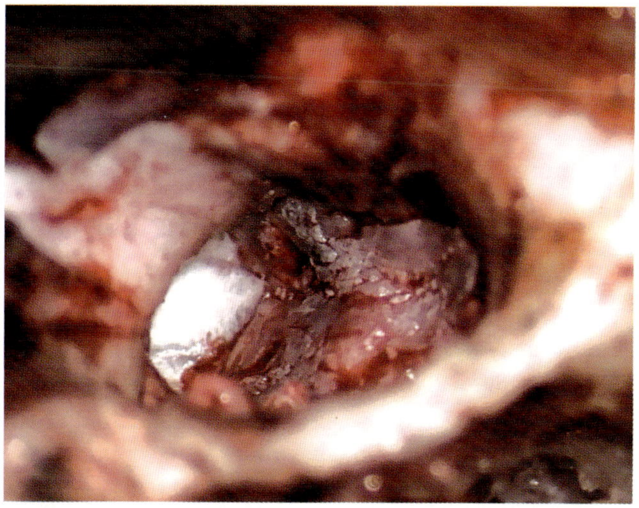

Fig. 7.19: Replacement of tympanomeatal flap onto posterior canal wall (left ear).

As drilling progresses medially, it is even more critical to avoid trapping oneself into a deep narrow hole.

Constant suction and irrigation should be employed during drilling to cool the bone and remove bone dust that may accumulate in the operative field. This is especially important when thinning the bone of the fallopian canal, as overheating may result in facial paresis. Similar caution should be taken to avoid overheating and drying of bone when drilling over the sigmoid sinus and dura.

When performing revision mastoidectomy, the mastoid defect should be digitally palpated to approximate the margins of the previously drilled cavity. Periosteal cuts are made horizontally along the temporal line just above the superior margin of the drilled cavity, and the vertical limb is created behind the posterior edge of the opened cavity. It is good practice to assume exposed dura and uncovered sigmoid when elevating the musculoperiosteal flaps. If there are any concerns, the Bovie should be avoided and a scalpel used instead to raise flaps under micro-otoscopic guidance.

Sufficient thinning of the posterior canal wall is a crucial step in ICW mastoidectomy. Inadequate thinning can lead to an artificially contracted mastoid that may impede visualization and access as dissection progresses deeper. The true thickness of the canal wall can be appreciated by gently elevating the soft tissues of the posterior canal skin. In an extremely well-pneumatized temporal bone, the posterior canal wall may contain air cells too; thus, extra care must be taken to avoid creating an inadvertent dehiscence.

The main clues that help identify the tegmen's position include the loss of air cells as drilling progresses superiorly and transition to a higher pitched "tinny" sound on the drill. As the tegmen is skeletonized, the underlying dura appears slightly pink under its bony covering. It is important to remember that the level of the tegmen does not remain constant from its lateral to medial extent. It may be variable with tendency toward a mild bulge inferiorly into the mastoid midway into the antrum.

The sigmoid sinus is variable in its depth, and can sometimes be encountered at a relatively superficial position after just a few bur strokes on the mastoid cortex. The surgeon must be aware of this inherent variability to avoid potential injury to the sinus. If preoperative CT imaging of the temporal bones is available, the expected location of the sigmoid sinus can be confirmed prior to surgery.

If the horizontal semicircular canal is not readily recognized in the antrum, it is often the case where tegmen may not have been properly identified and/or posterior canal wall adequately thinned, leading to antral entry in a relatively inferior position. This puts the facial nerve and horizontal canal at great risk for injury. It is never necessary to drill on the floor of the antrum to locate the horizontal canal, and inadvertent entry can result in permanent sensorineural hearing loss. Occasionally, a spiculated pattern of bone may overlie the smooth dome of the horizontal canal, but the canal itself is usually quite apparent beneath this.

The bony protective covering of the fallopian canal is usually preserved when performing routine mastoidectomy unless disease or injury necessitates neural decompression. The best way to avoid iatrogenic injury to the facial nerve is to actively identify it by direct visualization. Stimulating dissectors may be used to confirm the location of the nerve. Use of intraoperative facial monitoring can greatly enhance the safety of mastoidectomy.

MASTOIDECTOMY IN CHILDREN

The temporal bone in children is essentially fully developed as in adults with the main difference being the mastoid tip, which does not achieve adult size and location until about 5–6 years of age.[6] The stylomastoid foramen thus sits at a relatively superficial location, which can put the facial nerve at greater risk for surgical trauma. Drilling must be undertaken in a cautious manner, and it is advisable to avoid use of the Bovie electrocautery for soft tissue work around the tip due to potential for thermal injury to the nerve.

POSTOPERATIVE CARE

A pressure mastoid dressing is typically applied for the initial 24-hour period. The dressing helps to catch drainage or oozing from the incision, which is typically minimal with meticulous hemostasis during surgery. The pinna is expected to protrude slightly in the immediate postoperative period, and reassurance to the patient is usually sufficient.

With CWD mastoidectomy, blood-tinged drainage is expected for several days via the meatus due to the more extensive dissection and soft-tissue work carried out. Ototopical drops containing steroid and antibiotic are applied for a few weeks to keep the packing moist and uninfected. Dry ear precautions must be maintained to avoid any interference with healing.

Activity restrictions are not usually necessary for mastoidectomy alone. Instructions are given based on any concomitant tympanoplasty and middle ear ossicular work performed.

Long-term follow-up and routine debridement of a CWD mastoid cavity is necessary to avoid excessive accumulation of cerumen and debris. Recurrent disease must be monitored for, with greater propensity to occur in ICW procedures.

COMPLICATIONS OF MASTOIDECTOMY

Dural Tear

The middle fossa dura is usually protected by the bony tegmen. The tegmen should be thinned using a diamond bur to reduce risk of inadvertent dural injury. Cutting burs have greater tendency to lacerate the dura if the tegmen bone is violated. A small area of iatrogenic tegmen dehiscence, although not ideal, is usually inconsequential. Larger areas should be repaired, as there is concern of encephalocele development with prolonged pulsations through the defect. If dura has been violated, with or without cerebrospinal fluid leak, layered repair must be performed. Soft tissue covering using fascia or perichondrium in combination with a firm scaffold such as bone, cartilage, hydroxyapatite disk, or cement is applied both intra- and extradurally. Repair can usually be undertaken via the transmastoid exposure, but occasionally, conversion to the middle fossa approach may be necessary.

The posterior fossa dura generally remains completely covered during routine mastoidectomy except in endolymphatic sac surgery or skull base tumor excision. Dural tears in this region are hard to patch, and often require fat packing for resolution. A lumbar drain may be required in the postoperative period.

Labyrinth Injury

Iatrogenic injury to the horizontal semicircular canal can result in vertigo and permanent sensorineural hearing loss, especially with violation of the endosteum. This can be minimized by immediate repair of the defect by plugging with bone wax. In cases of horizontal canal fistula due to cholesteatoma, matrix should be left behind if its removal opens into the perilymphatic space as this carries high risk of a dead ear. CWD mastoidectomy should be performed either primarily or as a staged procedure in these instances. If palpation of the horizontal canal fistula reveals endosteum and it is deemed safe to remove the overlying matrix, the area can be covered with soft tissue or bone wax, with option to retain ICW mastoid cavity. Systemic steroids and antibiotics should be considered when there is concern of otic capsule violation, to reduce any resultant bacterial or chemical labyrinthitis.

Sigmoid Sinus and Jugular Bulb Injury

Bone removal over the sigmoid sinus and jugular bulb should be performed using a diamond bur under constant irrigation to prevent injury to these low-pressure high-volume venous structures. Caution must be taken due to their variance of location within the mastoid. A high-riding jugular bulb can be located just inferior to the posterior semicircular canal. The sigmoid sinus can course far anteriorly and laterally especially in poorly-pneumatized mastoids. Minimal bleeding can usually be controlled by digital pressure and use of Adrenalin or thrombin-soaked gelatin sponge. However, small tears may require packing with oxidized cellulose hemostatic agents. The bleeding site can be more easily tamponaded by squeezing packing under a bony ledge to apply pressure on the sinus or bulb.

Facial Nerve Injury

The facial nerve is rarely dehiscent along its mastoid segment (1–5%), in contrast to its inherent dehiscence rate along the tympanic segment (50–75%).[15-18] Injury to the nerve during mastoidectomy tends to occur around the second genu, situated posterolateral to the pyramidal process. Inadvertent slippage of the drill especially with cutting burs that can skip on bone may cause facial injury. In the setting of chronic ear disease and cholesteatoma, drilling or dissection around an exposed nerve must be undertaken with extreme caution. Stimulating dissectors are helpful to map out the expected course of the nerve; however, it is no substitute for thorough knowledge of facial nerve anatomy.

Facial nerve injury can occur as a result of neural disruption, complete transection, or thermal injury. Treatment is dictated by the degree of injury. Minor trauma of the nerve sheath or exposure of (without entry into) epineurium has low tendency to cause clinical facial paresis and can often be observed without negative sequelae. If less than 40% diameter of the facial nerve is injured, decompression of the adjacent segments with incision of epineurium is typically recommended to allow for neural edema in the postinjury phase. If greater than 40% diameter of the facial nerve is injured, resection of injured segment with primary reanastomosis or interposition nerve grafting tends to yield better results for long-term facial function.

Thermal injury can be prevented by constant irrigation during mastoidectomy. Excessive transmission of heat energy to the facial nerve can cause paresis or paralysis.

In general, delayed facial paresis will usually resolve in due time. Steroids are often administered to aid with facial nerve recovery. Complete paralysis, even if delayed onset, should be monitored closely with serial electrical testing to guide need for re-exploration. The classic guideline of 90% degeneration on facial electroneuronography within 2 weeks of mastoidectomy should prompt re-exploration. Decision to re-explore is based in part on intraoperative findings during the initial surgery, mechanism of injury, and if anything was done immediately to mitigate the injury caused.

REFERENCES

1. Kangsanarak K, Fooanant S, Ruckphaopunt K, et al. Extracranial and intracranial complications of suppurative otitis media. Report of 102 cases. J Laryngol Otol. 1993;107:999-1004.
2. Petit JL. Traite des maladies chirurgicales. Paris; 1774.
3. Schwartze HH, Eysell CG. Ueber die künstliche Eröffnung des Warzenfortsatzes. Arch Ohrenheilkunde. 1873;7:157-87.

4. Berrettini S, Ravecca F, de Vito A, et al. Modified Bondy radical mastoidectomy: long-term personal experience. J Laryngol Otol. 2004;118(5):333-7.
5. Sanna M, Facharzt AA, Russo A, et al. Modified Bondy's technique: refinements of the surgical technique and long-term results. Otol Neurotol. 2009;30(1):64-9.
6. Lambert PR, Dodson EE, Hashisaki GT. Intact canal wall versus canal wall down mastoidectomy. In: Lalwani AK, Grundfast KM (Eds). Pediatric Otology and Neurotology. Philadelphia, PA: Lippincott-Raven; 1998. p. 663.
7. Brackmann DE. Tympanoplasty with mastoidectomy: canal wall up procedures. Am J Otol. 1993;14:380.
8. Glasscock ME, Miller GM. Intact canal wall tympanoplasty in the management of cholesteatoma. Laryngoscope. 1976; 86:575.
9. Sheehy JL, Brackmann DE, Graham MD. Cholesteatoma surgery: residual and recurrent disease: a review of 1024 cases. Ann Otol Rhinol Laryngol. 1977;86:451.
10. Yoon TH, Park SK, Kim JY, et al. Tympanoplasty, with or without mastoidectomy, is highly effective for treatment of chronic otitis media in children. Acta Otolaryngol Suppl. 2007;558:44-8.
11. Nilssen ELK, Wormald PJ. Facial nerve palsy in mastoid surgery. J Laryngol Otol. 1997;111(2):113-6.
12. Syms CA, Syms MJ, Sheehy JL. Mastoidectomy—intact canal wall procedure. In: Brackmann DE, Shelton C, Arriaga MA (Eds). Otologic Surgery, 3rd edition. Philadelphia, PA: Saunders Elsevier; 2010. pp. 195-207.
13. Arriaga MA. Mastoidectomy—canal wall down procedure. In: Brackmann DE, Shelton C, Arriaga MA (Eds). Otologic Surgery, 3rd edition. Philadelphia, PA: Saunders Elsevier; 2010. pp. 209-20.
14. Marchioni D, Molteni G, Presutti L. Endoscopic anatomy of the middle ear. Indian J Otolaryngol Head Neck Surg. 2011;63(2):101-13.
15. Takahashi H, Sando I. Facial canal dehiscence: histologic study and computer reconstruction. Annals Otol Rhinol Laryngol. 1992;101(11):925-30.
16. Martino ED, Sellhaus B, Haensel J, et al. Fallopian canal dehiscences: a survey of clinical and anatomical findings. Eur Arch Otorhinolaryngol. 2005;262(2):120-6.
17. Selesnick SH, Lynn-Macrae AG. The incidence of facial nerve dehiscence at surgery for cholesteatoma. Otol Neurotol. 2001;22(2):129-32.
18. Moody MW, Lambert PR. Incidence of dehiscence of the facial nerve in 416 cases of cholesteatoma. Otol Neurotol. 2007;28(3):400-4.

CHAPTER

8 Surgery for Temporal Bone Cancer

Brent J Benscoter

INTRODUCTION

Temporal bone malignancy is a rare disease diagnosed and treated infrequently even in busy otolaryngology and otology practices. The key to patient outcome is early identification and diagnosis in hopes of treating the tumor before medial spread.[1] Accurate staging and preoperative planning are critical to obtaining an adequate resection. Historically temporal bone malignancy had an extremely poor prognosis, but advances in surgery and postoperative radiation treatment have greatly improved survival rates.

TUMOR PATHOLOGY

Lesions of the temporal bone can arise as primary temporal bone tumors or may spread to the temporal bone from adjacent structures. The parotid gland is in close proximity to the anterior temporal bone, and small communications such as the fissures of Santorini and the foramen of Huschke exist within the cartilaginous external auditory canal allowing a break in the natural barrier.[2] Tumor spread into and from the temporal bone occurs via other natural openings in the complex bony foramina including the stylomastoid foramen, carotid canal, jugular foramen, eustachian tube, and petrotympanic fissures. Knowledge of these avenues of spread is important in preoperative planning to perform an adequate resection.

Primary temporal bone lesions are primarily epidermal tumors. The most common pathology is squamous cell carcinoma, occurring in 86% of diagnoses, followed by basal cell carcinoma.[3] Other pathology includes ceruminous carcinoma, adenocarcinoma, adenoid cystic carcinoma, and mesenchymal tumors such as rhabdomyosarcoma, though this is not an exhaustive list.[4]

A large number of tumors invade the temporal bone from an extratemporal source, most of which are of salivary origin. Both benign and malignant tumors can invade the adjacent temporal bone relatively easily. There have been rare reports of ectopic rests of salivary tissue within the middle ear, though this is not the norm.[5] Benign tumors of the parotid gland rarely truly invade the temporal bone but have been reported. The most common malignant parotid neoplasm requiring temporal bone resection is adenocarcinoma, followed by adenoid cystic carcinoma and mucoepidermoid carcinoma.[6] An intraparotid or scalp lymph node may also invade the temporal bone, commonly from metastatic lesions originating on the auricle, anterior scalp, or face.

PRESENTATION

The most common symptoms of primary temporal bone tumors are aural discharge and otalgia, each of which occurs in 80% of patients at presentation. This is followed by hearing loss (both conductive and sensorineural), which occurs in 71% of patients. Other symptoms such as facial palsy, canal mass/lesion, tinnitus, swelling, or bloody otorrhea can occur each at a rate of approximately 25%.[7] Aural discharge is a common symptom of many otology conditions, making the diagnosis challenging. Practitioners must have a high index of suspicion in any adult patients with otorrhea and otalgia. All patients with a worrisome lesion should undergo meticulous microscopic examination of the ear, biopsy of any suspicious lesions, and imaging.

Temporal bone involvement from adjacent structures such as the parotid gland often presents with more vague symptoms, which go unnoticed for a significant amount of time. Benign tumors of the parotid gland often cause symptoms of a facial mass, trismus, or invasion into the parapharyngeal space prior to temporal bone invasion.[6] In fact, the temporal bone can be remodeled by the tumor without true invasion. These tumors may not require a true temporal bone resection if adequate resection can be obtained through standard parotidectomy techniques.

Temporal bone involvement by malignant temporal bone lesions may also present slowly, manifesting with a painless mass most frequently in 75% of patients. Often patients will not seek care until invasion into the ear canal causes otorrhea, or deeper invasion to the parapharyngeal space and skull base cause cranial nerve deficits to the facial nerve and/or the lower cranial nerves.

DIAGNOSIS

One should have a low threshold to biopsy any painful, draining, or protuberant lesion of thc car canal. While technically possible to biopsy a lesion in the office, consideration should be given to imaging prior to deep tissue biopsies. Without an idea of the extent of the lesion, one could unexpectantly encounter uncontrolled bleeding or injury to the facial nerve, carotid artery, or jugular bulb. False-negative biopsies are common due to inflammation or secondary infection. If initial biopsy results are negative but one has a high-index of suspicion for cancer, deeper tissue biopsies should be performed in the operating room.

Audiologic testing is important in assessing the status of the middle and inner ear. Conductive hearing loss can be due to obstructive lesions of the ear canal or due to erosion of the tympanic membrane and/or ossicles. Sensorineural hearing loss suggests otic capsule involvement. Symptoms of tinnitus, dizziness, or vertigo can also suggest inner ear involvement. Finally, an audiogram can assess the hearing of the contralateral ear, which can influence hearing rehabilitation.

Radiographic imaging of the temporal bone with both magnetic resonance imaging (MRI) and computed tomography (CT) are crucial to determine the extent of the disease, tumor proximity to vital structures, and accurate staging.[8] CT with and without contrast more accurately evaluates the bony anatomy and potential destruction, and is often the initial imaging obtained. Studies have shown that CT can achieve 98% accuracy in predicting pathological involvement in temporal bone resection specimens.[9] Thin axial cuts with coronal reconstructions should be obtained to help in determining if soft tissue exists in the middle ear, which may indicate medial spread through the tympanic membrane. Images without contrast show the best bony detail while contrasted images can help with determining tumor extent. CT imaging of the neck and parotid gland should also be considered depending on patient presentation. CT limitations include the inability to distinguish scarring and mucosal inflammation from tumor. Positron emission tomography (PET) may be helpful in this scenario.[10]

Magnetic resonance imaging with and without gadolinium contrast can provide valuable information regarding soft-tissue involvement of both the lateral soft tissues and the brain medially. MRI may also show enhancement of the facial nerve and may give a rough estimate of neuronal involvement.

Angiography should be performed in all cases where the carotid artery is at risk of involvement, injury, or sacrifice. Four-vessel angiography can show arterial stenosis and contour irregularity, which may suggest carotid involvement. When carotid artery resection is anticipated, cerebral blood flow analysis should be performed to determine resectability. While PET scanning and functional MRI are options, xenon-CT is the best modality to predict occlusion.[11] There is a high risk of perioperative stroke after carotid sacrifice when cerebral blood flow is <30mL/100g/min, or the patient develops neurologic symptoms. Venous outflow is also important, as patency of the confluence of sinuses is necessary for ipsilateral venous outflow if the sigmoid-jugular system is sacrificed.

STAGING

Accurate staging is of utmost importance in preoperative planning. Unfortunately, a lack of uniformity has made the study of temporal bone cancer difficult. The most commonly used staging system is from the University of Pittsburgh, which incorporates TNM-staging similar to other cancers of the head and neck[9] (Table 8.1). Changes have been proposed such as one by Moody and colleagues, which would upstage patients with facial nerve paralysis or paresis to T4 status.[12] The University of Cincinnati staging is an alternate system incorporating both radiologic and clinical involvement.[7] Validation of the various paradigm systems is pending, and a standardized system is still needed to better compare patient outcomes. All of these staging systems focus on primary cancer of the temporal bone and do not specifically relate to cancers of the salivary gland or pinna that spread to the temporal bone. However, staging criteria and decisions regarding surgical resection are similar. The most important factors in determining resection ability and dramatically decreasing prognosis are tumor involvement outside the bounds of the external ear canal, and spread medial to the tympanic membrane. Once the tumor has entered the middle ear, and even more importantly if it has invaded the facial nerve, the prognosis drops dramatically. This is partially due to the increased difficulty in obtaining a sound en bloc resection.

SURGICAL TREATMENT

Treatment of temporal bone malignancy is a complicated problem. Surgery with postoperative radiation is the mainstay of treatment. Often patients are elderly with

Table 8.1: Staging

The University of Pittsburgh Tumor Lymph Node Metastasis Staging System for Squamous Cell Carcinoma of the External Auditory Canal.[9]

T status:

T1—Tumor limited to external auditory canal without bony erosion or evidence of soft-tissue extension

T2—Tumor with limited external auditory canal bony erosion (not full-thickness) or radiographic finding consistent with limited (<0.5 cm) soft-tissue involvement

T3—Tumor eroding osseous external auditory canal (full-thickness) with limited (<0.5 cm) soft-tissue involvement, or tumor involving middle ear or mastoid, or patients presenting with facial paralysis

T4—Tumor eroding cochlea, petrous apex, medial wall of middle ear, carotid canal, jugular foramen, or dura, or with extensive (>0.5 cm) soft-tissue involvement

N status:

Nodal involvement and stage can be classified as it is for other cancers of the head and neck. Involvement of lymph nodes is a poor prognostic finding and automatically places patient in advanced stage.

N1—Single ipsilateral lymph node, size less than 3 cm

N2—Single ipsilateral node, size 3–6 cm

N2b—Multiple ipsilateral nodes, all less than 6 cm

N2c—Bilateral or contralateral nodes, all less than 6 cm

N3—Nodes involved greater than 6 cm

M status:

Distant metastasis indicates poor prognosis and immediately places patient in stage IV.

M0—No evidence of distant metastasis

M1—Evidence of distant metastasis present

multiple other medical problems leading the practitioner to desire a "less is more" approach. However, without aggressive treatment there is a high incidence of spread and almost certain death. Symptoms from the tumor will certainly worsen, and additional morbidity will develop as the tumor extends into the otic capsule and skull base. These grave symptoms include worsening pain, otorrhea, dizziness, hearing loss, dysphagia, and voice changes due to lower cranial nerve deficits and carotid or cavernous sinus involvement. Even in cases with distant malignant spread, palliative surgery can often alleviate some suffering, understanding that the goal of surgery is not for cure.

Temporal bone resection for primary tumors of the external auditory canal (EAC) that spread anteriorly should also include a parotidectomy.[13] Along the same lines, tumors that originate from the parotid gland but spread posteriorly into the temporal bone should include a temporal bone resection with the planned parotidectomy.

Management of the neck should be performed concurrently with the temporal bone resection. Primary temporal bone cancers rarely metastasize to the cervical lymph nodes. Parotid gland tumors that encroach on the temporal bone, however, frequently metastasize to the jugulodigastric lymph node chain, necessitating the need for lymphadenectomy.[14]

Sleeve Resection

The sleeve resection involves making medial and lateral incisions of the ear canal with an adequate margin around the tumor. This should only be performed for nonaggressive or benign pathology truly confined to a small portion of the cartilaginous external ear canal. The resulting defect is a large meatoplasty with exposed underlying soft tissue. It is often reconstructed with a split-thickness skin graft. Again, this is only indicated for benign or nonaggressive tumors and is rarely used today.

Lateral Temporal Bone Resection

A lateral temporal bone resection (LTBR) resects the entire bony and cartilaginous ear canal en bloc. The medial limit of resection is the promontory, facial nerve, and stapes. It is indicated for tumors confined to the EAC without extension through the tympanic membrane or bony ear canal. This falls into the Pittsburgh staging systems T1 and T2.

Incision/Soft-Tissue Dissection

Step 1: The main variant in planning the incision is whether or not the pinna will be sacrificed. If the tumor

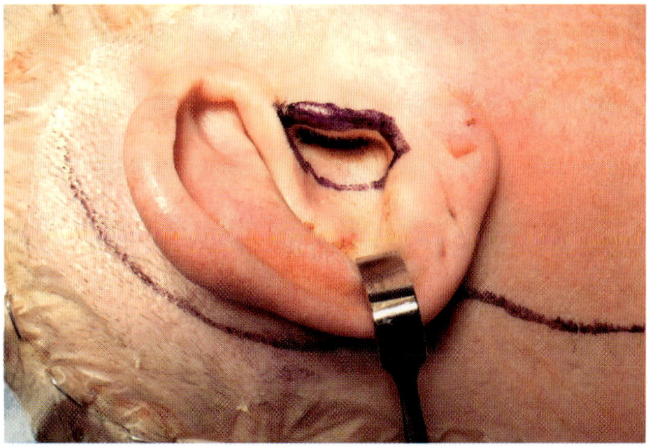

Fig. 8.1: Incision drawn for lateral concha incision.

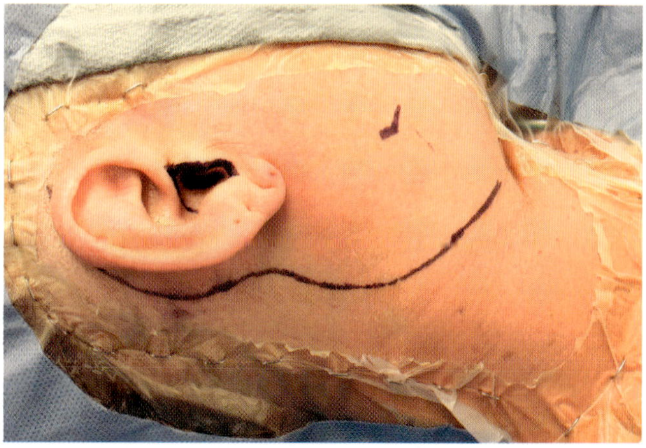

Fig. 8.2: Incision drawn into neck for planned neck dissection. The angle of the mandible is also marked.

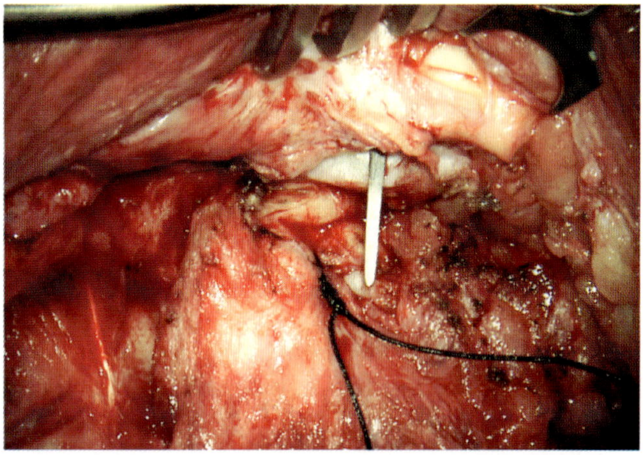

Fig. 8.3: Ear canal overclosure after tragal-conchal incision to prevent tumor spillage (note instrument entering from lateral ear canal).

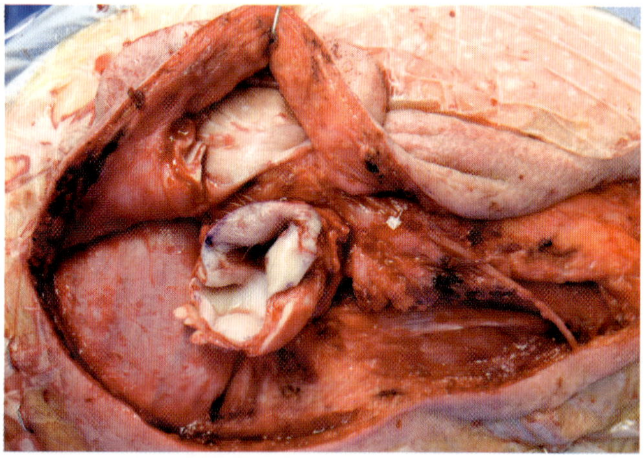

Fig. 8.4: The skin flap is elevated anteriorly exposing the parotid fascia and sternocleidomastoid muscle. The temporoparietal fascia is left intact over the temporalis muscle.

remains confined to the ear canal and the pinna can be saved, a circumferential incision laterally at the level of the conchal cartilage is made (Fig. 8.1). A postauricular incision is then made which is extended up to the scalp and inferiorly into the neck (Fig. 8.2). It should be kept in mind that the primary blood supply to the pinna will be based anteriorly, so the superior curve anteriorly should be as flat and posterior as possible.

Step 2: The ear canal skin is sutured closed to prevent tumor spillage (Fig. 8.3).

Step 3: The skin flap is dissected forward to expose the parotid gland. A flap is raised along the parotid fascia, similar to a parotidectomy (Fig. 8.4). Superiorly care should be taken to remain lateral to the temporoparietal fascia, as this may be required for reconstruction. Care should be taken to avoid injury to the temporal branch of the facial nerve.

Step 4: If a parotidectomy is to be included in the resection, the facial nerve is dissected from the stylomastoid foramen to the pes anserinus. This helps to obtain the depth of the facial nerve, which will again be identified from the mastoid side during the bony resection.

Step 5: If the pinna requires sacrifice, a preauricular incision is added leaving a rather large soft-tissue defect. The pinna will be resected en bloc with the specimen.

Bony Resection

Step 1: A complete mastoidectomy is performed with identification of the tegmen mastoideum, sigmoid sinus, antrum, and horizontal semicircular canal (Fig. 8.5).

Step 2: A hook is used to separate the malleus-incus joint (Fig. 8.6). The incus is removed to allow visualization of the horizontal segment of the facial nerve.

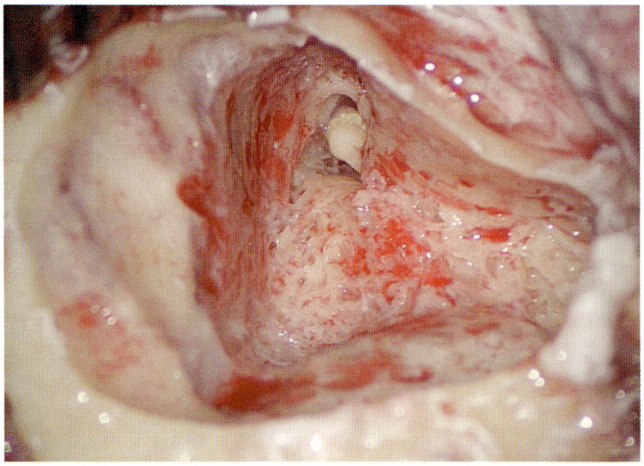

Fig. 8.5: Mastoidectomy performed with identification of the sigmoid sinus, tegmen mastoideum, and antrum.

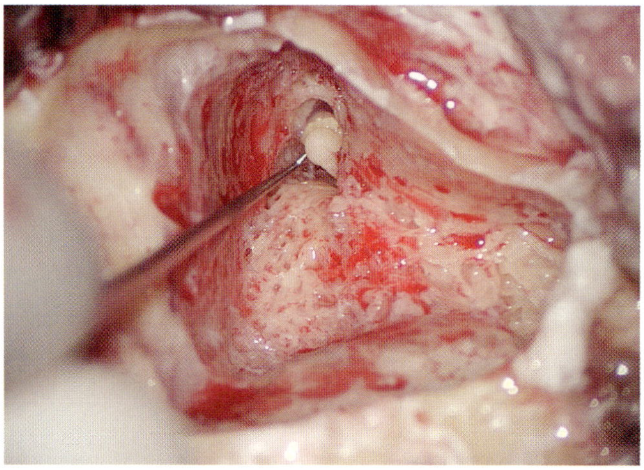

Fig. 8.6: A hook is used to separate the malleus-incus joint. Removing the incus allows a direct view of the horizontal segment of the facial nerve.

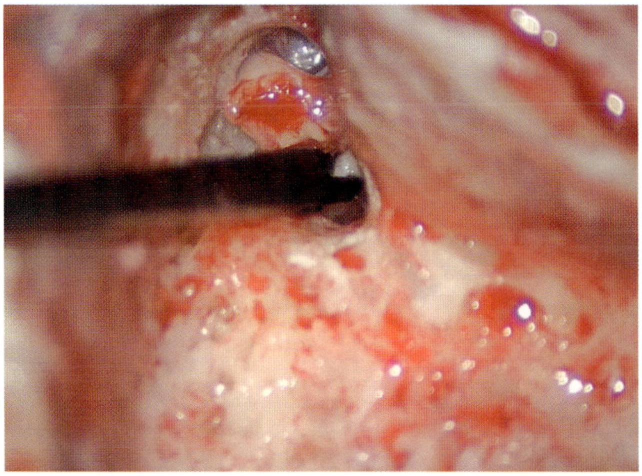

Fig. 8.7: Microscissors are used to section the tensor tympani tendon.

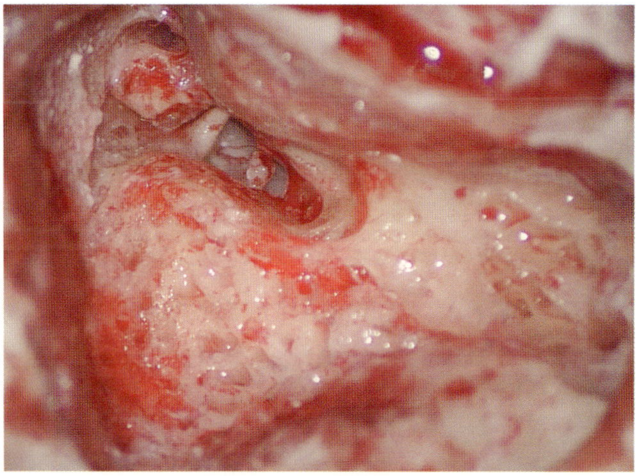

Fig. 8.8: The facial recess is drilled away to enter the middle ear, leaving the bony ear canal and tympanic annulus intact. The incus buttress has been removed.

Step 3: Microscissors are used to section the tensor tympani tendon. This will free the tympanic membrane from all deep attachments (Fig. 8.7).

Step 4: A facial recess is performed to enter the middle ear between the corda tympani nerve and the facial nerve. We find that it is easiest to take down the incus buttress immediately to allow wide opening of the facial recess (Fig. 8.8). Care should be taken to avoid thinning the posterior ear canal excessively as tumor may have invaded the bone superficially from the other side. One should also avoid disrupting the tympanic membrane or tympanic annulus as this serves as a barrier for tumor spillage.

Step 5: An extended facial recess is performed by sacrificing the corda tympani nerve. The facial nerve is followed inferiorly to the stylomastoid foramen. Dissection is continued anteriorly around the inferior portion of the bony ear canal to the glenoid fossa (Fig. 8.9). Preoperative CT examination can help determine the position of the jugular bulb and carotid artery to avoid injury when drilling around the inferior portion of the ear canal. These structures are usually fairly medial to the inferior tympanic annulus, but occasionally they can be located quite laterally.

Step 6: Attention is then turned to the superior portion of the mastoid cavity. Drilling continues anteriorly through the zygomatic air cells with the anterior limit being the glenoid fossa (Fig. 8.10). Usually the head of the malleus is removed, and the surgeon must be careful to avoid disrupting the underside of the pars flaccida.

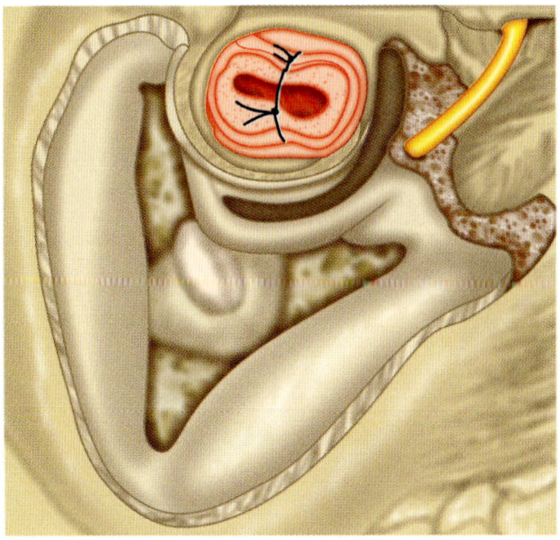

Fig. 8.9: An extended facial recess is performed by sacrificing the corda tympani nerve. The facial nerve is followed to the stylomastoid foramen. Dissection is continued around the inferior portion of the bony ear canal.

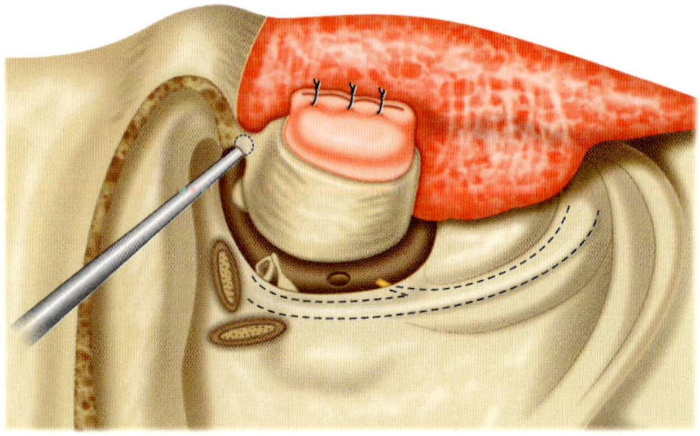

Fig. 8.10: The zygomatic air cells are drilled lateral to the ossicles to the superior glenoid fossa.

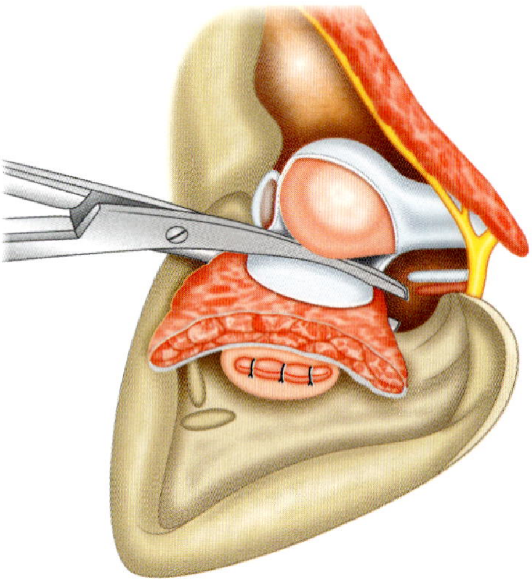

Fig. 8.11: Sharp scissors are used to remove the soft-tissue off of the glenoid fossa.

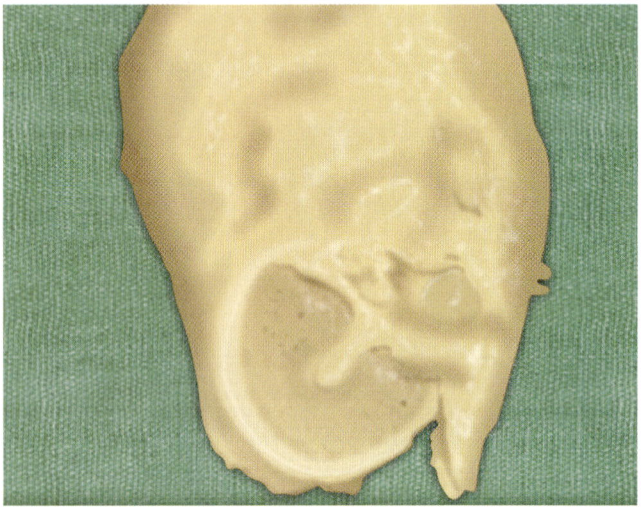

Fig. 8.12: Representative specimen after a lateral temporal bone resection. The tympanic membrane is removed with the bony ear canal.

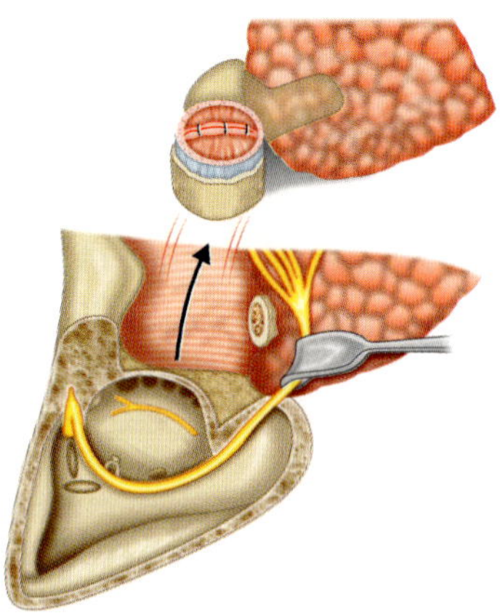

Fig. 8.13: If appropriate, the parotid gland is removed in continuity with the temporal bone resection.

Step 7: Now, the ear canal is only attached at its anterior attachments to the glenoid fossa and anterior tympanic bone. This can be fractured with gentle anterior pressure or with a small osteotome, making sure to angle the tip away from the carotid artery. Sharp scissors can be used to dissect the remaining soft tissue off of the glenoid fossa (Fig. 8.11). Ideally, the specimen should be a complete ring of bone with the tympanic membrane intact (Fig. 8.12).

Step 8: The parotid gland is removed in continuity if the tumor has spread into the parotid soft tissues (Fig. 8.13).

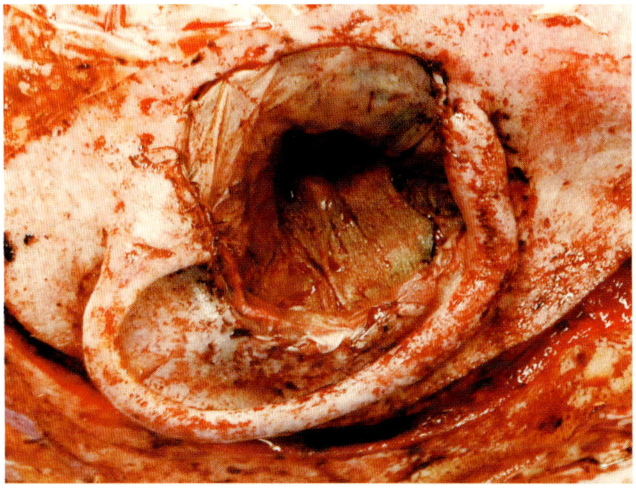

Fig. 8.14: Split thickness skin grafts can be used for reconstruction. They are sewn to the lateral pinna margin and are draped into the mastoid cavity over middle ear structures.

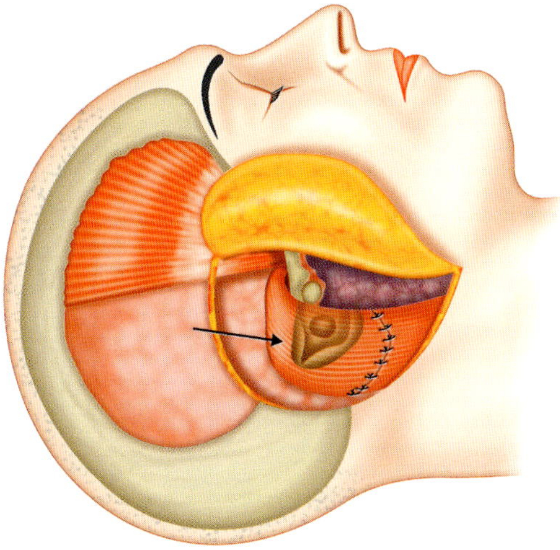

Fig. 8.15: The posterior portion of the temporalis muscle can be rotated down to provide vascularized tissue to cover the bone and eliminate dead space.

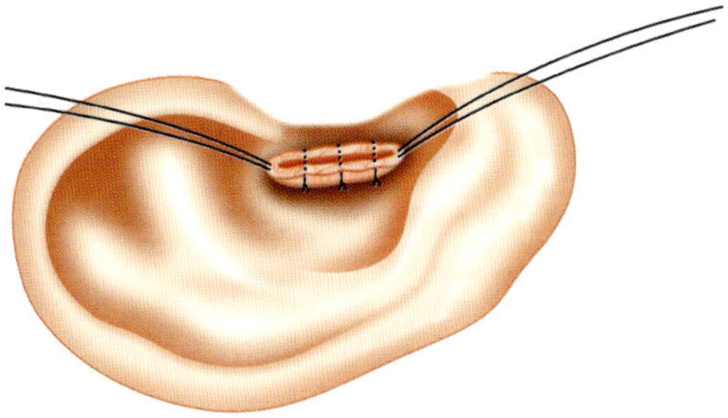

Fig. 8.16: The lateral ear canal may be overclosed with interrupted sutures.

Closure/Reconstruction

The main goals of reconstruction include eliminating dead space and providing the most optimal facial nerve outcome. Planning ahead during resection with careful soft-tissue dissection can leave many options available. For a LTBR, the remaining defect is a large mastoid cavity. Attempts to reconstruct the hearing are not performed.

Step 1: The Eustachian tube is packed with fascia or muscle to obliterate the connection to the nasopharynx.

Step 2: Split thickness skin grafts can aid in healing and can be sewn to the epidermis of the meatus (Fig. 8.14). They line the cavity and cover the middle ear structures. Postoperative debridement is necessary, and often radiation therapy causes some necrosis to the nonvascularized skin.

Step 3: Alternatively, soft tissue can be used to obliterate the mastoid cavity. A temporal-parietal fascia flap, a postauricular soft-tissue flap, or the posterior portion of the temporalis muscle (Fig. 8.15) may be rotated in for closure. This vascularized tissue has the benefit of ensuring more optimal healing with less chance of necrosis.

Step 4: Over-sewing of the EAC can be an option (Fig. 8.16).

Subtotal Temporal Bone Resection

Once tumors are beyond T3 staging per the Pittsburgh staging system, meaning that the facial nerve or middle ear is involved, a more aggressive approach is necessary. The dissection typically continues into the otic capsule, with the internal auditory canal and petrous carotid artery serving as the medial margin. Residual hearing and vestibular function would be sacrificed with otic capsule dissection. Adjustments can be made to either technique to remove portions of the dura, sigmoid sinus, parotid gland, and mandible as needed.

Incision/Soft-Tissue Dissection

Step 1: A postauricular incision is made, with the incision extended inferiorly into the neck, taking care to avoid the marginal mandibular nerve (Fig. 8.1). A neck dissection is performed to identify the great vessels of the neck. The jugular vein and the internal carotid artery are marked with vessel loops.

Step 2: With parotid and facial nerve involvement, the distal branches of the facial nerve are identified and tagged. The involved parotid gland is then dissected off the masseteric fascia from anterior to posterior, leaving it attached to the ear canal (Fig. 8.17). If the parotid gland

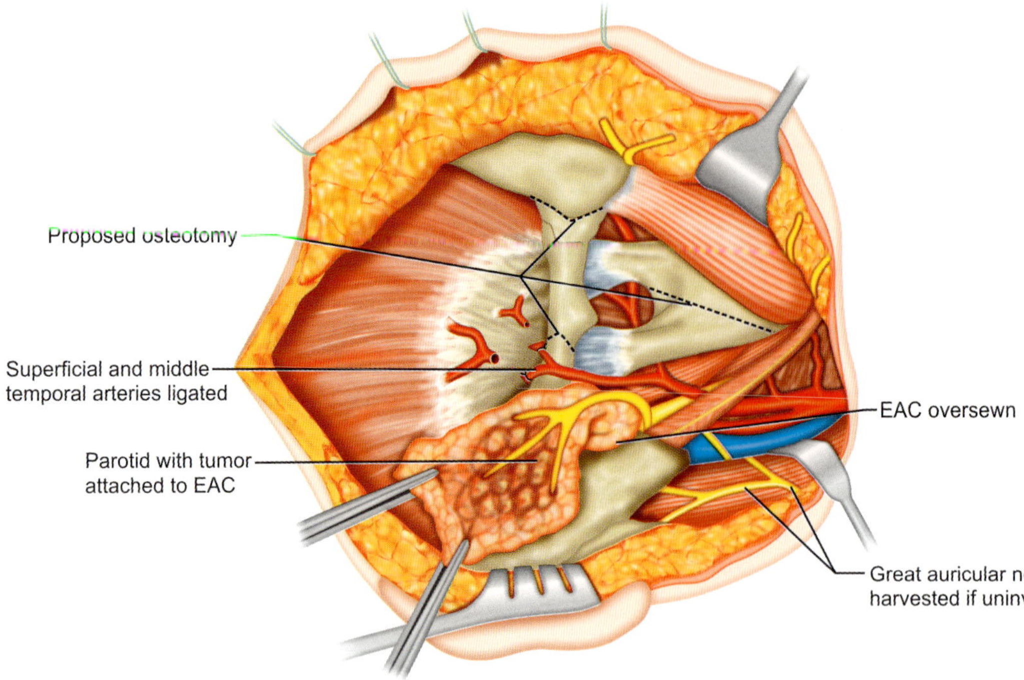

Fig. 8.17: With parotid gland and facial nerve involvement, the distal segments of the facial nerve are identified. The parotid gland is then reflected posteriorly off of the masseteric fascia.

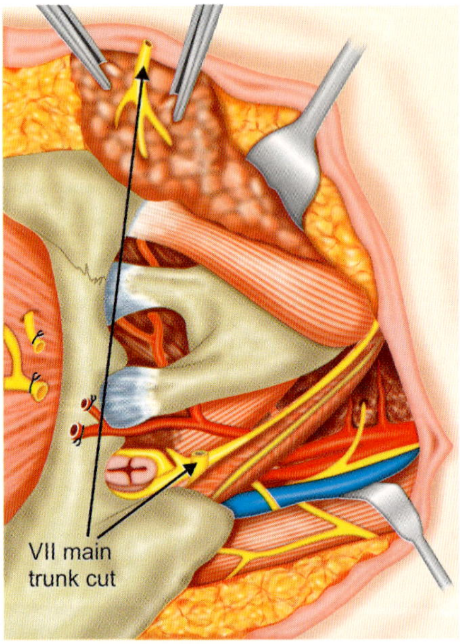

Fig. 8.18: If the parotid gland is to remain, the facial nerve is identified (and sacrificed if needed). The parotid can be reflected anteriorly to expose the masseteric fascia.

is to remain, the facial nerve should be identified (and sacrificed if needed). The parotid gland is then reflected anteriorly (Fig. 8.18).

Step 3: The zygoma is transected along with the ascending ramus of the mandible. These are brought posteriorly as part of the specimen.

Step 4: The inferior portions of the temporal bone must be freed of its muscular attachments (sternocleidomastoid and posterior digastric).

Bony Resection

Step 1: A temporal craniotomy is performed to identify the tegmen mastoidium as well as to ensure that the tumor has not invaded the brain parenchyma. The temporal lobe is retracted extradurally to expose the petrous bone (Fig. 8.19).

Step 2: A large mastoidectomy is performed removing all bone off of the sigmoid sinus and jugular bulb (Fig. 8.20).

Step 3: A labyrinthectomy is then performed, and the facial nerve is identified in the perigeniculate region. The facial nerve is generally sacrificed in this location (Fig. 8.21).

Step 4: Bone is completely removed over the posterior and middle fossa dura (Fig. 8.22).

Step 5: Bone is further removed in zygomatic root to the temporomandibular joint. The condyle of the mandible is resected depending on tumor invasion.

Step 6: The facial recess is widely opened including sacrifice of the facial nerve. This exposes the middle ear (Fig. 8.23).

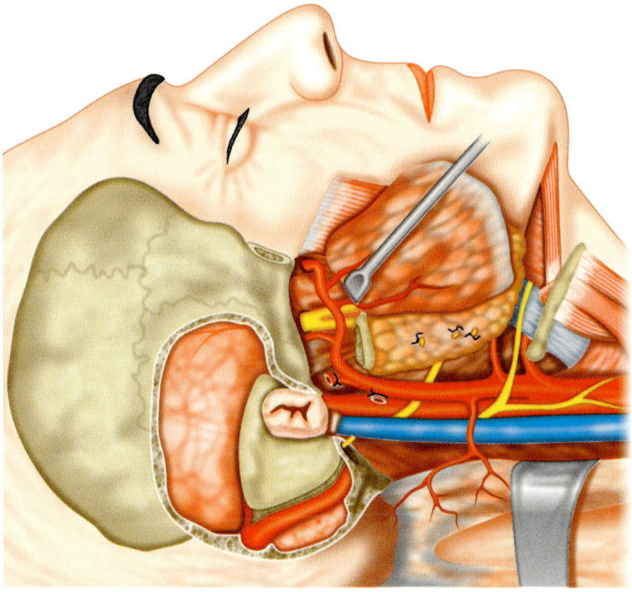

Fig. 8.19: A lateral craniotomy is made in the tegmen mastoideum to identify the dura. The temporal lobe is retracted extradurally to free the superior temporal bone.

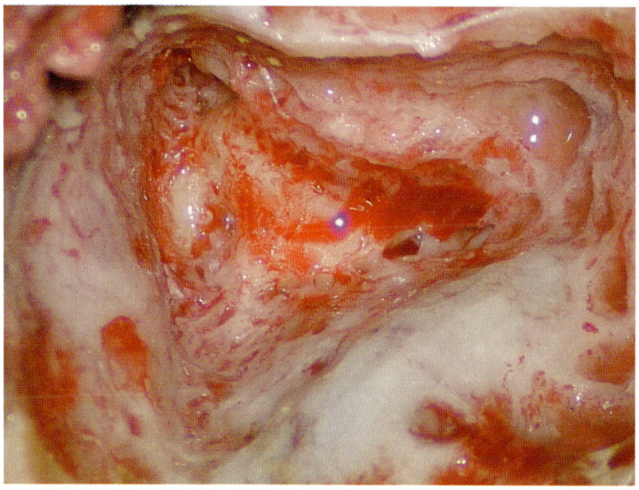

Fig. 8.20: A large mastoidectomy is performed removing all bone off of the sigmoid sinus and jugular bulb.

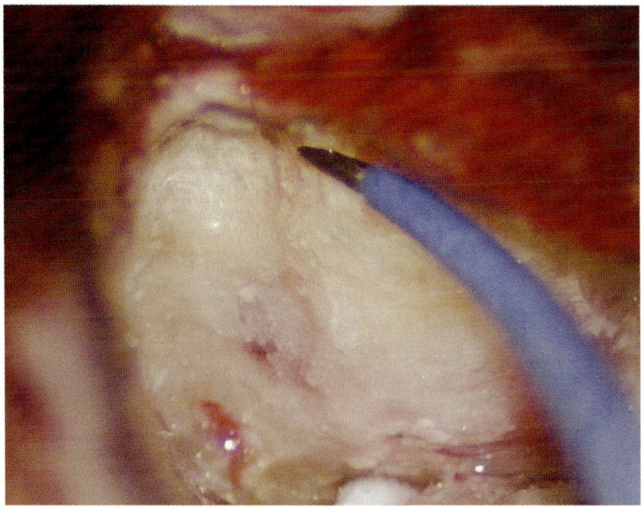

Fig. 8.21: A labyrinthectomy is then performed, and the facial nerve is identified in the perigeniculate region (note instrument).

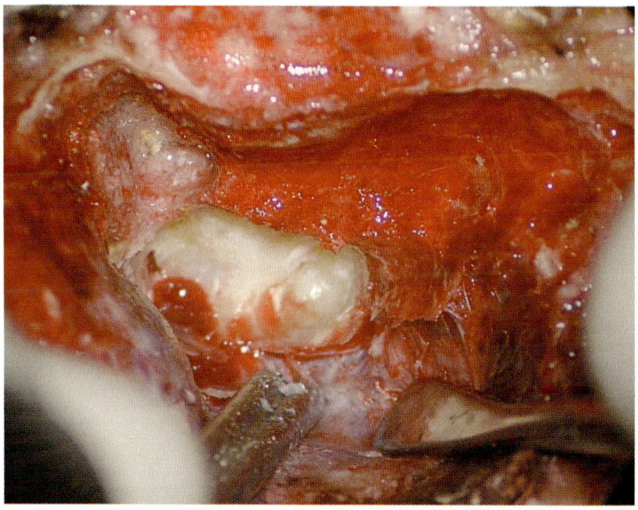

Fig. 8.22: Bone is completely removed over the posterior and middle fossa dura.

Step 7: The cochlea is drilled out exposing the dura over the internal auditory canal (Fig. 8.24).

Step 8: Bone is then removed from over the internal carotid artery anteriorly with a diamond drill, completing the bony resection.

Step 9: Additional resection: If the jugular bulb requires resection, the jugular vein should first be tied off in the neck. If dural entry is planned, the sigmoid sinus can be ligated with sutures via small dural incisions anterior and posterior to the vein (Fig. 8.25). Upon opening the jugular bulb, the openings of the inferior petrosal vein should be packed with surgical.

Step 10: If warranted, and if proximal and distal margins are negative via frozen section pathology, the facial nerve can be grafted from the area of the geniculate ganglion to the pes anserinus (Fig. 8.26).

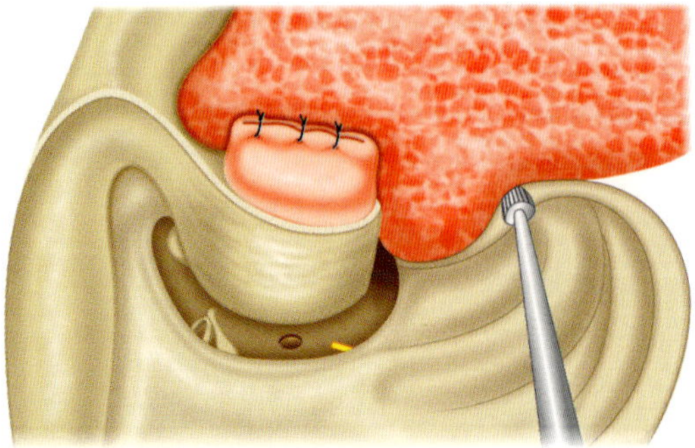

Fig. 8.23: The facial recess is widely opened including sacrifice of the facial nerve. This exposes the middle ear.

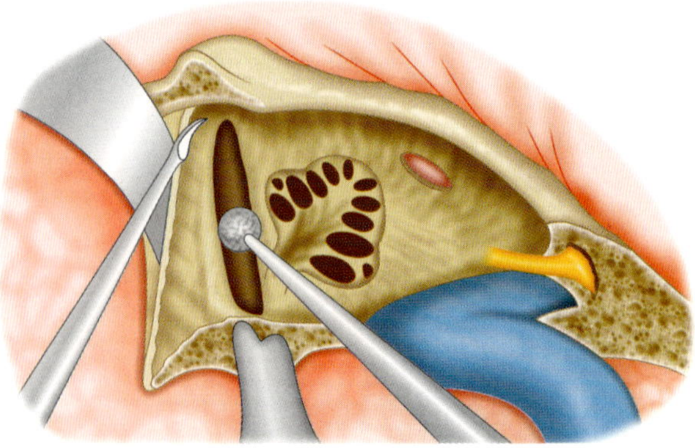

Fig. 8.24: The cochlea is drilled out exposing the internal auditory canal laterally.

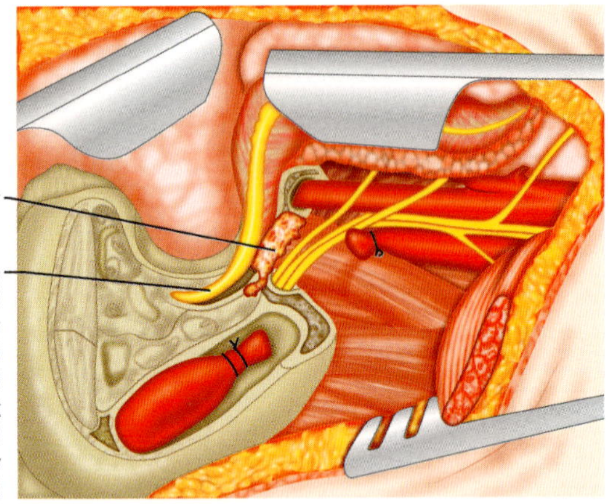

Fig. 8.25: If the jugular bulb requires resection the jugular vein should first be tied off in the neck. If dural entry is planned, the sigmoid sinus can be ligated with sutures via small dural incisions anterior and posterior to the vein.

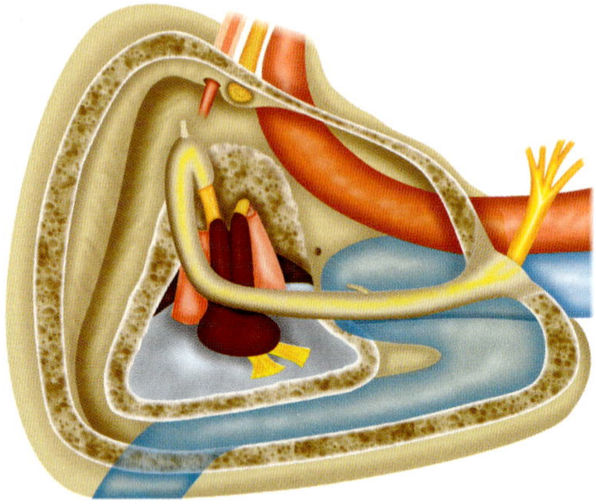

Fig. 8.26: The facial nerve is jump-grafted from pathologically free margins.

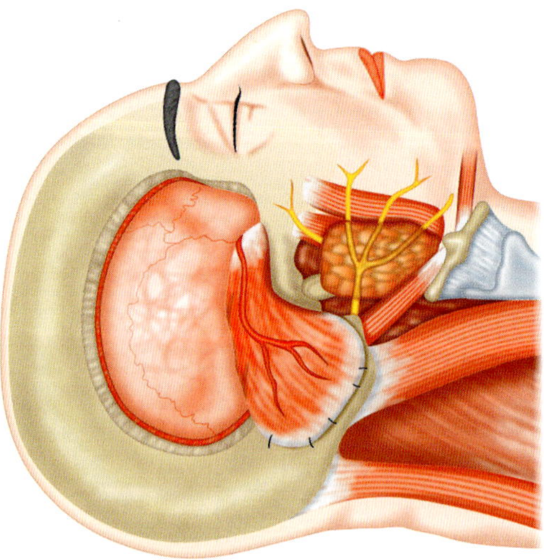

Fig. 8.27: The entire temporalis muscle can be used to provide vascularized bony covering. Extra length may be obtained by sectioning the zygoma.

Closure/Reconstruction

Closure of temporal bone defects can be quite challenging. The three goals of reconstruction after a subtotal temporal bone resection (STBR) or total temporal bone resection (TTBR) include (1) preventing a cerebrospinal fluid leak, (2) eliminating dead space, and (3) providing the most optimal facial nerve outcome.

Step 1: If the dura was entered, a watertight closure must be achieved. This can be done with pericranium, fascia, or other commercially available dura substitutes.

Step 2: After ear canal oversew, larger vascularized tissue is preferred over a free abdominal fat graft due to the risk of radiation necrosis. The temporalis muscle should remain well-vascularized from the deep temporal artery and can fill in a relatively large defect (Fig. 8.27). Note that extra length can be gained by removing the zygomatic arch.

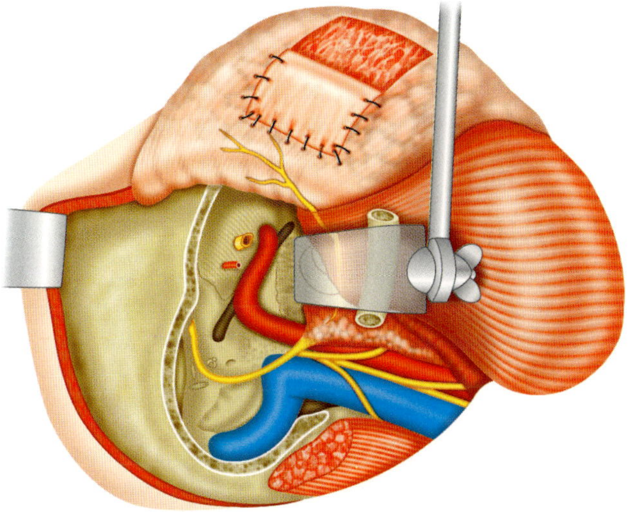

Fig. 8.28: The middle meningeal artery is divided via the temporal craniotomy, as is the greater superficial petrosal nerve and the third division of the trigeminal nerve.

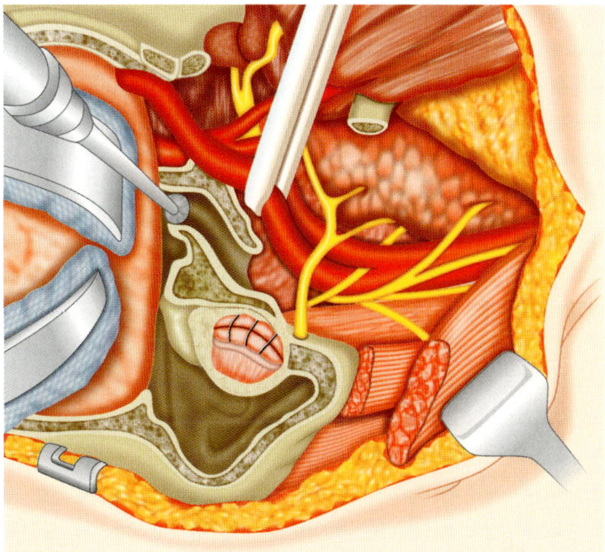

Fig. 8.29: A total temporal bone resection is performed by resecting the petrous apex, with or without carotid sacrifice to the cavernous sinus.

Step 3: A trapezius, latissimus, or pectoralis major muscle rotational flap can fill larger defects and is helpful when the entire pinna is resected. For even larger defects, a microvascular free tissue transfer may be performed.

Step 4: Details of facial reanimation are discussed in the facial nerve chapter. For cable grafting, the great auricular nerve may be used, but one must be absolutely certain that there is no encroachment of tumor around the harvest site. Because of this concern and the need for a longer graft, the sural nerve can be harvested from the lower leg.

Total Temporal Bone Resection

Total temporal bone resection is indicated when the tumor involves the anterior petrous apex or carotid artery. The TTBR refers to the additional removal of the entire petrous apex, with or without sacrifice of the internal carotid artery up to the cavernous sinus. With sacrifice of the carotid artery comes significant morbidity and mortality, even if the patient is deemed “acceptable” in the preoperative evaluation. Because of this, and the lack of well-documented survival benefit, the procedure is rarely performed today.[14]

Step 1: Bone and soft-tissue resection is performed as noted above with a STBR.

Step 2: The middle meningeal artery is divided via the temporal craniotomy, as is the greater superficial petrosal nerve and the third division of the trigeminal nerve (Fig. 8.28).

Step 3: Bony dissection is continued further forward drilling through the petrous apex (Fig. 8.29). Often the sixth cranial nerve is sacrificed. Bone is removed over the carotid artery, following the horizontal segment toward the cavernous sinus.

Step 4: The carotid artery can be ligated and removed depending on tumor involvement.

Step 5: Adjustments to the procedure are made if invasion of the dura is suspected. Dissection can continue in an intradural manner understanding that cerebrospinal fluid leak rate is greatly increased and will require a more substantial reconstruction. Even a limited involvement of the inferior temporal gyrus and cerebellum can be resected if needed, though the benefits on survival are likely small if any.

ADJUVANT THERAPY

All patients with tumors T2 or greater per the Pittsburgh scale should undergo postoperative external beam radiation. Staging should be anticipated preoperatively and confirmed intraoperatively. Some recommend postoperative radiation in all cases of temporal bone malignancy.[15] Radiation therapy should not be delayed over 6 weeks if possible. Patients should continue to be seen during radiation for meticulous care of the wound and/or mastoid cavity as osteoradionecrosis can cause delays in therapy and may be catastrophic. Radiation doses typically range from 5,000 to 6,000 rad and should include the operative site as well as the nodal drainage pattern.[14]

Chemotherapy has historically not been shown to provide benefit, and surgery and radiation continue to be the mainstays of treatment. In T4 temporal bone squamous cell carcinoma, adding chemotherapy to surgery and radiation has been shown to have potential benefit, by improving survival to that of T3-staged patients. There was no proven benefit if the tumor involved the dura, pyramidal apex, carotid canal, or lymph nodes.[16]

Brachytherapy catheters can be inserted into residual tumors at the time of resection if total tumor removal is expected to cause significant morbidity or death.[17]

PROGNOSIS

Patients staged with T1 lesions treated with a LTBR have an excellent 5-year survival rate of 95%. Some advocate adjuvant therapy in all temporal bone cancers, though evidence for T1 disease is equivocal. More extensive T2 and T3 lesions treated with surgery and radiation have an 85% chance of 5-year survival. Patients with extensive disease that require a TTBR have survival rates of 50% at one year and essentially 0% chance of survival at 2 years.[4,17] Patients with recurrent disease have significantly shorter overall survival and disease-free interval.[18] Advanced age, the presence of tumor of epithelial origin, and pathologically positive lymph nodes are significantly predictive of poor survival.[19]

CONCLUSION/PEARLS

- The most important way to improve patient outcome is diagnosis at an early stage. Practitioners should have a low threshold to biopsy any suspicious lesion that persists for > 2 weeks after medical treatment.
- Imaging with both CT and MRI provide evidence of possible bony erosion and soft-tissue involvement, respectively.
- Preoperative staging should be used to plan the appropriate surgical resection.
- The most important factor in patient prognosis is invasion beyond the external ear canal into the middle ear.
- There is extremely limited role for a sleeve resection. This should only be performed on benign lesions or extremely small lesions with low malignant potential located exclusively in the cartilaginous ear canal.
- LTBR should be completed with care taken to avoid tumor spillage.
- T4 lesions requiring TTBR, especially those that require carotid artery sacrifice, can be performed but have shown little survival benefit.
- Reconstruction of tissue defects should be considered during surgical resection, but should not limit or influence the completeness of surgical resection.
- The primary focus of surgery should be to provide as oncologically sound of a resection as possible. Hearing restoration, vestibular function, and facial nerve outcome are secondary benefits only.

REFERENCES

1. Bacciu A, Clemente IA, Piccirillo E, et al. Guidelines for treating temporal bone carcinoma based on long-term outcomes. Otol Neurotology. 2013;34(5):898-907.
2. Prasad M, Kraus D. Acinic cell carcinoma of the parotid gland presenting as an external auditory canal mass. Head Neck. 2004;26:85-8.
3. Brackmann DE, Arriaga MA. Posterior fossa skull base neoplasms. In: Cummings C, Fredrickson J, Krause C, Schuller D (Eds). Cummings Otolaryngology—Head and Neck Surgery, 4th edition. St. Louis, Mosby; 2005.
4. Marsh MM, Jenkins HA. Temporal bone neoplasms and lateral cranial base surgery. In: Cummings C, Fredrickson J, Krause C, Schuller D (Eds). Cummings Otolaryngology—Head and Neck Surgery, 4th edition. St. Louis: Mosby; 2005.
5. Peters BR, Maddox HE, Batsakia JG. Pleomorphic adenoma of the middle ear and mastoid with posterior fossa extension. Arch Otolaryngol Head Neck Surg. 1988;114:676-8.
6. Leonetti JP, Smith PG, Anand V, et al. Subtotal petrosectomy in the management of advanced parotid neoplasms. Otolaryngol Head Neck Surg. 1993;108:270-6.
7. Pensak ML, Gleich LL, Gluckman JL, et al. Temporal bone carcinoma: contemporary perspectives in the skull base surgical area. Laryngoscope. 1996;106:1234-7.
8. Glenn L. Innovations in neuroimaging of skull base pathology. Otolaryngol Clin North Am. 2005;38:613-29.
9. Arriaga M, Curtin H, Takahashi H, et al. Staging proposal for external auditory meatus carcinoma based on preoperative clinical examination and computed tomography findings. Ann Otol Rhinol Laryngol. 1990;99:714-21.
10. Shintani SA, Foote RL, Lowe VJ, et al. Utilizing of PET/CT imaging performed early after surgical resection in the adjunct treatment planning from head and neck cancer. Int J Radiat Oncol Biol Phys. 2008;70(2):322-9.
11. Janecka IP, Sekhar LN, Horton JA. General blood flow evaluation. In: Cummings CW, Fredrickson J, Krause C, Schuller D (Eds). Otolaryngology—Head and Neck Surgery Update II. St. Louis: Mosby; 1990. pp. 54-63.
12. Moody SA, Hirsch BE, Myers EN. Squamous cell carcinoma of the external auditory canal: An evaluation of a staging system. Am J Otol. 2000;21:582-8.
13. Zhang T, Li W, Dai C, et al. Evidence-based surgical management of T1 or T2 temporal bone malignancies. Laryngoscope. 2013;123:244-8.
14. Arriaga MA, Leonetti JP. Malignancies of the temporal bone—limited temporal bone resection. In: Brackmann DE, Shelton C, Arriaga MA (Eds). Otologic Surgery, 3rd edition. Philadelphia, PA: Saunders Elsevier; 2010.

15. Masterson L, Rouhani M, Donnelly NP, et al. Squamous cell carcinoma of the temporal bone: clinical outcomes from radical surgery and postoperative radiotherapy. Otol Neurotol. 2014;35(3):501-8.
16. Nakagawa T, Kumamoto Y, Natori Y, et al. Squamous cell carcinoma of the external auditory canal and middle ear: an operation combined with preoperative chemoradiotherapy and a free surgical margin. Otol Neurotol. 2006; 27:242-9.
17. Prasad S, Janecka IP. Malignancies of the temporal bone: radical temporal bone resection. In: Brackmann DE, Shelton C, Arriaga MA, et al. (Eds). Otologic Surgery. Philadelphia, PA: Saunders; 1994.
18. Gidley PW, Roberts DB, Sturgis EM. Squamous cell carcinoma of the temporal bone. Laryngoscope. 2010;120(6): 1144-51.
19. Mantravadi AV, Marzo SJ, Leonetti JP, et al. Lateral temporal bone and parotid malignancy with facial nerve involvement. Oto HNS. 2011;144(3):395-401.

CHAPTER

9 Treatment of Labyrinthine Disorders

John J Zappia, Daniel R Pieper

INTRODUCTION

The inner ear is subject to a variety of disorders. Many are self-limited or readily treated medically but some require more aggressive therapies. Some of these more aggressive therapies are disease specific, such as posterior semicircular canal occlusion (PSCO), and others, such as labyrinthectomy, have broader treatment potential. This chapter reviews many of the treatment options for these labyrinthine disorders.

ENDOLYMPHATIC SAC SURGERY

Meniere's Disease

Meniere's disease is an idiopathic disorder of the inner ear consisting of the tetrad of vertigo, hearing loss (usually fluctuant), tinnitus, and aural fullness. The pathophysiology is purported to be endolymphatic hydrops based on histologic studies. Not all patients experience the full tetrad of symptoms. Generally these patients are labeled with the more generic term, endolymphatic hydrops. The terms "cochlear" Meniere's disease and "vestibular" Meniere's have been used for patients with only aural or only vestibular symptoms, respectively.

Meniere's disease is responsive to medical therapy in 70% of patients. The most common medical regimen centers on sodium control, consisting of a low-sodium diet and the use of a diuretic. Other medical treatment philosophies (either separate from, or in conjunction with, sodium control) include use of betahistine/histamine, altering middle ear pressure dynamics (PE tube, Meniette), allergy treatment, and dietary modification/avoidance—mostly commonly dairy.

In those where standard medical therapy does not control symptoms, multiple options are available. The options can generally be classified as conservative versus ablative and/or in office versus surgical. The conservative options include oral or intratympanic (IT) steroid treatment and endolymphatic sac surgery. Labeling them as conservative does not suggest that they are without risk, but that ablation of the vestibular function is not intended. The most common ablative treatments include IT gentamicin, labyrinthectomy, and vestibular neurectomy.

Endolymphatic Sac Surgery

Endolymphatic sac surgery was introduced by Portmann in the 1920s.[1] It was popularized in the 1960s. The technical variations include simple decompression of the endolymphatic sac, wide decompression of the endolymphatic sac and sigmoid sinus, endolymphatic sac to mastoid shunt and endolymphatic sac to subarachnoid shunt.

Telischi et al.[2] looked at the long-term success of endolymphatic-subarachnoid shunt. They found that of 234 patients that had been followed for at least 10 years, 63% needed no further surgery, 17% went on to revision endolymphatic sac surgery, and 20% went on to a more destructive procedure. Brackmann and Nissen[3] reported that the endolymphatic sac to mastoid shunt was equal to the endolymphatic sac to subarachnoid shunt. Gianoli et al.[4] looked at the results of endolymphatic sac decompression and reported 85% complete or substantial vertigo control 2 years after surgery.

In a 1981 Danish study looking at the efficacy of endolymphatic sac surgery,[5] it was found that vertigo was controlled in 70% of patients in both active surgery group and "control" simple mastoidectomy group. Interestingly, there were two divergent conclusions from this. One was that endolymphatic sac surgery is of no more value than placebo and should not be part of treatment consideration in Meniere's disease. The second conclusion is that both the simple mastoidectomy and the "active" surgery resulted in 70% control and have a role.[6]

Questions did arise about the mechanism of action of the surgery, given the apparent "success" of the simple mastoidectomy. The potential mechanism of the surgery

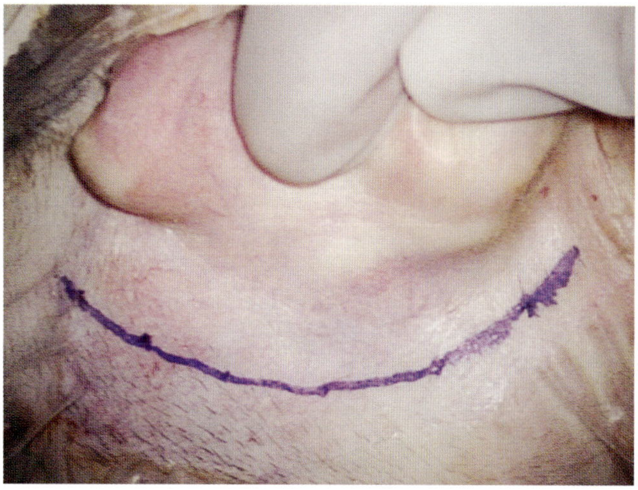

Fig. 9.1: Position of planned postauricular incision in a right ear.

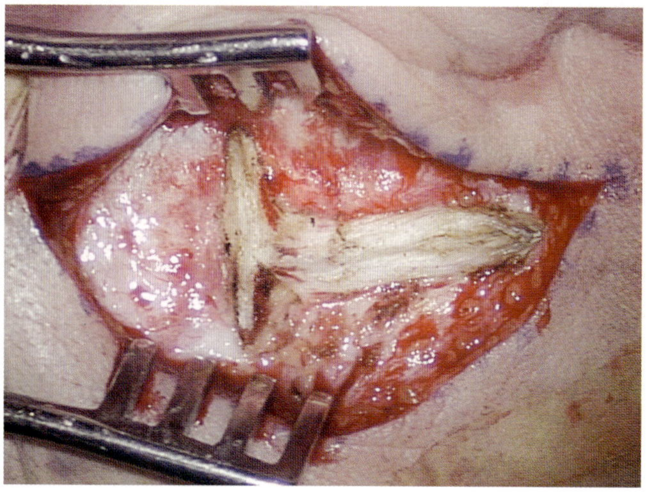

Fig. 9.2: Periosteal "T" incision with horizontal limb over linea temporalis and vertical limb extending down to the mastoid tip.

has been postulated to be bony decompression, shunting/drainage of fluid, placebo, general anesthesia, alteration of blood supply, inflammatory response, and vibration from drilling. The majority, but not all, of those treating patients with Meniere's disease continue to consider endolymphatic sac surgery as a viable treatment option.

The surgery is performed as an outpatient. Although the complication rate is low, the risks include hearing loss, dizziness, facial nerve injury, cerebrospinal fluid leak. Patients may experience some disequilibrium postoperatively, but it is usually very limited. This significantly distinguishes endolymphatic sac surgery from ablative procedures typically requiring several weeks of disequilibrium and recuperation. Postoperatively, temporary hearing loss and fullness in the treated ear due to the collection of blood and fluid in the mastoid and middle ear will occur. The results are occasionally immediate but can take several weeks to be realized.

It is important to reinforce with the patient that the integrity of the ear has been maintained and that ongoing medical treatment will be necessary. If there is incomplete control, further ablative procedures can be considered. In select patients who have initial prolonged success and later failure, revision endolymphatic sac surgery can be contemplated.

Endolymphatic Sac Surgical Procedure

In most cases, general endotracheal anesthesia is utilized, although it can be done under local anesthesia with sedation. The patients receive perioperative antibiotics and preoperative intravenous dexamethasone for postoperative nausea.

Step 1

After induction of anesthesia, the patient is placed in a supine position with the affected ear up. The periauricular area is prepped and draped in the usual manner. One percent lidocaine with 1:100,000 epinephrine is infused in the postauricular area.

Step 2

A standard postauricular incision is made about 5 mm behind the auricular crease (Fig. 9.1).

Step 3

A "T"-shaped incision is made in the periosteal layer with the horizontal limb along the linea temporalis and the vertical limb along the axis of the mastoid bone (Fig. 9.2).

Step 4

Soft tissue is then elevated to expose the lateral mastoid bone surface and self-retaining retractors are placed (Fig. 9.3).

Step 5

A cortical mastoidectomy is initiated with a large cutting burr. The sigmoid sinus and tegmen are identified for orientation. As the drilling progresses medially, care is always taken to ensure the drilling is superior, along the

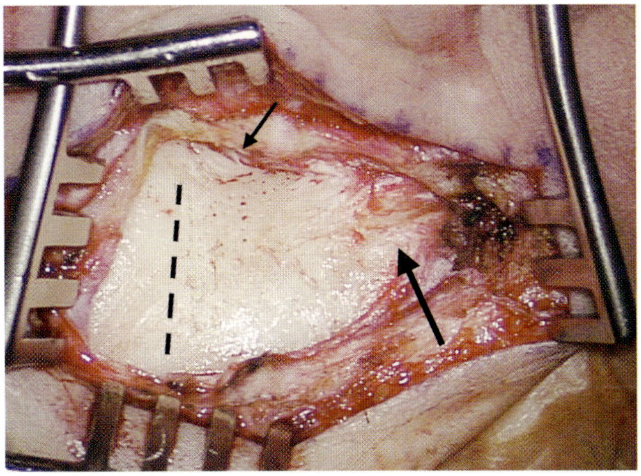

Fig. 9.3: The lateral mastoid bone surface can be seen after the incisions (small arrow shows spine of Henle; large arrow shows mastoid tip; dotted line shows linea temporalis).

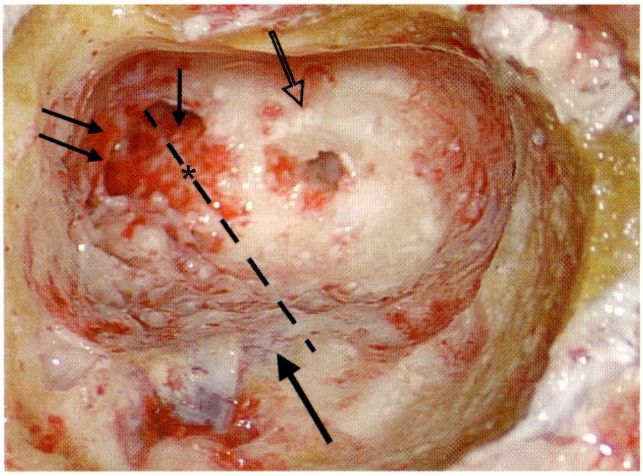

Fig. 9.4: Completed mastoidectomy (horizontal semicircular canal shown by asterisk; tegmen shown by double arrow; short process of the incus shown by small arrow; sigmoid sinus shown by large arrow; facial nerve shown by hollow arrow; Donaldson's line shown by dotted line).

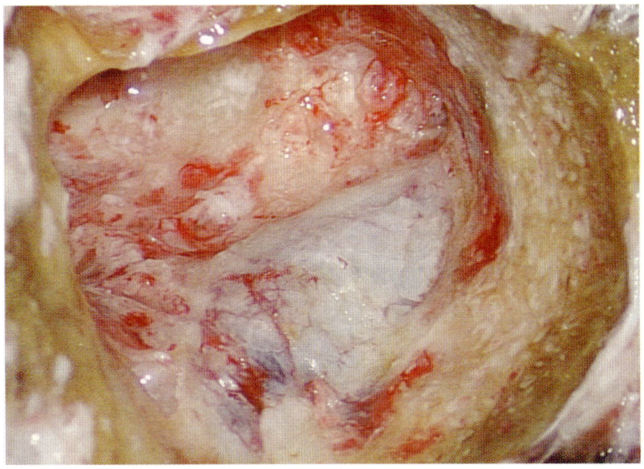

Fig. 9.5: Generous exposure of the sigmoid sinus in preparation for the decompression.

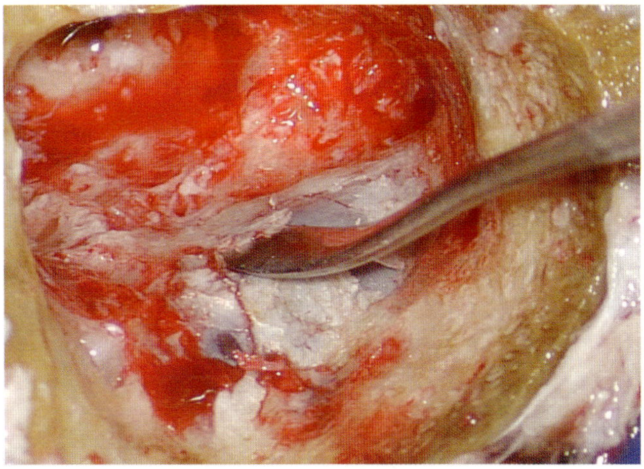

Fig. 9.6: The beginning of the decompression with the thinned bone over the sigmoid sinus being gently elevated with a Freer elevator.

tegmen, to keep the facial nerve and horizontal semicircular canal safe. The antrum is identified and the horizontal semicircular and short process of the incus are visualized (Fig. 9.4). Generous irrigation during the procedure is performed with particular attention to the prevention of bone collection in the epitympanum and middle ear. Occasional conductive hearing loss postoperatively is theorized to be due to bone matter collection around the ossicular chain.

Step 6

Donaldson's line is visualized posteriorly to define the upper limit of the exposure necessary. Although not absolutely necessary, the inferior mastoid air cells are generally opened widely and the vertical segment of the facial nerve is identified (Fig. 9.4).

Step 7

The bone over the sigmoid sinus and the posterior fossa dura into the retrofacial area is thinned with a diamond burr (Fig. 9.5).

Step 8

The final layer of bone is removed with either a Freer or annular elevator (Fig. 9.6).

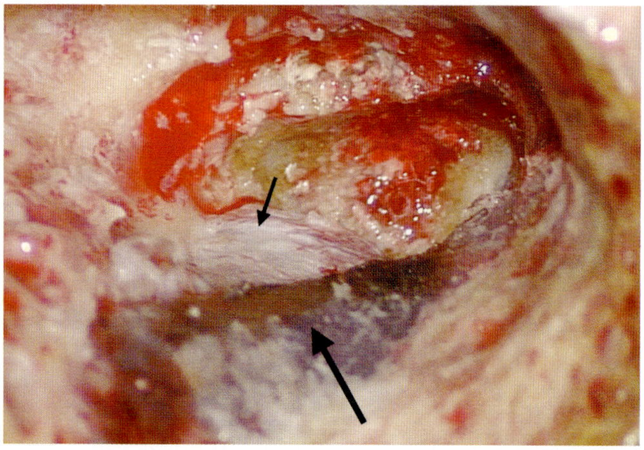

Fig. 9.7: The sigmoid sinus and the endolymphatic sac after bony decompression (endolymphatic sac shown by small arrow; sigmoid sinus shown by large arrow).

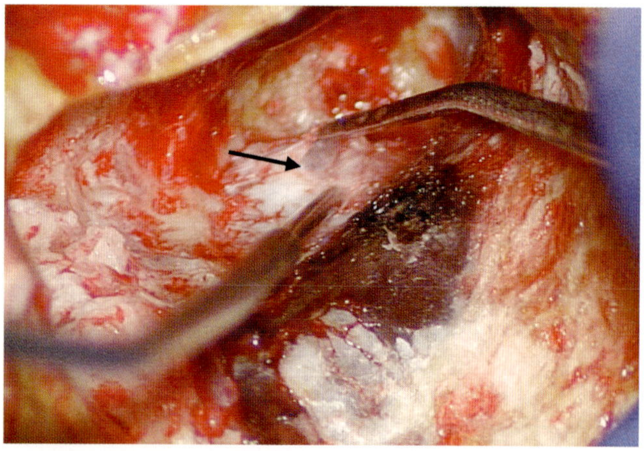

Fig. 9.8: The lumen of the endolymphatic sac being opened with an annulus elevator (endolymphatic sac lumen shown by arrow).

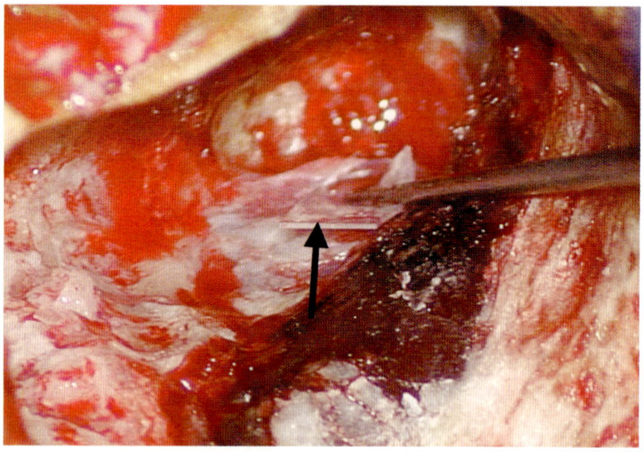

Fig. 9.9: Silastic shunt being placed in the endolymphatic sac (Silastic shunt shown by arrow).

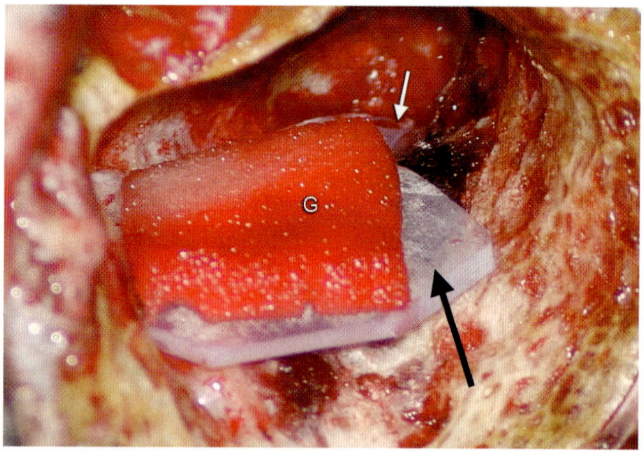

Fig. 9.10: Protective Silastic over exposed sigmoid sinus (thick Silastic shown by large arrow; Silastic shunt in background shown by small arrow; Gelfoam–G).

Step 9

The sigmoid sinus and the endolymphatic sac overlying the posterior fossa dura in the retrofacial area are widely exposed/decompressed (Fig. 9.7). This would complete the decompression procedure.

Step 10

For the mastoid shunt, the endolymphatic sac inferior to the posterior semicircular canal is incised with a sickle knife. The lumen is probed and the opening enlarged with an annulus elevator (Fig. 9.8).

Step 11

Although there are different possibilities, the simplest shunt is a piece of thin Silastic fashioned into a T shape. The horizontal portion is placed within the sac and the vertical stem is extended into the mastoidectomy defect (Fig. 9.9).

Step 12

The wound is copiously irrigated with saline solution. The middle ear is also irrigated to remove all bone dust. A piece of thick Silastic can be placed over the exposed sigmoid sinus to protect it should subsequent surgery be necessary (Fig. 9.10).

Step 13

The deep layers of the wound are closed with 3-0 Vicryl suture and the skin is reapproximated with glue or 5-0 fast absorbing gut. A standard mastoid dressing is placed.

Most patients are discharged postoperatively, but observation overnight is available for the occasional patient with pain or nausea issues. The patient is seen 1 week postoperatively and then at 2 months if there are no concerns. The patient is counseled preoperatively and reminded postoperatively about the importance of continued medical therapy.

INTRATYMPANIC THERAPY

Introduction

Although there have been many medications delivered intratympanically, steroids and the aminoglycoside, gentamicin, are currently the most common. The most common diagnoses for these interventions are Meniere's disease and sudden sensorineural hearing loss (SSNHL).

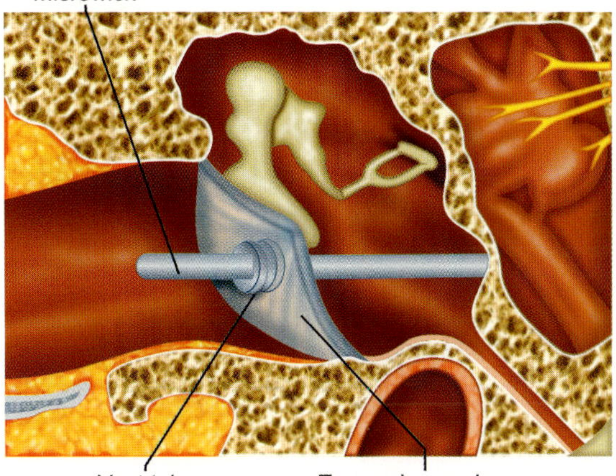

Fig. 9.11: A microwick used for intratympanic therapy.

Intratympanic Steroid Therapy

Steroid usage has been more often studied in SSNHL and the most often referenced article on the benefit of oral steroids in SSNHL is Wilson et al.[7] Their double-blind, placebo-controlled study reported a 61% response in treated patients and 32% in control. They observed that a primarily mid-frequency hearing loss was extremely favorable and that a severe/profound loss was unfavorable for recovery. Although vertigo was not studied directly, it was observed that patients with severe/profound hearing loss were more likely to have vertigo. Not all studies have confirmed this benefit and, although steroids are generally considered the treatment of choice, there is some controversy in their usage.

Intratympanic (IT) steroids have been used as initial therapy, adjuvant therapy, and rescue therapy for failure of oral therapy in SSNHL. Reports are strongly suggestive of their benefit but findings are not unanimous. One of the most inclusive studies was a randomized, double-blind, placebo-controlled multi-institutional report that suggested that IT steroids were equal to oral steroids for treatment of SSNHL.[8] Steroid (oral or IT) responsiveness is less studied but frequently utilized in Meniere's disease.

The technique for IT therapy varies. Most commonly a needle is used to penetrate the drum. Also used is a myringotomy with placement of a tube or wick. Protocols vary from a single injection[9] up to daily injections for 8 days.[10] With the microwick (Fig. 9.11), either repeated applications of topical drops or continuous infusions are utilized for periods up to 4 weeks.[11] Presently the two most common medications are dexamethasone and methylprednisolone. There is some evidence that methylprednisolone reaches higher concentration in the inner ear[12] but discomfort is more likely. Various concentrations are possible. In our clinic, a 10 mg/mL dexamethasone solution is used, as it is relatively comfortable and it is a standard solution that is readily available.

Intratympanic steroids are always the treatment of choice for patients in whom oral steroid therapy is contraindicated, i.e. diabetics. It is frequently used in conjunction with oral therapy in most other situations. It would also be considered the treatment of choice in patients with a definite history of IT steroid responsiveness. For SSNHL, a series of two to three injections over 2 weeks is considered, although the protocol is modified depending on the patient situation, severity of loss, evidence of response, and use of concomitant oral steroids. For the Meniere's patients, more often a single injection is performed either as part of initial therapy or during a "flair up".

During IT treatment, the patient will typically experience pressure during the injection and only occasionally true pain. Although the solution is warmed by hand before injecting, it will be below body temperature and result in temporary dizziness beginning several seconds after the initiation of the injection. Some solution will invariably drain into the patient's mouth. Although rare, there is a risk of hearing loss and tympanic membrane perforation with IT therapy.

Intratympanic Steroid Treatment Protocol

The expected sensation of fullness and temporary dizziness during the injection are discussed and the potential risks are carefully reviewed with the patient.

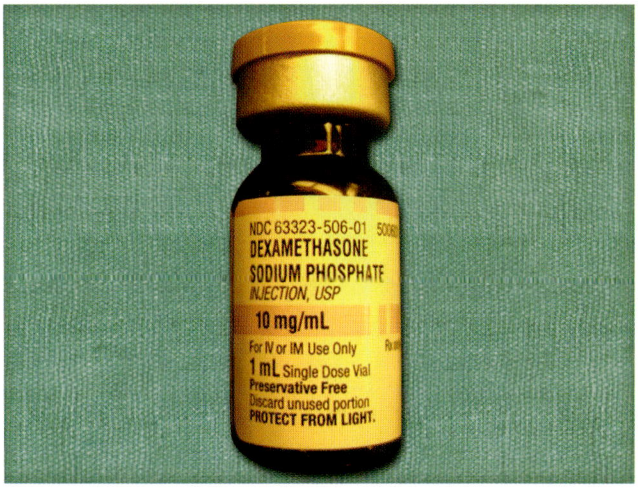

Fig. 9.12: The dexamethasone solution used for intratympanic therapy.

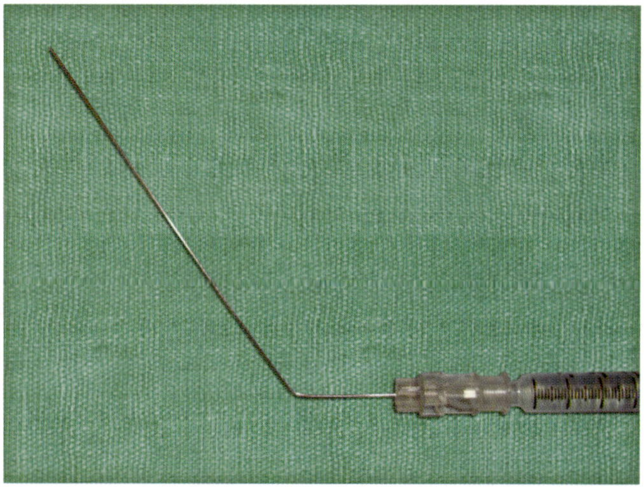

Fig. 9.13: The syringe and the attached 27G 3.5 in spinal needle bent appropriately for injection.

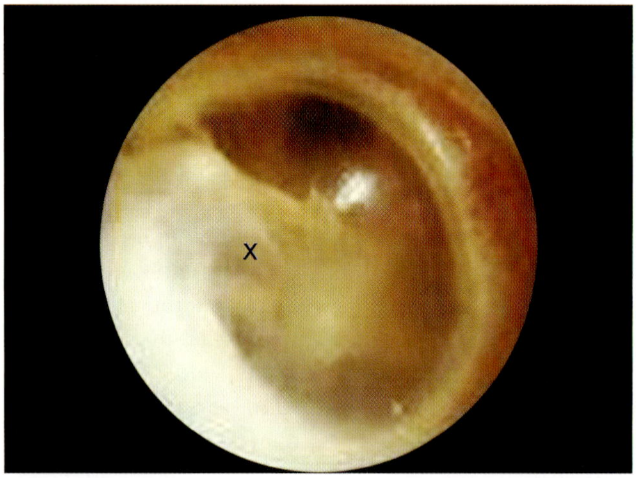

Fig. 9.14: The target area of injection in the right tympanic membrane (x shows target area).

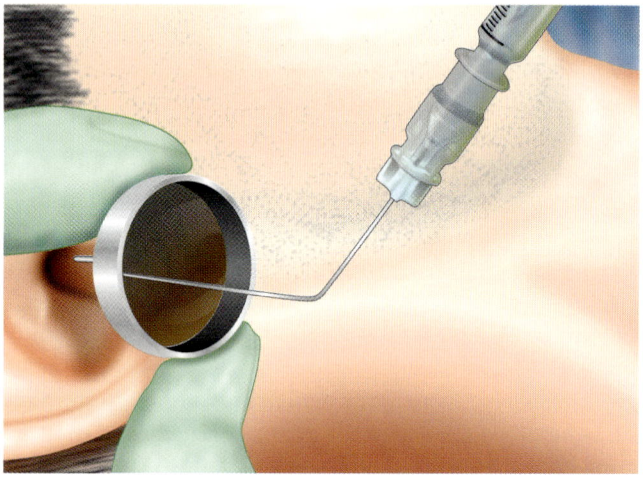

Fig. 9.15: The tuberculin syringe and spinal needle in position for the injection.

Step 1

Stock dexamethasone (10 mg/mL) is utilized (Fig. 9.12). One milliliter is drawn up in a 1.0 cc tuberculin syringe.

Step 2

A 27G 3.5 in spinal needle is attached for use in the injection. At about 1 cm from the hub, the needle is bent at a 30° angle with the bevel of the needle away from the syringe (Fig. 9.13).

Step 3

The patient is placed in a supine position with the head rotated slightly away from the affected ear. A minimal amount of phenol is applied to the tympanic membrane immediately posterior to the long process of the malleus, closer to the short process than the umbo (Fig. 9.14).

Step 4

With the syringe above and the bevel of the needle down (Fig. 9.15), the needle is passed through the anesthetized area of the tympanic membrane. If done carefully, a middle ear seal is maintained.

Step 5

The dexamethasone solution is slowly infused. The droplets can usually be seen dripping down behind the tympanic membrane and filling the middle ear from posteriorly. Care is taken to inject slowly so no air collects in the posterior tympanum around the windows. The air-fluid level will be seen rising and, with an appropriate seal around the needle, it will rise past the injection site to completely fill the middle ear. As mentioned above, the patient will typically experience fullness as the injection occurs and will also usually taste some of the solution as it overflows into the Eustachian tube orifice. Dizziness will usually begin within seconds of the initiation of the injection and will last several minutes until the solution in the middle ear reaches body temperature.

Step 6

The needle is left in the tympanic membrane for approximately 1 minute to maintain the seal and the pressure. Once the needle is withdrawn, pressure is released and some fluid will drain into the ear canal.

Step 7

The patient is instructed to keep their head position and avoid swallowing. They are kept in the supine position for 30 minutes.

Most patients will have a sense of pressure in the ear for approximately 1 day. The perforation is usually sealed within 2 weeks, if not sooner. For those requiring repeat treatment, the injection site is frequently open at the subsequent injections, eliminating the need for anesthesia. The patient is instructed to keep water out of the treated ear for 1 week after treatment. The hearing will typically be rechecked at 2 weeks from the initial injection unless the patient reports normal hearing. If this is the case the hearing is checked at that time and treatment discontinued if hearing has, in fact, returned to normal.

Intratympanic Gentamicin Therapy

Meniere's disease is reviewed in the endolymphatic sac section and is the most common indication for gentamicin IT therapy. IT gentamicin is an in office ablative possibility considered in medical failures. Steroids (oral and IT) have a role as discussed above.

Before any ablative treatment is considered, careful evaluation is necessary. A patient must understand not only the likely benefit but the potential risks and expected recovery. The decision to proceed is based on the life limitation, which is extremely variable patient to patient. Evaluation will include a videonystagmography (VNG) and frequently an electrocochleogram (ECoG) to document the ipsilateral problem, but more importantly to identify any potential contralateral problems that may alter the decision-making process. An MRI of the brain is imperative in the evaluation of any significant unilateral otologic process.

The first aminoglycoside, streptomycin, was introduced clinically in the 1940s. Soon after introduction otologic complications were being recognized.[13] Intramuscular streptomycin was described in 1948.[14] Schuknecht reported on IT streptomycin in 1956[15] and intramuscular streptomycin in 1957.[16] Gentamicin was introduced in 1964 with a more favorable toxicity profile. Beck and Schmidt reported on IT gentamicin in 1978 renewing interest in its benefits.[17] In 1993, Nedzelski[18] reported on a large series somewhat ushering in the recent era.

The exact mechanism of aminoglycoside ototoxicity is not completely understood. Theories include (1) inhibition of ornithine decarboxylase with impairment of cellular repair process, (2) binding to phosphoinositides with disruption of signaling across membranes, (3) superoxide production from mitochondrial gene translation error, (4) blockage of transduction of hair cells, (5) damage mediated via reductions in glutamate decarboxylase.

The aminoglycosides have variable relative ototoxicity with neomycin, kanamycin, and amikacin being differentially cochleotoxic and primarily affecting the outer hair cells in the basal turn of the cochlea. Streptomycin, gentamicin, and tobramycin are differentially vestibulotoxic, affecting the hair cells of the cristae and the maculae with destruction of the endolymph producing dark cells. The treatment mechanism is likely from both ablation of sensorineural epithelium and reduction of dark cell activity.

Although streptomycin had been used some in the past, gentamicin is the entity now used for IT therapy. Probably the most important reason for this is relative clinical availability. Also, gentamicin is relatively less cochleotoxic and the solution is generally more comfortable. Gentamicin is available in a 40 mg/mL standard solution. In this form, it is acidic and a local irritant and can be physically uncomfortable on contact. When this acidic solution is buffered with a sodium bicarbonate solution to a physiologic pH, the result is a final concentration of 25–30 mg/mL and a generally better tolerated entity.

Treatment protocols and goals vary. There are two basic treatment philosophies. In ablation treatment, the goal is complete elimination of vestibular function in the treated ear. The treatment can either be aggressive, with only monitoring of vestibular function after completion of the protocol, or more moderate, with monitoring of

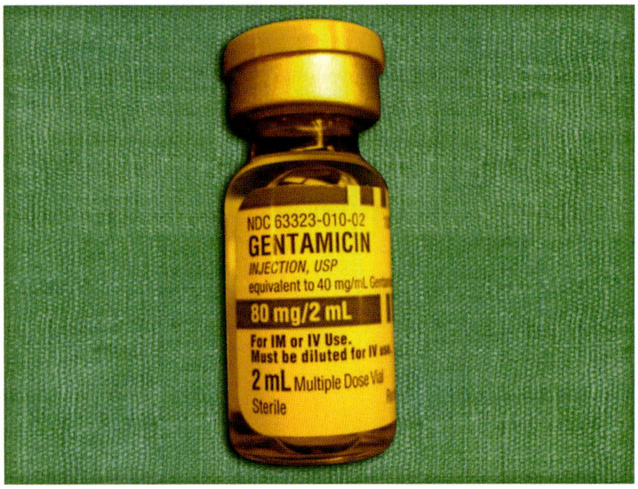

Fig. 9.16: The gentamicin solution used for intratympanic therapy.

vestibular function until ablation is achieved. In titration therapy, the second treatment philosophy, vestibular, and auditory functions are carefully monitored and treatment is continued until dizziness is eliminated.

The physiology of the gentamicin helps to understand treatment expectations and protocols. The half-life of gentamicin in perilymph is approximately 12 hours. The concentrations of the gentamicin increase in outer hair cells over several days. The onset of vestibular symptoms is typically 2–7 days after the injection.

Depending on the protocol, the endpoint of treatment can be completion of a set protocol, abolition of caloric function, onset of disequilibrium/oscillopsia, hearing loss, or presence of nystagmus. Generally, the ablative protocols have a higher vertigo control rate and higher incidence of sensorineural hearing loss. The simpler protocols include one[19] or two injections.[20] Soderman et al.'s titration protocol is daily gentamicin injections until unsteadiness or nystagmus occur.[21] Hirsch and Kamerer's protocol is 1 dose/week until disequilibrium occurs, hearing loss occurs, or treatment achieves control of vertigo.[22]

Success of IT gentamicin treatment can be measured in multiple ways, including employability or patient satisfaction but most commonly is measured by vertigo reduction. Studies report vertigo control 73–100%. Although some of the initial reports were more optimistic, the reported incidence of hearing loss is 15–50%.

Post-treatment disequilibrium is a significant part of treatment and the pretreatment discussion. As mentioned above, it will generally occur 2–7 days after the injection and can range from mild to temporarily debilitating. As with steroids, the risk of perforation and further hearing loss are reviewed. In this case, though, the risk of hearing loss is much greater and occurs primarily because of the solution and not the actual injection. Failure of therapy and the risk of persistent disequilibrium are important risks to consider.

Intratympanic Gentamicin Treatment Protocol

Once gentamicin IT therapy has been chosen, the patient is scheduled for three injections, each 1 week apart. Audiogram, videonystagmography (VNG), electrocochleogram, and MRI are carefully reviewed. If there is any evidence of contralateral disease, ablative therapy must be carefully reconsidered. As with IT steroid treatment, the expected sensation of fullness and temporary dizziness during the injection, as well as the potential risks, are carefully reviewed with the patient.

Step 1

The gentamicin 40 mg/mL stock solution (Fig. 9.16) buffered to physiologic pH and resultant 26 mg/mL is utilized.

Step 2

The remainder of the injection procedure is the same as with dexamethasone discussed above.

At the completion of the injection, the patient is counseled about the onset of disequilibrium and seen in 1 week. The second of the three planned injections is scheduled in 1 week. It is deferred if sensorineural hearing loss or excessive postinjection dizziness is noted. Basic vestibular exercises are generally started at the time of the second injection. The patient is seen 3 weeks after the last injection and an audiogram is performed. Further injections can be considered at any time in the future if vertigo recurs.

VESTIBULAR ABLATIVE SURGERY

Introduction

The most common indication for vestibular ablative surgery is Meniere's disease, which is described in the endolymphatic sac surgery section. These procedures are useful in other processes such as labyrinthitis, incomplete unilateral vestibular loss, delayed endolymphatic hydrops, post-traumatic and occasional postsurgical patients such as stapedectomy. Ablative procedures can either be the first surgical intervention or have a role in failure of more conservative interventions such as endolymphatic sac surgery or IT therapy.

Most commonly, candidates for ablative surgery are those who are limited by the condition and have failed a more conservative therapy, either medical or surgical. Others come to surgery because they are unable to complete medical therapy either because of intolerance of medical intervention or because they have difficulty with adherence to medical or dietary recommendations.

Concomitant medical problems can create treatment dilemmas either because of medication considerations/conflicts or the potential exacerbating effects of the medical condition(s). As well, these patients will create greater risk associated with anesthesia, surgery and recovery.

Life disruption is defined on a patient to patient basis. Life disruptiveness and candidacy for surgery are somewhat, but not exactly, related to the frequency and severity of vertigo. The patient's occupation, age and psychological tolerance are important factors in considering ablative procedures or surgery in general.

Classification of hearing loss is an important consideration. In the majority of patients, labyrinthectomy will not be recommended and will not be chosen unless the patient has severe hearing loss. Classically, the audiologic cutoff for consideration is the 50/50 rule—hearing with a speech reception threshold (SRT) above 50 dB and word discrimination below 50%.

All other factors being equal, preservation of the labyrinth is a priority. Preservation of the cochlea and cochlear nerve has the obvious value of immediate preservation of hearing but also preserves the possibility of hearing rehabilitation in the future, with cochlear implantation for example. On the other hand, there are occasional patients with good measurable hearing but with significant distortion or sensitivity who request and benefit from the elimination of hearing.

Evaluation for second diagnoses, both otologic and nonotologic, is imperative. Minimum evaluation will include an MRI scan of the brain and posterior fossa, VNG, and, in Meniere's disease, electrocochleography. A second diagnosis would usually be considered a contraindication to vestibular ablation although there are exceptions, depending of the life disruptiveness, and the perceived odds of improvement postsurgically.

Labyrinthectomy

Labyrinthectomy was first reported in 1904 by Lake[23] and popularized in the 1940s and 1950s. The procedure can be performed transcanal or transmastoid. The transmastoid approach is more commonly performed and allows for more direct visualization and removal of the neuroepithelial elements and as a result has a somewhat higher success rate. The operating time will generally be greater for the transmastoid approach though.

Vertigo control is 85–100% and patients consistently report quality of life improvement.[24] Failure is reported to be result of secondary diagnoses such as contralateral Meniere's, incomplete removal of all neuroepithelial elements and neuroma formation. One labyrinthectomy postsurgical result that is not often discussed, but many patients report as one of the most positive results of the surgery, is the elimination of the need for restrictive diet and medication.

The most common postoperative complication is persistent disequilibrium. This can be due to incomplete compensation, presence of secondary diagnoses, and incomplete surgical ablation. Even patients with postoperative disequilibrium tend to report significant functional improvement, but the disequilibrium can be limiting and interfere with personal and occupational function. Facial nerve injury and CSF leak are uncommon but significant potential complications.

Transmastoid Labyrinthectomy Procedure

General endotracheal anesthesia is utilized. The patients receive preoperative intravenous dexamethasone for postoperative nausea and perioperative antibiotics. Facial nerve monitoring is routinely utilized.

Step 1

The first five steps and four figures are identical to endolymphatic sac surgery (Figs. 9.1 to 9.4).

Step 2

After initiation of the mastoidectomy, the sigmoid sinus and tegmen can be identified for orientation. In a well pneumatized mastoid, this may not be necessary. As the drilling progresses medially, care is always taken to ensure the drilling is superior along the tegmen to keep the facial nerve safe. The antrum is identified and the horizontal semicircular canal and short process of the incus are visualized (Fig. 9.4). Care must be taken in this area with a cutting burr as the facial nerve can be injured if the burr catches and rolls forward. For safety, a diamond burr can be used in this area in reverse mode. The inferior mastoid air cells are opened and the vertical segment of the facial nerve is identified with a large diamond burr and left covered by bone (Fig. 9.4).

Step 3

Because the facial nerve is immediately below the horizontal semicircular canal, the canal is bivalved from superiorly (Fig. 9.17).

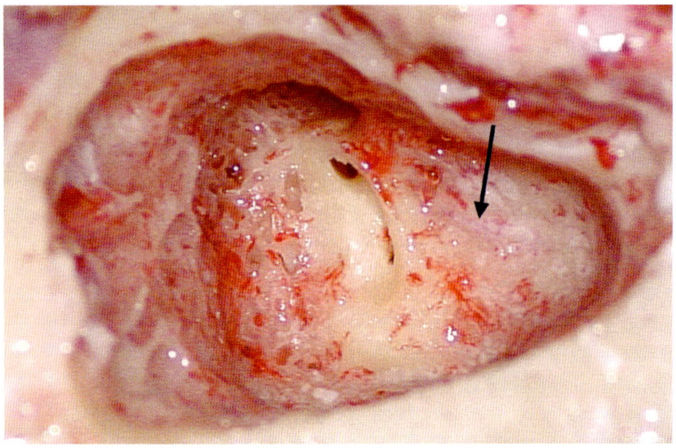

Fig. 9.17: Open lumen of the horizontal semicircular canal (facial nerve shown by arrow).

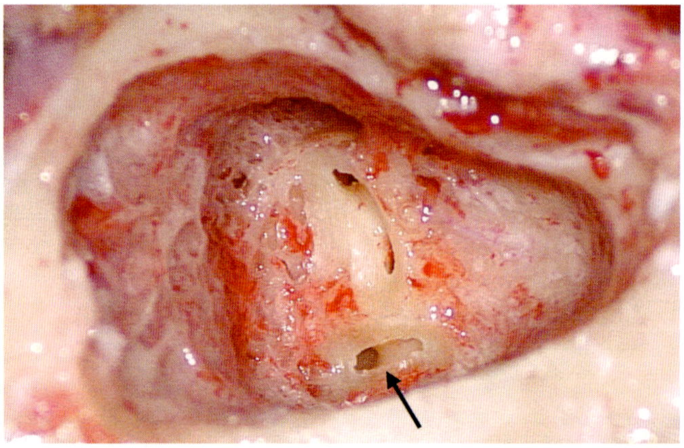

Fig. 9.18: Opening of the posterior semicircular canal (lumen of the posterior canal shown by arrow).

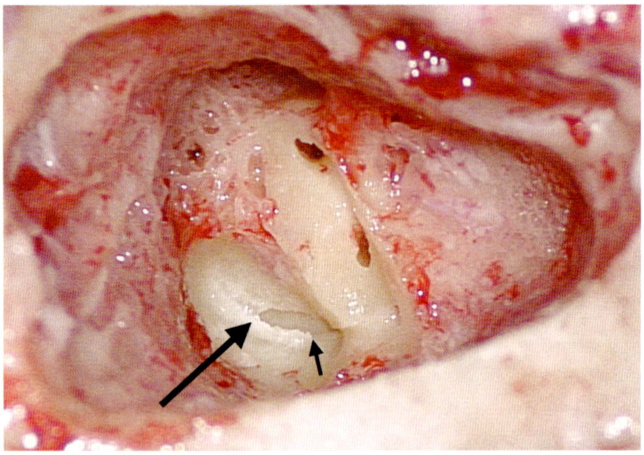

Fig. 9.19: Identification of the common crus (common crus shown by small arrow; posterior limb of superior semicircular canal shown by large arrow).

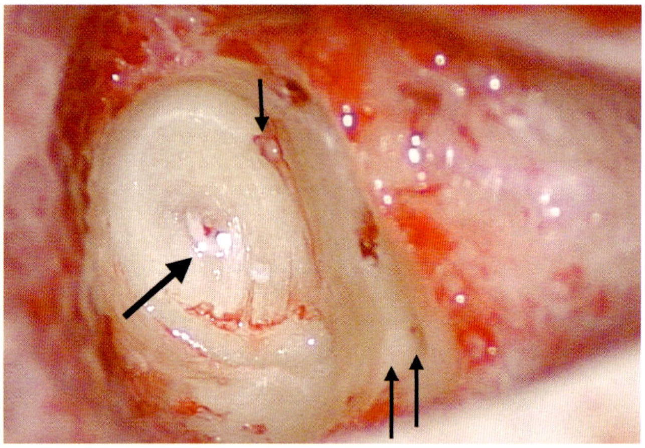

Fig. 9.20: Completely exenterated superior semicircular canal (subarcuate artery shown by large arrow; ampullated end of superior canal shownby small arrow; posterior semicircular canal lumen shown by double arrow).

Step 4

Once the horizontal canal lumen is opened, drilling is continued posteriorly to identify the posterior semicircular canal, whose lumen is then opened (Fig. 9.18). A well with protective bone around, or cup, is created to protect the adjacent structures.

Step 5

The superior limb of the posterior canal is traced medially to identify the common crus and the posterior limb of the superior semicircular canal (Fig. 9.19).

Step 6

The superior canal is then opened in its entirety from posterior to anterior and its ampullated end is visualized (Fig. 9.20). Some bleeding from the subarcuate artery may be encountered but is easily controlled with the diamond bur. Just lateral and inferior to the superior canal's ampullated end, the horizontal semicircular canal's ampullated end is identified and opened.

Step 7

Attention is turned posteriorly and the inferior limb of the posterior canal is opened (Fig. 9.21) to its ampullated end with the vertical segment of the facial nerve under direct vision.

Step 8

The semicircular canal openings are connected and the vestibule is opened widely (Fig. 9.22). Care is taken not to disrupt the deep wall of the vestibule and risk cerebrospinal fluid leak.

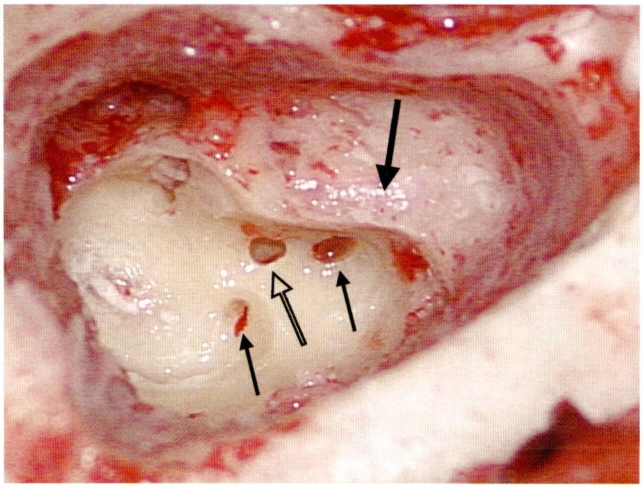

Fig. 9.21: Opening of posterior semicircular canal (lumen of the posterior canal shown by small arrows; lumen of the horizontal semicircular canal shown by hollow arrow; facial nerve shown by large arrow).

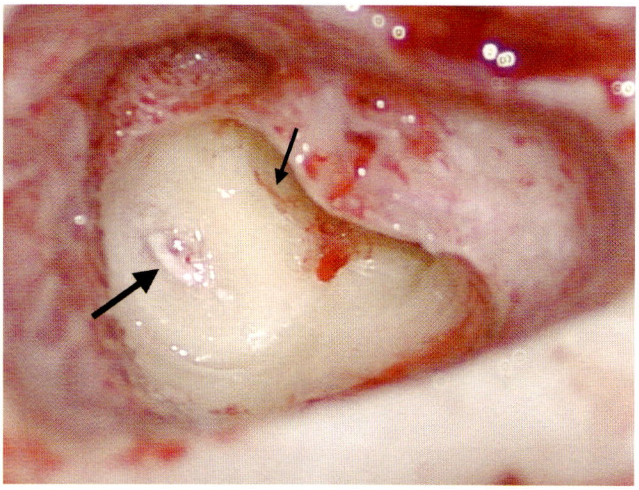

Fig. 9.22: Completed labyrinthectomy (subarcuate artery shown by large arrow; open vestibule shown by small arrow).

Step 9

With gentle manipulation (generally with a joint knife) and suction, the vestibular neuroepithelial elements of the maculae and semicircular canals are carefully removed.

Step 10

The wound is copiously irrigated with a saline solution. The deep layers of the incision are closed with 3-0 Vicryl. The skin is approximated with skin adhesive. A standard mastoid dressing is placed and the patient is awakened.

The patient is admitted postoperatively. Postoperative disequilibrium is experienced in most patients. In some patients with extreme preoperative ipsilateral vestibular weakness, the symptoms will be limited or absent. On the first postoperative morning, a vestibular therapist will meet with the patient to instruct in vestibular therapy. The dressing is removed on the first postoperative morning. The patient is discharged home when fluid intake is assured and ambulation is safe—usually 1-4 days.

No strenuous activity is recommended for 3 weeks postoperatively. The patient may resume driving and return to work when they feel confident—usually 3-6 weeks. For those with Meniere's disease, they are reminded that their medical regimen is no longer necessary.

Transcanal Labyrinthectomy Procedure

General anesthesia is most commonly chosen but the procedure can be performed under local anesthesia with sedation. Perioperative intravenous antibiotics are given for infection prophylaxis and preoperative intravenous dexamethasone for control of postoperative nausea.

Step 1

The patient is placed in the supine position with the affected ear up. One percent lidocaine with 1:100,000 epinephrine is injected circumferentially around the auricle and in the external canal meatus. The periauricular area is prepped and draped in the usual manner.

Step 2

Under the operating microscope, the external auditory canal is injected with additional 1% lidocaine with 1:100,000 epinephrine. A 6 o'clock longitudinal canal incision is made extending laterally from the annulus. A transverse incision is made 5 mm lateral to the annulus on the posterior canal (Fig. 9.23).

Step 3

The tympanomeatal flap is widely elevated. After elevation superiorly, a Bellucci scissor is used to create a 12 o'clock longitudinal incision to complete the flap incisions. Flap elevation is then extended to the annulus. The annulus is carefully elevated and the middle ear space is entered (Fig. 9.24).

Step 4

Usually, a portion of the posterior-superior annulus needs to be removed with a curette or microdrill to allow

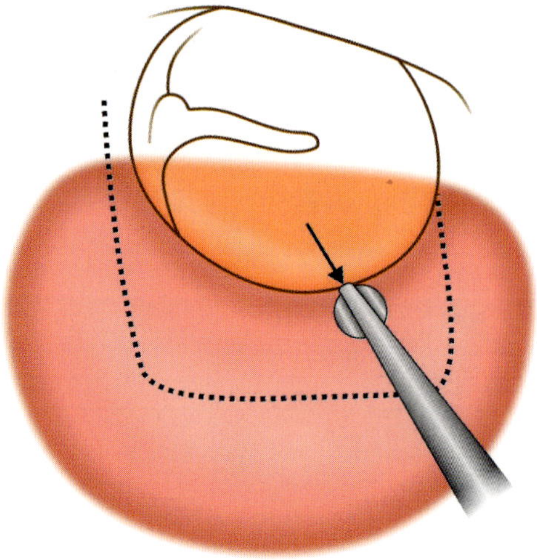

Fig. 9.23: Tympanomeatal incisions in a right ear.

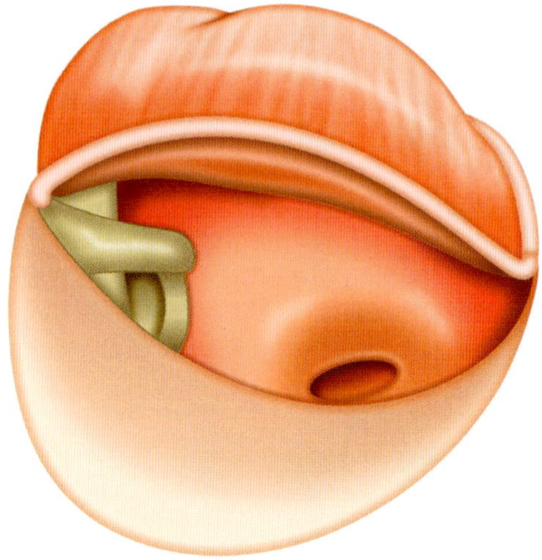

Fig. 9.24: View of the middle ear after tympanomeatal incision elevation.

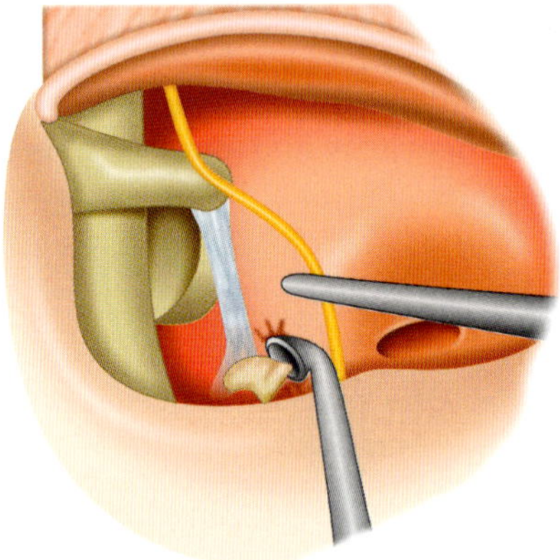

Fig. 9.25: A portion of the posterior/superior annulus generally needs to be removed to allow complete visualization of the necessary middle ear structures.

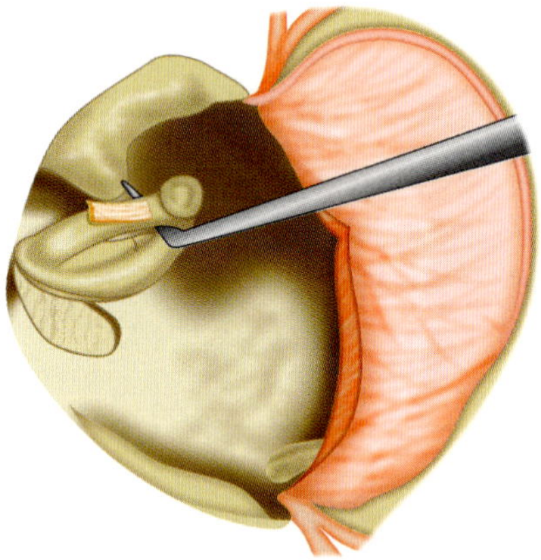

Fig. 9.26: Removal of stapes after incudostapedial joint separation.

complete visualization of the oval window area and the inferior aspect of the horizontal facial nerve (Fig. 9.25).

Step 5

The incudostapedial joint is separated and the stapedial tendon is transected. The stapes is removed with a right angle hook (Fig. 9.26).

Step 6

A microdrill is used to open the oval window inferiorly down to the RW (Fig. 9.27).

Step 7

With a small suction and right angle, an attempt is made to remove the neuroepithelial elements in the vestibule (Fig. 9.28). During removal of the semicircular canal elements, care must be exercised, particularly superiorly, as the bone layer between the vestibule and the underside of the horizontal segment of the facial nerve may be thin and put the nerve at risk. Care must also be taken with the medial wall of the vestibule that abuts the internal auditory canal and puts the patient at risk of a cerebrospinal fluid leak if disrupted.

Step 8

The vestibule can be packed with gentamicin soaked Gelfoam. The middle ear is then packed with Gelfoam. The tympanomeatal flap is placed back in its anatomic position. The external ear canal is packed with Gelfoam and a cotton ball is placed in the external auditory meatus.

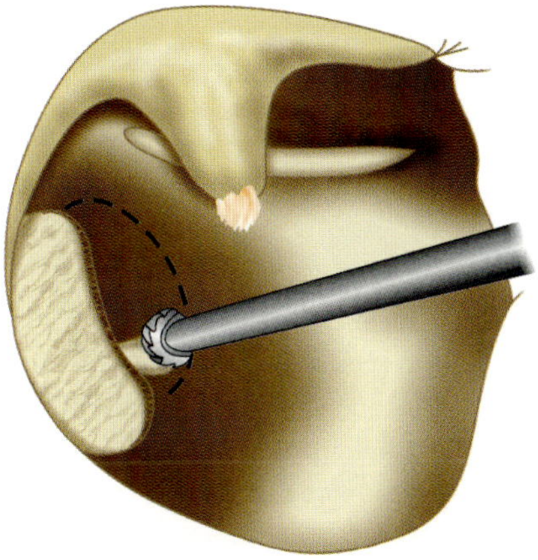

Fig. 9.27: After removal of the stapes, a small bur is used to remove the bone between the round and oval windows.

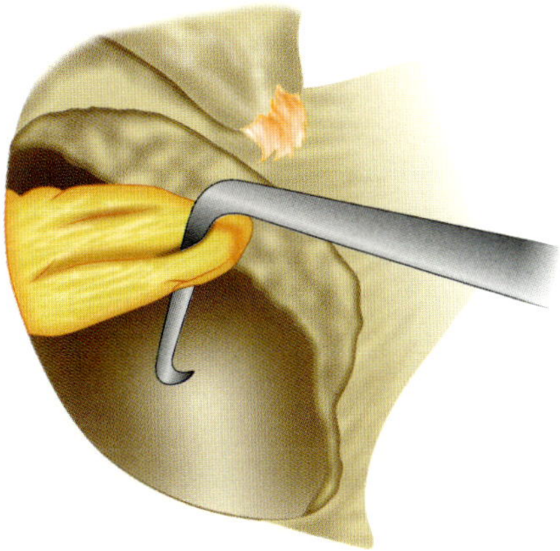

Fig. 9.28: A right angle hook is used to probe for the neuroepithelial elements of the vestibule and semicircular canals.

The expected hospitalization and recovery are similar to transmastoid labyrinthectomy.

Vestibular Neurectomy

Clinical considerations for vestibular neurectomy are similar to those associated with labyrinthectomy and discussed earlier. The surgery is typically considered after failure of adequate medical and nonablative therapy. It is an important option in patients with useful hearing. One issue to be emphasized with vestibular neurectomy in Meniere's patients is that ongoing medical therapy is indicated, as the labyrinth is left intact and the aural symptoms are still treatment dependent. Having said that, it is noted that postoperatively a moderate portion of patients have fewer problems with the aural symptoms.

VIIIth neurectomy was apparently first attempted by Fedor Krause in 1898.[25] Division of VIIIth nerve for vertigo was first reported by Parry in 1902.[25] McKenzie was credited with the first selective vestibular neurectomy in 1936.[26] The procedure was refined and reintroduced with in the 1960s by Bill House who performed the first microsurgical vestibular neurectomy. At the time of its reintroduction, the middle fossa approach was most commonly used. Access to the nerves after the trifurcation of the VIIIth cranial nerve was a benefit with respect to isolating and protecting the cochlear nerve. Initially only the superior nerve was addressed but later both branches of the vestibular nerve were identified and transected. Vertigo control was good but hearing loss and postoperative facial nerve weakness were significant risks. An additional limitation of this approach is the increased risks in patients over the age of 60 due to the amount of temporal lobe retraction.

The retrosigmoid approach is generally the most direct access to the cerebellopontine angle and the VIIIth nerve. The major concerns have been that the VIIIth nerve is unified and that separation of the vestibular and cochlear portions can be difficult at times. The second major concern of the retrosigmoid (or suboccipital) approach is the risk of postoperative headaches. For a standard retrosigmoid approach, the risk of headaches is reported as high as 50% in some series and the headaches can be debilitating. Residual bone dust intracranially, associated with drilling of the internal auditory canal, was thought to be one of the possible causes of the headaches, although the risk seems to be very high even in procedures where no intracranial drilling was performed. A more likely factor was theorized to be the exposed dura after the closure adhering to the overlying tissue. The incidence was reduced with placement of fat over the dural closure at the completion of the procedure or a cranioplasty with plating or bone cement. A final concern regarding this approach is the amount of cerebellar retraction necessary to access the cerebellopontine angle.

The retro labyrinthine approach avoided some of the issues with the two approaches. This approach posterior to the labyrinth and anterior to the sigmoid sinus avoided much of the brain retraction related issues of the middle cranial fossa and the postoperative headache risk of the retrosigmoid approach. The risk of hearing loss and VIIth nerve injury was reportedly reduced. The most significant issues in the approach were the somewhat limited visualization of the VIIIth nerve laterally, the limited working space, and the risk of postoperative cerebrospinal fluid (CSF) leak.

The translabyrinthine approach had been more popular in the past, but with the generally good success rate of transmastoid labyrinthectomy alone, there has been less interest. This approach also negates one of the fundamental reasons for considering vestibular neurectomy—hearing preservation.

The retrosigmoid approach for the vestibular neurectomy is the most common and as a result will be the focus of this discussion. The approach is named for its location immediately behind the sigmoid sinus but is also defined by the lateral sinus as its superior limit. This approach generally is considered the simplest, gives the best view of the cerebellopontine angle and requires the least operative time. As mentioned, the inability to identify the VIIIth nerve lateral to its trifurcation into cochlear and vestibular portions is one of the criticisms of the approach although there is usually a relatively well-defined plane between the vestibular and cochlear portions of the nerve. In an effort to address the three major concerns, we now perform the procedure endoscopically. The limited incision and small craniectomy significantly reduce the general postoperative discomfort and the risk of long-term headaches, as well as the risk of cerebrospinal fluid leak. The use of the endoscope after CSF drainage minimizes the amount of cerebellar retraction necessary.

Disequilibrium is typical postoperatively but normal or near normal stability is achieved in most patients. Some long-term disequilibrium occurs in up to 30% of patients although only occasionally do patients not report significant overall functional benefit. Thedinger and Thedinger[27] suggest possibilities for persistent postoperative disequilibrium or recurrent dizziness include incomplete nerve section, neuroma formations, unsatisfactory compensation processes, vestibular dysfunction in the contralateral ear, nerve regeneration, and possible nonotologic vertigo. Cerebrospinal fluid leak, wound infection, and meningitis are possible, and each has been reported in about 5% of retrosigmoid patients, although the incidence has been reduced with the endoscopic approach. Stroke and intracranial bleeding are possible in any intracranial procedure. Postoperative headaches, which had been a significant risk with retrosigmoid surgery in the past, have been minimized with the endoscopic approach.

Surgical results tend to be better when there is a clear single diagnosis. In Meniere's disease, the vertigo control rate is over 90%. The success rate in other diagnoses is generally less. Hearing preservation can be difficult to assess but the risk of hearing loss is generally noted to be 5% or less immediately postoperatively. There does tend to be degradation of hearing over time, possible due to the surgery, but the natural history of Meniere's disease is a likely factor.

Endoscopic Retrosigmoid Vestibular Neurectomy Procedure

The procedure is performed under general anesthesia. The patients receive preoperative intravenous dexamethasone for postoperative nausea and perioperative antibiotics.

Step 1

The patient is placed in the supine position with the head turned away and affected ear up. The head is secured in a three prong Mayfield head holder. The course of the transverse sinus is approximated by extending a line from the root of zygomatic arch to the occipital protuberance, or inion. The sigmoid sinus course is estimated to run along the route of the posterior mastoid groove and a line is drawn. The intersection of these two lines corresponds very closely to the transverse-sigmoid junction. An approximately 4 cm incision is outlined that is 1/3 above the mark and 2/3 below. The incision slants from anterior-superior to posterior-inferior (Fig. 9.29).

Step 2

Facial nerve and auditory brainstem response (ABR) monitoring electrodes are placed. The ABR stimulating probe is placed in the external auditory canal.

Step 3

The postauricular area is generously injected with 1% lidocaine with 1:100,000 epinephrine. The area is prepped and draped in the usual sterile manner preserving the marked incision. Mannitol is given prior to incision, and the patient is hyperventilated to $Paco_2$ of 26 torr to reduce intracranial pressure.

Step 4

Once the skin is scored, monopolar cautery is used to control bleeding and carry the incision down to the cranial bone. The asterion is identified. The asterion is the junction of the lambdoid, parietomastoid, and occipitomastoid sutures and the junction of the parietal, occipital, and the mastoid portion of the temporal bone. It is used as a rough surface marker for the junction of the sigmoid and transverse sinus. Once identified, the sigmoid-transverse sinus junction will mark the superior-anterior limit of the craniotomy.

Step 5

Drilling is initiated over the estimated position of the sinus junction. Once dura is encountered, the characteristic

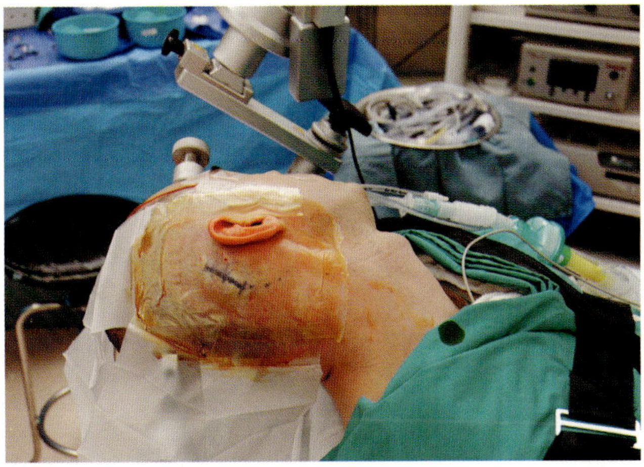

Fig. 9.29: The planned incision for the right endoscopic suboccipital approach.

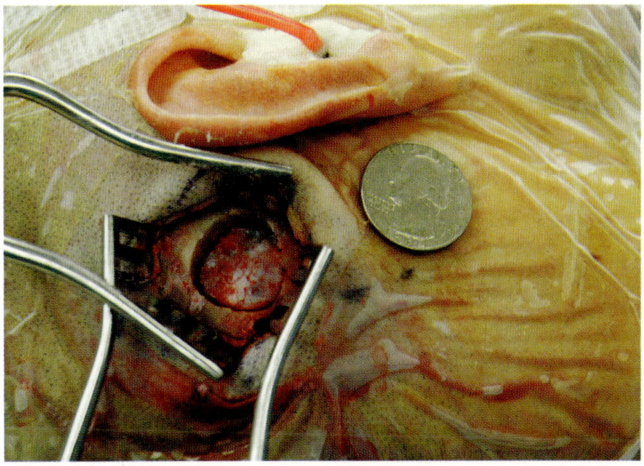

Fig. 9.30: Limited craniotomy shown relative to the size of a quarter.

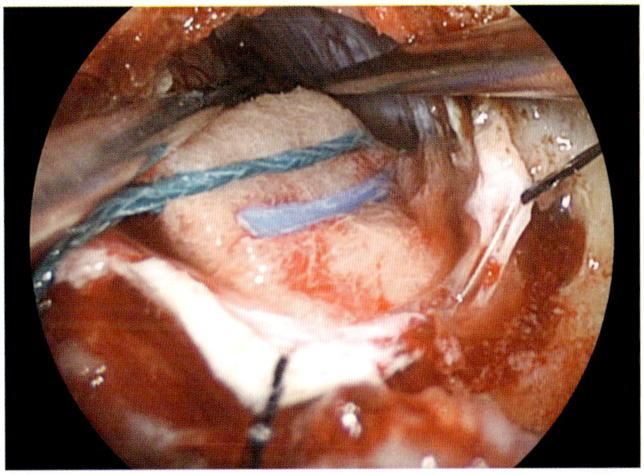

Fig. 9.31: Dural incision 3 mm posterior to the sinuses with the pledget used to gently retract the cerebellum ventrally while the dissection proceeds medially.

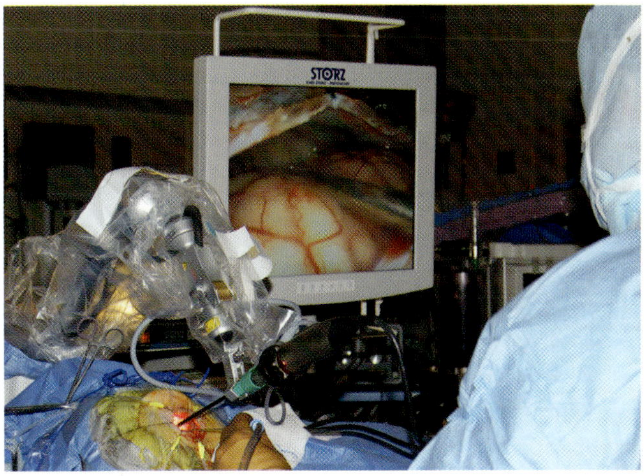

Fig. 9.32: The surgical setup after the introduction of the endoscope.

blue hue of a cranial sinus is identified. If none is seen, then drilling is directed anterior and superior exposing dura along the way. Once the sigmoid-lateral sinus junction is identified, an approximately quarter-size craniectomy is created (Fig. 9.30). It is helpful to expose several millimeters of the sinuses to give flexibility to the dura during opening, the procedure and closure. Large and medium diamond burrs are used to complete the bony opening to prevent damage to the dura or sinuses. A Kerrison rongeur can be used to complete the deep aspect of the opening and give several extra millimeters of dural exposure for the same size craniotomy.

Step 6

The dura is palpated to grossly assess intracranial pressure. If soft, it is incised parallel to and 3 mm away from the exposed sinuses. With a cottonoid on the cerebellum, the cerebellopontine angle is gently approached (Fig. 9.31).

Step 7

Dissection is advanced ventral to the cerebellar hemisphere along the petrous bone to the basilar cisterns. Either the cisterna magna inferiorly or the prepontine cistern more superiorly are entered to drain cerebrospinal fluid and further decompress the posterior fossa pressure. The cerebellum will fall readily away from the petrous face after this maneuver, thereby avoiding the need for any retractor.

Step 8

With gentle dissection, occasional cautery of small bridging vessels, and dissection of some arachnoid bands,

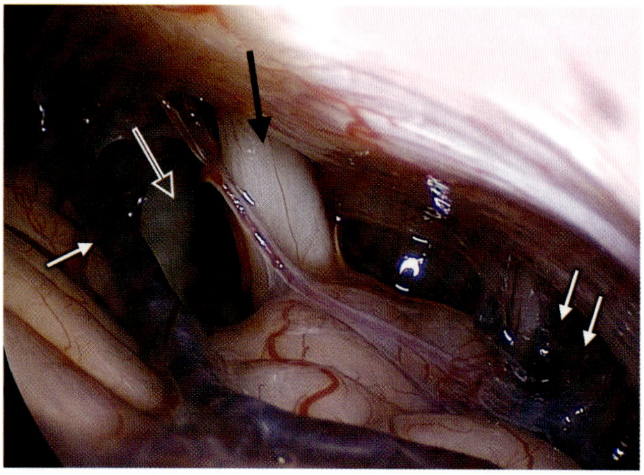

Fig. 9.33: Endoscopic view of the cerebellopontine angle after release of CSF (petrosal vein shown by small arrow; lower cranial nerve roots shown by small arrows; VIIIth nerve shown by solid arrow; Vth nerve shown by hollow arrow).

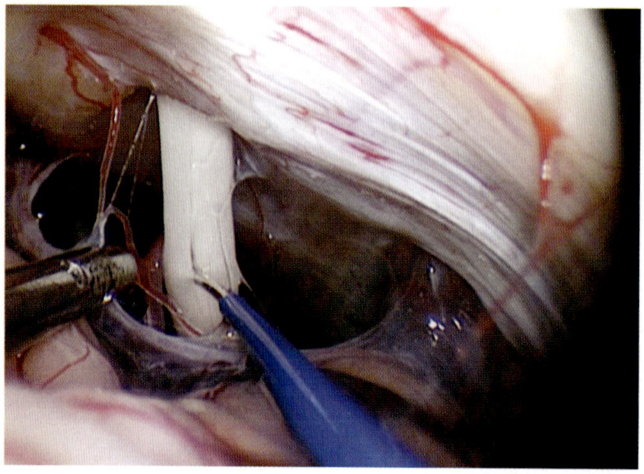

Fig. 9.34: Dissection of the VIIIth nerve along the vestibular-cochlear plane.

the cerebellopontine angle will be readily exposed and the pertinent structures visualized. Once this has been accomplished, a 2.7 or 4 mm rigid endoscope 0° is placed in an appropriate position and secured with a pneumatic arm (Fig. 9.32).

Step 9

A generous view of the cerebellopontine angle is obtained (Fig. 9.33). The VIIIth cranial nerve will be seen exiting the ventral pontomedullary junction (root entry zone), traversing the cerebellopontine angle, and entering the porous of the internal auditory canal. The Vth cranial nerve will be seen superior and medial and the lower cranial nerve (IX, X, XI) roots will be seen inferiorly. It is important to identify the adjacent cranial nerves to assure orientation.

Step 10

There is generally a small blood vessel traversing the lateral aspect of the VIIIth nerve along the division of the cochlear division inferiorly and the vestibular division superiorly (Fig. 9.33). The cochlear division is generally whiter because of the greater number of fibers (31,000) than the greyer appearing vestibular with about 18,000 fibers. Care must be taken during the procedure as the VIIth nerve and nervus intermedius will lie hidden immediately ventral (behind) the readily identified VIIIth nerve. Additionally, the anterior-inferior cerebellar artery will course between the VII/VIII complex and must be preserved.

Step 11

Sharp dissection is used to initially develop the longitudinal plane between the nerve divisions with care to protect the VIIth nerve on the medial side (Fig. 9.34). The division is completed with a blunt annulus elevator. The superior vestibular portion is then transected with a microscissor. The cut ends are pushed away from each other to minimize risk of reconnection (Fig. 9.35).

Step 12

The surgical area is gently irrigated with warm saline. A Valsalva maneuver is completed to check for hemostasis. The endoscope is withdrawn. The dural incision is carefully closed with interrupted 4-0 nylon sutures. The exposed bone of the craniotomy is aggressively coated with bone wax to control any bleeding and seal any adjacent air cells.

Step 13

A layer of artificial dura is cut to overlay the exposed dura and dural closure. Hydroxylapatite bone cement is used to fill the cranial defect (Fig. 9.36). We typically avoid using mesh for the bone closure as there has been a tendency to extrude through the thinner skin of the postauricular area over time. The wound is again irrigated. The patient's $Paco_2$ is allowed to return to normal. The deep layers are carefully reapproximated with absorbable sutures. The skin is approximated with skin adhesive.

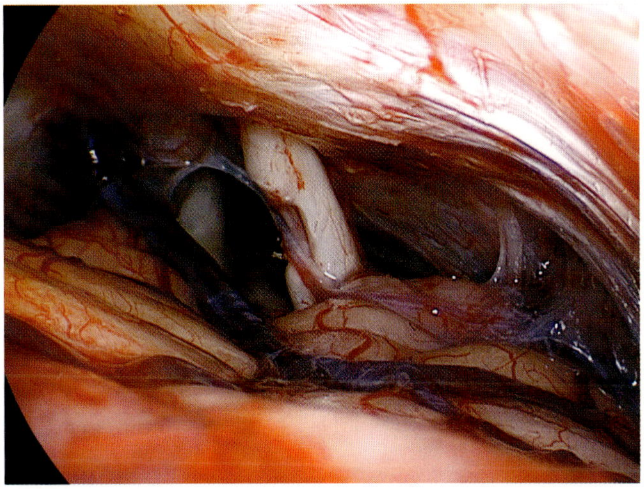

Fig. 9.35: Postneurectomy view with the anterior-inferior cerebellar artery branch running between the cut ends of the vestibular (superior) portion of VIII.

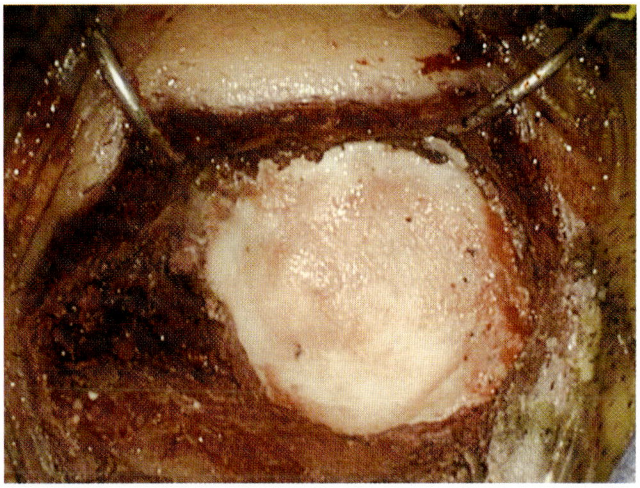

Fig. 9.36: Bone cement drying in the craniotomy defect prior to skin closure.

Step 14

The ABR ear canal probe and the facial nerve and ABR monitoring electrodes are removed. The patient is taken out of the Mayfield head holder and a mastoid dressing is placed. The patient is allowed to awaken from the anesthetic.

VIIth nerve function is assessed as soon as possible. The patient is observed in the neurologic intensive care unit overnight. As with labyrinthectomy, postoperative dizziness is expected. On the first postoperative morning, a vestibular therapist will meet with the patient to instruct in vestibular therapy. The dressing is removed on the first postoperative morning. The patient is discharged home when ambulation is safe—usually 1-4 days.

The postoperative dizziness, along with fatigue, usually dominates the recovery period. The patient is instructed to avoid Valsalva, heavy lifting, and nose blowing for 3 weeks. Driving and work may resume when the patient feels competent—usually 3-6 weeks.

SURGERY FOR BENIGN PAROXYSMAL POSITIONAL VERTIGO

Introduction

Benign paroxysmal positional vertigo (BPPV) is a peripheral vestibular disorder characterized by episodes of vertigo precipitated by changes in head position. The episodes are generally short lived. An occasional patient will experience a more prolonged feeling of vertigo at the time of onset. Some of those affected with have a persistent feeling of disequilibrium between the positioning-induced symptoms. There are no associated aural or neurologic symptoms. It is a relatively common cause of dizziness and in many vestibular clinics is noted to be the most frequently identified entity.[28] Interestingly, in a population study in 2000,[29] BPPV was identified in 9% of random patients over the age of 65.

The diagnosis is usually straightforward and in most patients BPPV can be suspected from the history alone. On physical examination, the Dix-Hallpike maneuver is confirmatory (Fig. 9.37). The three features of a positive response include geotropic rotary nystagmus, a slight delay in onset after reaching the head down position (latency) and reduced nystagmus and dizziness upon repetition (fatigability).

In most patients, the actual cause of BPPV is unknown. In <5%, a cause (e.g. trauma, surgery, and SSNHL) can be associated with the onset of symptoms. Post-traumatic forms are more frequently bilateral and are generally more difficult to treat. BPPV can be associated with otologic surgery such as stapedectomy or endolymphatic sac procedures. Its incidence is higher in certain inner ear disorders such as Meniere's disease. One must be careful in existing Meniere's patients to recognize the different description of the vertigo spells to suspect the new diagnosis.

The symptoms of BPPV were originally theorized by Schuknecht[30] to be due to cupulolithiasis—the collection of deposit on the cupula of the semicircular canal. This

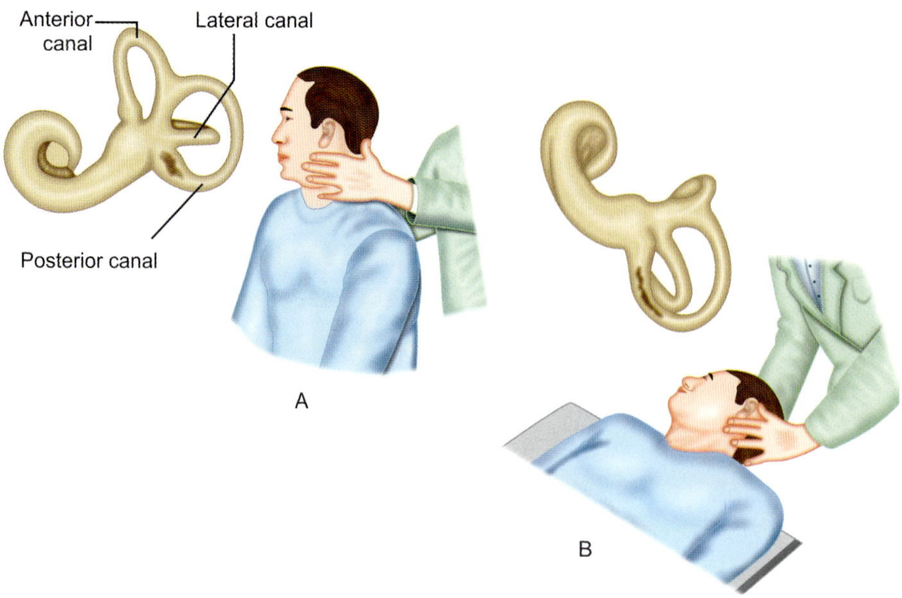

Fig. 9.37: Dix-Hallpike maneuver for identifying right posterior canal benign paroxysmal positional vertigo. The patient's head is turned 45° to the right while sitting up (position A). The patient is then lowered to a supine position with the head extended causing canaliths to fall further into the posterior canal (position B). The result is a geotropic rotatory nystagmus to the right.

would turn the motion sensing organ into a gravity sensing organ. Although it may explain some patients' symptoms, it did not seem to either explain the temporary nature of the dizziness in most patients or the latency of symptoms after moving the head in a stimulating way. Also, there have been studies identifying the particles in temporal bones of those without BPPV.[31]

In 1979, Hall et al.[32] introduced the theory of canalithiasis, proposing that particles floating in the semicircular canal were responsible for the BPPV symptoms. The movement of these particles with head position changes would better account for the latency of symptoms, as there is inertia to their initial movement, and the temporary nature of the symptoms, as the dizziness should subside once the particles had settled in a dependent position. There is significant evidence for this theory although the particles have been seen in patients without BPPV symptoms.[33]

Benign paroxysmal positional vertigo can be quite variable in its severity and duration. A portion of patients experience spontaneous resolution and do not come to medical attention. Many patients will need subsequent treatment after successful intervention, with the recurrence rate after an initial episode reported as high as 50%.[34]

Generally, there seems to be three forms. The single episode form can be self-limited or require clinical intervention, but the affected individual has no further events. In the chronic form, no manner of conservative treatment is successful in controlling the symptoms. The most frustrating is the recurrent form. Each episode will usually respond to intervention but recurrences are the hallmark.

The term BPPV generally refers to the condition involving the posterior semicircular canal. It can occur in the lateral canal and, although its existence is somewhat controversial, has been reported in the superior canal. BPPV can be bilateral, which tends to create a more symptomatic situation and will generally make it more difficult to treat.

One must remember that there is a differential diagnosis for positional dizziness. Postural hypotension, cervical vertigo, vertebrobasilar insufficiency, disabling positional vertigo, and central nervous system abnormalities must be considered. There are usually features that can differentiate these entities from BPPV such as nonvestibular symptoms and dizziness not exclusively associated with movement. Lack of response to appropriate treatments is also a reason to consider an alternate or associated diagnosis. Central nervous system entities, such as posterior fossa tumors, are rare but important considerations.

Treatment of BPPV is usually straightforward. As some patients recover spontaneously, time can be considered a treatment option. For the majority of patients, though, intervention is recommended. A particle repositioning maneuver is the most common treatment and is very successful. Most physicians utilize a form of the Epley maneuver (Fig. 9.38). This can be completed within a

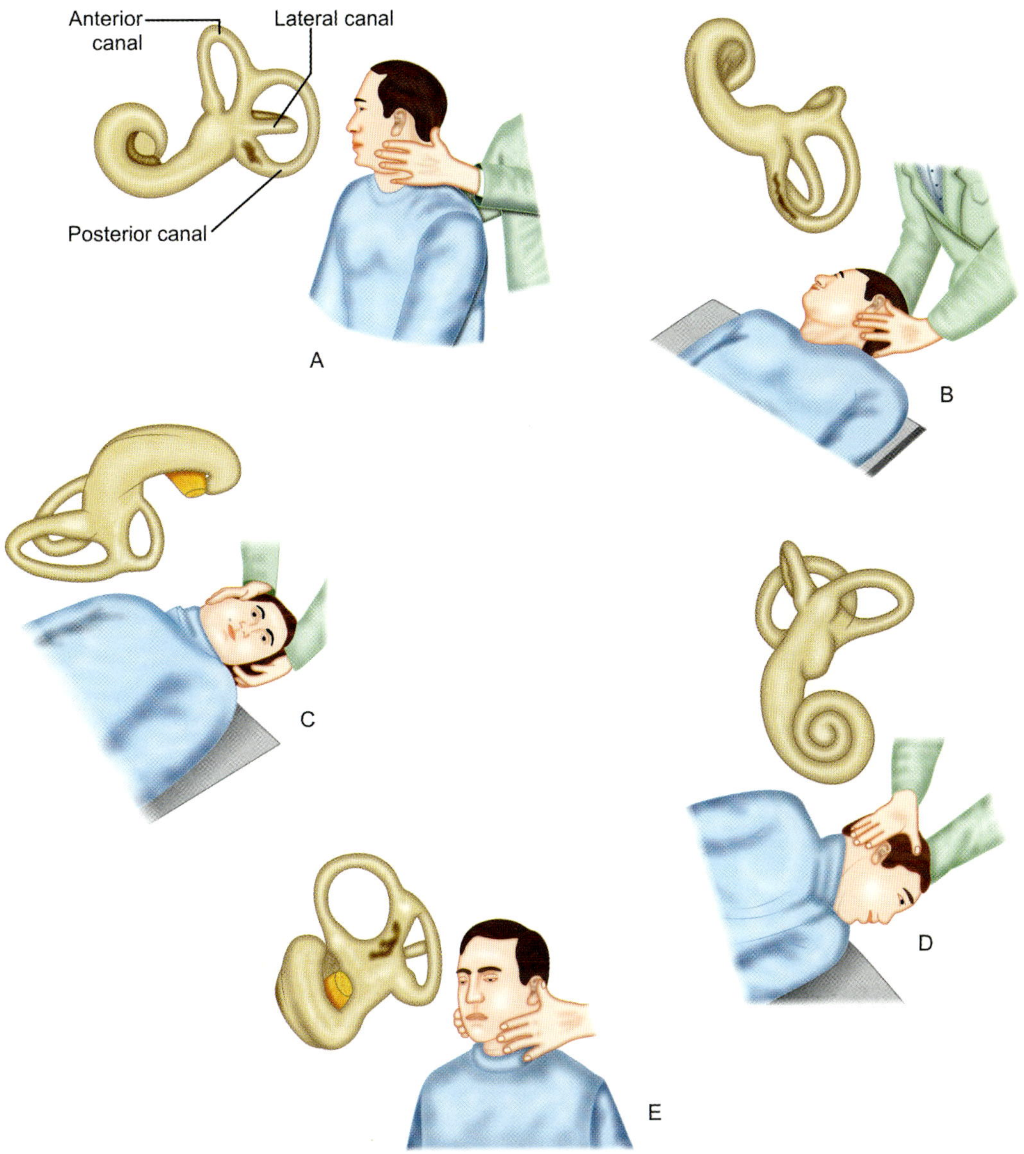

Fig. 9.38: Particle repositioning maneuver for treatment of right posterior canal BPPV. This diagram shows the head position and the coinciding position of the labyrinth and particles within the posterior canal. Positions A and B, a Dix-Hallpike maneuver is performed to the right. The head is rotated to the left 90° to position C, maintaining head extension. Debris approaches the common crus. The patient is rolled into position D with his/her left shoulder, head facing down. Debris enters the vestibule. The patient is then transferred to position E, the original sitting position, allowing the debris to settle in the vestibule.

few minutes and success rates for dizziness control are generally reported as >80%. Alternatively, the Semont maneuver (Fig. 9.39) is an option. Some physicians will use these maneuvers interchangeably while others will use an Epley maneuver for suspected canalithiasis and a Semont maneuver for suspected cupulolithiasis. The Brandt-Daroff exercises are also used. These are performed by the patient at home. Although they have been reported to be somewhat less successful than the office maneuvers, they are a possible alternative to the maneuvers. The Epley Omniax is a more aggressive repositioning option for those that do not respond to basic intervention.

Surgical Treatment of Benign Paroxysmal Positional Vertigo

For the occasional patient who does not respond to office treatment, and is symptomatic enough, surgery is possible. In the past, ablative surgeries such as labyrinthectomy and vestibular neurectomy were the primary options. More recently, the selective surgeries of singular

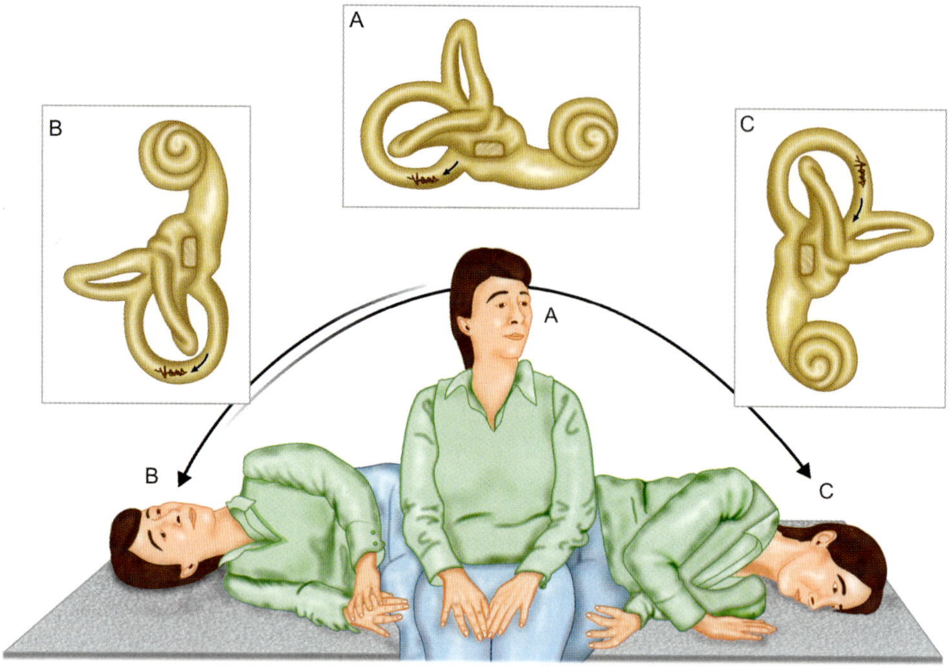

Fig. 9.39: Semont maneuver for right benign paroxysmal positional vertigo. The patient starts position A, in sitting position A with the head turned 45° to the left (away from affected labyrinth). The patient is quickly tilted into position B on their right shoulder with the nose pointing upward. The patient remains in position B for 3 minutes. Debris moves to the apex of the canal. The patient is quickly tilted through the seated position to position C laying on their left shoulder with the nose pointed to downward. Position C is held for 3 minutes. Debris exits the canal into the vestibule. The patient is brought back to position A gently.

neurectomy and posterior semicircular canal occlusion (PSCO) have become available.

Singular Neurectomy

First reported in 1974 by Gacek,[35] singular neurectomy was the first surgery specifically for BPPV. In his 1991 paper on the procedure, Gacek[36] reported complete vertigo control in 97% of 102 patients. In the remaining 3%, there was improvement of symptoms. Sensorineural hearing loss occurred in 4%. In a 2002 follow-up report of 252 singular neurectomy cases over a 29 year period, Gacek[37] reported similar results with complete control in 96.8% and sensorineural hearing loss (SNHL) in 3.7%. In 1990, Silverstein reported complete control of vertigo in 80% of 52 patients with an additional 17% being improved.[38] Sensorineural hearing loss occurred in 6%. In 1980, Epley[39] reported vertigo control in 73% (8/11) and some SNHL in 45% but significant SNHL in 18% (2/11). In his first four patients, Epley recognized the potential difficulty of the transcanal approach described by Gacek and developed a more inferior modified hypotympanotomy approach allowing drilling to occur at a further distance from the RW membrane, thus decreasing the risk of inadvertent damage. His results report 1 of 8 hypotympanotomy cases with moderate SNHL; all 8 had complete control of symptoms. These variable results suggest that success of this procedure is surgeon and experience dependent. The risk of SNHL is increased with variant singular canal course, presence of otosclerosis, and during revision surgery. Temporary postoperative disequilibrium is universal. As with any vestibular ablative procedure, long-term disequilibrium is a risk. The procedure is rarely utilized because of the overall infrequent need for surgical intervention in BPPV and the relative popularity of PSCO.

Single Neurectomy Procedure

The procedure is performed transcanal. The surgery can be performed under general anesthesia, but Gacek strongly preferred local with sedation.

Step 1

After introduction of anesthesia with the patient in the supine position, the patient's head is turned away with the affected ear up. The periauricular area is prepped and draped. The auricle and external canal are injected with 1% lidocaine with 1:100,000 epinephrine.

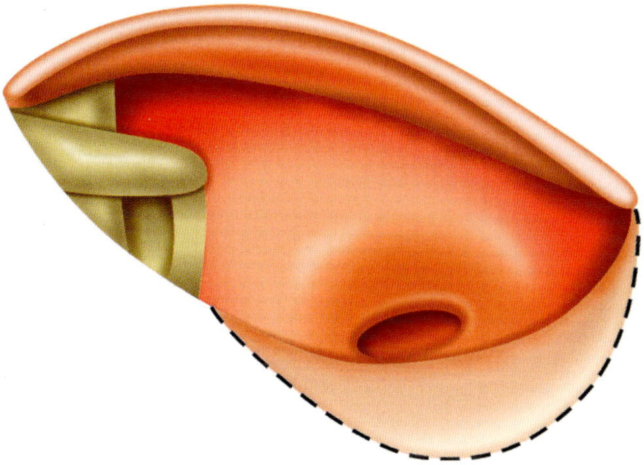

Fig. 9.40: Outline of annular bone that typically needs to be removed for singular neurectomy access.

Step 2

A tympanomeatal flap is created and elevated as in trans-canal labyrinthectomy (Figs. 9.23 and 9.24). An additional portion of the posterior annular area may need to be removed with either a curette or drill to allow adequate visualization of the RW and subiculum (Fig. 9.40).

Step 3

The RW overhang is drilled away to allow visualization of the RW.

Step 4

To access the singular nerve, a small diamond burr is used to create a depression immediately inferior to the RW. The nerve will usually be identified within 3 mm (Fig. 9.41). Gacek reports that the view of the singular nerve is obstructed by the RW in 20% of patients. In these situations, the nerve is disrupted blindly but the transection can be confirmed by the onset of nystagmus in the sedated patient.

Step 5

The middle ear is packed with Gelfoam, and the tympanomeatal flap is placed back in its anatomic position. The external canal is gently packed with Gelfoam.

Hospitalization will generally be 1–4 days. Vestibular therapy is initiated on the first postoperative day. Disequilibrium postoperatively is universal and usually temporary. For most patients, several weeks will be necessary to recover to a safe functional level.

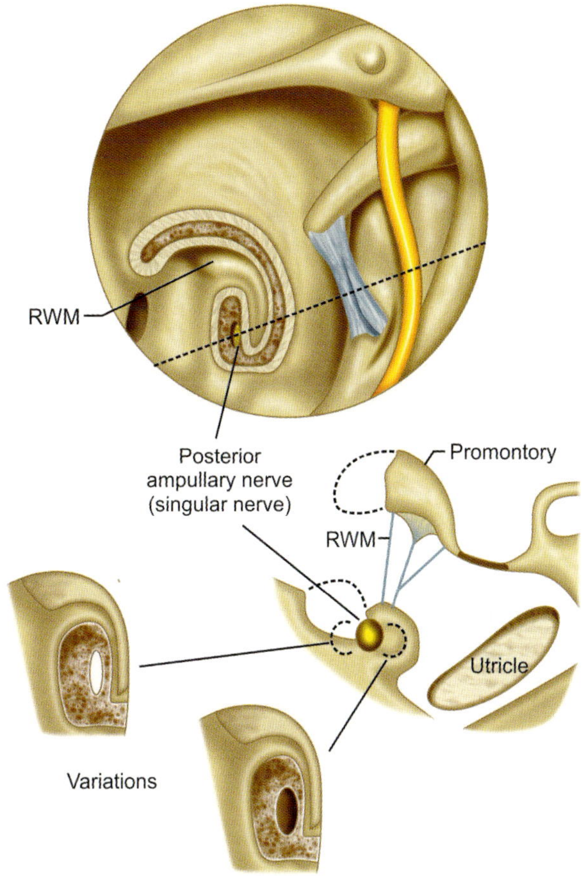

Fig. 9.41: Upper image shows the left ear with round window overhang removed, round window exposed and the drilled depression inferior to the round window exposing the singular nerve. The middle right image shows possible positions of the nerve in a section along the dotted line in the upper figure with the usual position of the singular nerve. The more favorable inferior location (left dotted line) and the less favorable superior position (right dotted line) are seen. The middle right image shows the surgical view of the singular nerve in the favorable position. The lower image shows the lack of surgical visualization of the singular nerve in the unfavorable position. (RWM: Round window membrane).
Courtesy: Richard R Gacek, MD

Posterior Semicircular Canal Occlusion

PSCO was first reported in 1990 as a treatment for BPPV.[40] It has generally been the surgery of choice for BPPV since its introduction. Control of vertigo is near 100%. Early papers, such as Zappia in 1996,[41] reported good results. One hundred percent (9 of 9) of patients had normalization of Dix-Hallpike maneuver postoperatively. In 2006, Shaia et al.[42] reported 100% normalization of Dix-Hallpike maneuver in 28 PSCO patients. In a 2007 literature review of 11 authors, Leveque et al.[43] reported complete

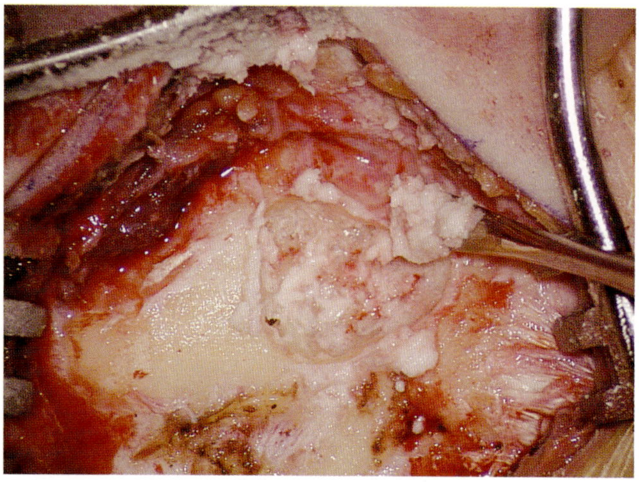

Fig. 9.42: Initial mastoidectomy. Bone pate is harvested and preserved for use later in the procedure.

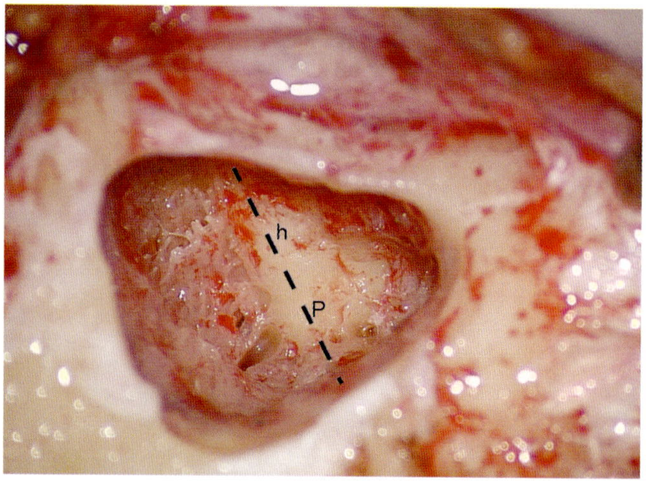

Fig. 9.43: Completion of limited mastoidectomy with exposure of the lateral aspects of the horizontal and posterior semicircular canals (h–horizontal semicircular canal; P–posterior semicircular canal; dotted line–Donaldson's line).

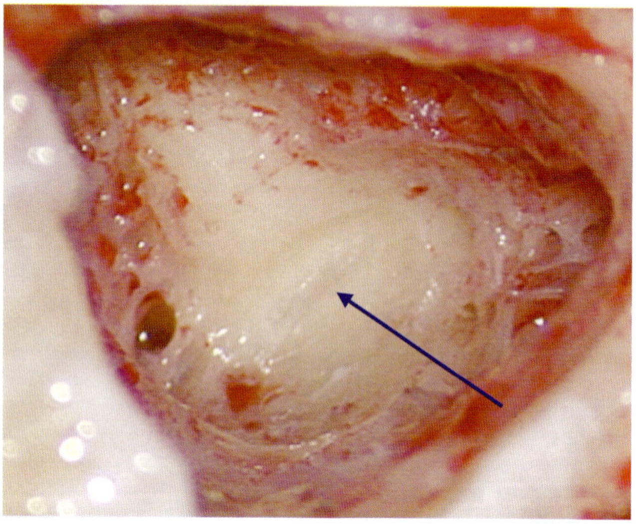

Fig. 9.44: Blue line of the posterior semicircular canal (arrow).

control in 94 of 97 cases and partial improvement in the remaining three. The most significant potential risk is sensorineural hearing loss. Walsh[44] and Zappia[41] reported no patients with long-term sensorineural hearing loss (SNHL) following the procedure. Leveque et al.'s review[43] identified sensorineural hearing loss in 2 patients and conductive hearing loss in 2 (of the 97 total) patients. Shaia more recently reported 1 of 28 patients with a >7.5 dB SNHL postoperatively.[42] As with singular neurectomy, temporary postoperative disequilibrium is universal with a risk of permanent balance dysfunction.

Posterior Semicircular Canal Occlusion Procedure

Perioperative antibiotics are given. Dexamethasone is given intravenously for the labyrinthine trauma and postoperative nausea. The surgery is performed under general anesthetic. Facial nerve monitoring is routinely utilized.

Step 1

The initial procedure is identical to steps 1–5 in the endolymphatic sac surgery section. Two additional items are necessary during the approach. First, a piece of temporalis fascia is harvested and, second, bone pate is collected during the mastoidectomy (Fig. 9.42).

Step 2

Donaldson's line is then followed posteriorly to identify the labyrinthine outline of the posterior semicircular canal that bisects it perpendicularly (Fig. 9.43).

Step 3

Small diamond burrs are used to blue line a 4 mm length of the posterior canal (Fig. 9.44). Excessive irrigation is avoided should the canal be inadvertently entered. The canal is thinned around the lateral 180°of the lumen.

Step 4

Once the bone is adequately thinned, the last layer is gently removed with a curved needle exposing the perilymph and the endothelium inside (Fig. 9.45).

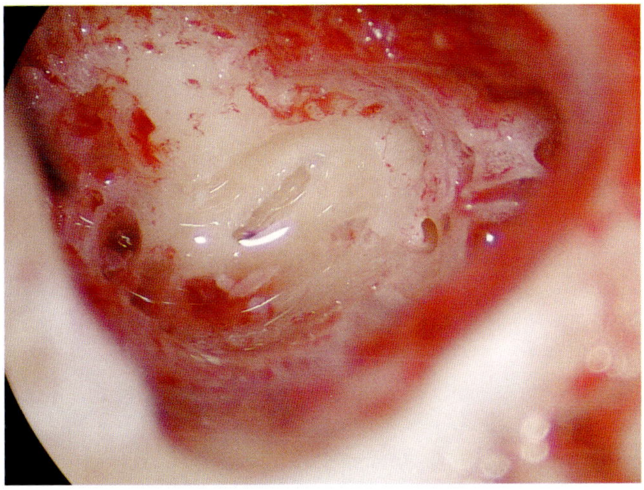

Fig. 9.45: Lumen of the open posterior semicircular canal.

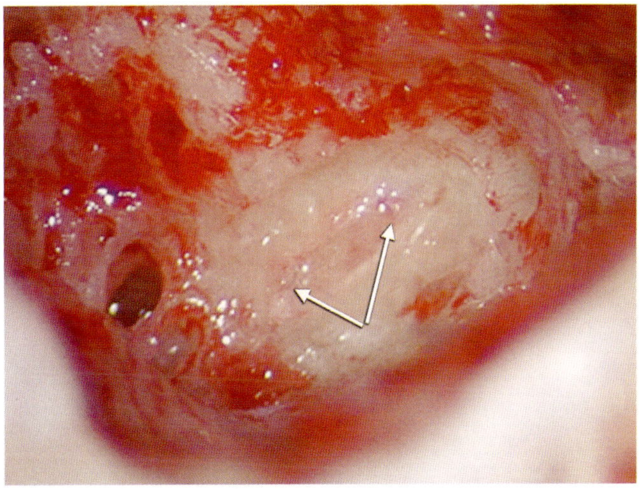

Fig. 9.46: Each open end of the posterior canal is occluded with a small piece of fascia (arrow shows fascia).

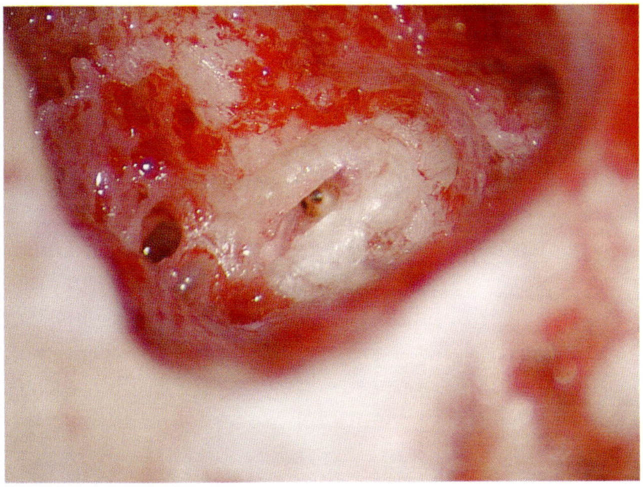

Fig. 9.47: The endothelium is transected with a single laser strike. The burn on the medial wall of the posterior canal lumen can be seen.

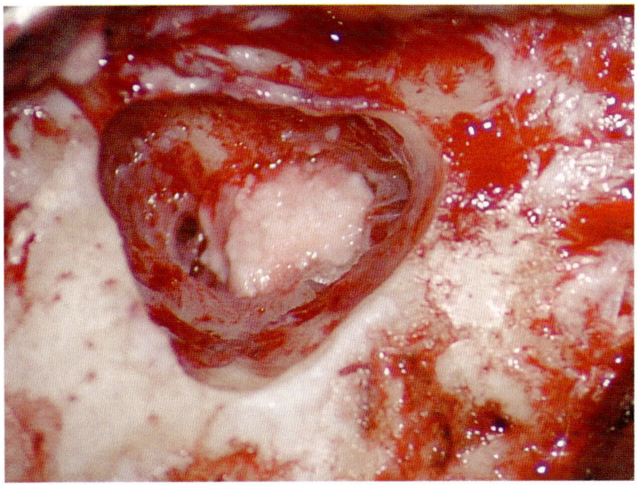

Fig. 9.48: Previously harvested bone pate over the repaired area.

Step 5

There are several methods of occluding the canal. Bone wax and bone pate have been used. Small pieces of tissue can be used to plug the open ends of the canal (Fig. 9.46).

Step 6

Although not always advocated, the endothelial membrane can then be transected with a single laser strike (Fig. 9.47).

Step 7

The canal is completely filled with tissue and bone pate is placed over this area (Fig. 9.48).

Step 8

Fascia is laid over the bone pate (Fig. 9.49). The mastoid cavity lateral to this is packed with saline soaked Gelfoam. Recently, a Porex plate designed to cover the lateral mastoid is placed to limit the amount of pressure that can be transmitted to the occlusion area, as this will result in a sense of dizziness.

Step 9

The incision is closed with absorbable suture in the subcutaneous layer and glue on the skin. A mastoid dressing is placed. The patient is gently awakened.

Invariably disequilibrium, marked by significant motion sensitivity, ensues. As with singular neurectomy,

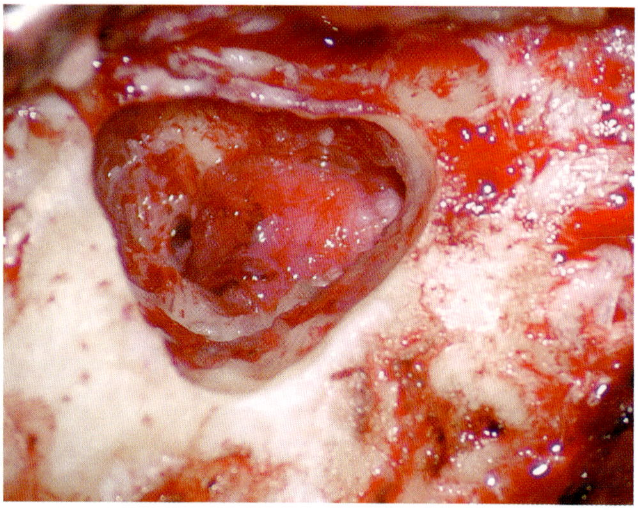

Fig. 9.49: Fascia over the occlusion area.

the hospitalization is of 1–4 days. Vestibular therapy is initiated on the first postoperative day to shorten the period of disequilibrium and maximize the possibility of total recovery. Even with the lateral mastoid plate, a portion of patients are bothered by the pressure induced dizziness created by manipulation of the auricle. A tympanostomy tube placed in the office will alleviate these symptoms by allowing the escape of pressure instead of its transmission to the repaired area.

SUPERIOR SEMICIRCULAR CANAL DEHISCENCE SURGERY

Introduction

Superior semicircular canal dehiscence (SSCD) is a relatively new clinical entity that was originally reported in 1998 by Minor et al.[45] It is defined as a lack of a complete bony covering over the superior semicircular canal (SSC) (Figs. 9.50A and B). It is increasingly recognized as a cause for a variety of otologic symptoms. SSCD's short history creates diagnostic extremes in that there are patients prior to 1998 who went undiagnosed to the present, where now the entity seems to be over recognized. Presently, SSCD is a well-recognized entity with definite treatment possibilities.

The clinical incidence of SSCD is uncertain. Histologically, Carey et al.[46] looked at 1,000 temporal bones from 596 individuals (404 bilateral and 192 single bones). SSCD was identified in 5 (0.5%) of temporal bones and 4 (0.7%) of individuals. The dehiscence was into the middle cranial fossa in 1 and the superior petrosal sinus in 4. They also looked at thinning (≤ 0.1mm) of bone over SSC and identified this in 14 (1.4%) of temporal bones and 10 (1.7%) of individuals. There was bilateral involvement in 6/12 (50%) bones.

Radiologically, the incidence is far higher. Williamson et al.[47] looked for SSCD in their review of 223 temporal bone CAT scans with 442 evaluable temporal bones. They found SSCD in 39 (9%) temporal bones and 30 (13%) individuals. Nine were bilateral, suggesting that radiologically 46% (18/39) of SSCDs are bilateral and that 30% (9/30) individuals with SSCD will be bilateral.

The symptoms are felt to be a result of the third window effect. If the vestibular portion of the inner ear is completely bone encased, the sound pressure/energy should be directed into the cochlea from the oval window because of the presence of the RW. In SSCD, some of this sound energy is shunted into the vestibular system.[48] This will result in the stimulation of the cupula of the SSC with corresponding dizziness and nystagmus. This can also result in loss of sound energy in the cochlea, resulting in hearing loss in the air conduction mechanism. The low frequencies are preferentially affected. The two active windows (round and SSCD) will also result in general decreased resistance and hypermobility of the stapes. There is enhanced sensitivity to bone conducted sound via the bony defect/dehiscence.

Clinical presentation varies and manifestations can generally be explained by the third window concept. Noise or pressure induced vertigo is a classic symptom. Disequilibrium is common. Low-frequency conductive hearing loss must be differentiated from ossicular problems particularly if it is the sole manifestation. Hyperacusis to bone conducted sounds can result in autophony, pulsatile tinnitus, as well as perception of eye movements, joints, and heel strike when walking. A portion of patients report a specific event associated with the time of onset including trauma, straining, or lifting.[49]

Physical examination will assist in the diagnosis. Dizziness can frequently be induced with application of external canal pressure (Hennebert's sign). Application of positive external canal pressure can result in torsional nystagmus up and away from the stimulated ear. Tuning fork testing will frequently result in the Weber lateralizing to the affected ear. Also, the affected individual will frequently perceive the tuning fork tone in the affected ear even when applied to a distant bony site such as the wrist or ankle.

A thin section CAT scan of the temporal bones is the test of choice for identification of SSCD. The orientation

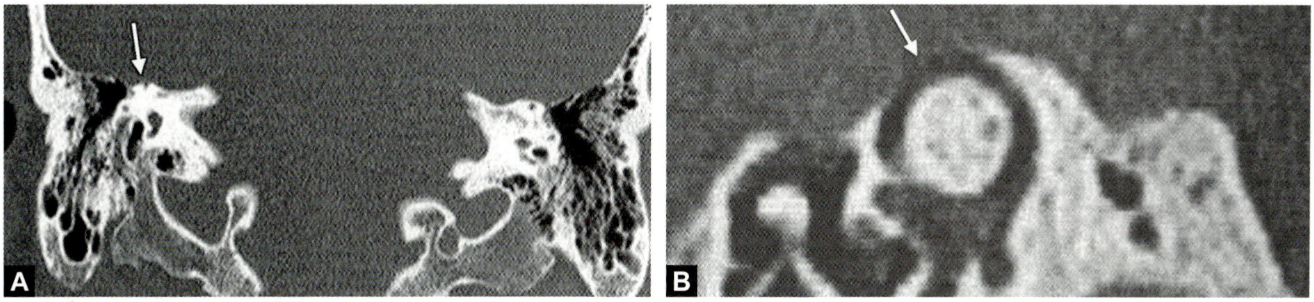

Figs. 9.50A and B: CAT scan of superior semicircular canal dehiscence. (A) Dehiscence of right semicircular canal can be seen on coronal view (arrow). (B) Obvious dehiscence seen in superior semicircular canal plane (arrow).

of the view seems to make a difference. Cloutier et al.[50] evaluated 346 consecutive temporal bone CAT scans and ultimately 581 ears in their review. They identified 58 ears (10%) with SCCD in the coronal plane (Fig. 9.50A) but only 23 (4%) when the image was viewed in the plane of the SSC (Fig. 9.50B). They concluded that if SSCD is not present if it is not seen in coronal plane and that if SSCD is present in coronal plane then SSC plane view is necessary to make diagnosis. Interestingly, they located medical information on 18 of the 21 individuals with radiologic SSCD and none had clinical SSCD symptoms.

Basic audiometric testing can reveal low-frequency conductive hearing loss. When this pattern of loss is present, acoustic reflexes will help to differentiate SSCD from other causes of conductive hearing loss. The acoustic reflex will be maintained in SSCD. A reduced threshold of activation (<70 dB) in cervical vestibular-evoked myogenic potential testing suggests a hyperexcitable ear and is consistent with SSCD.

The differential diagnostic considerations depend on the predominant symptoms present. For the autophony, patulous eustachian tube is possible but in SSCD the audible breath sounds are not present. Pressure-induced dizziness and sound sensitivity are possible in perilymphatic fistula (PLF), syphilis, and Meniere's disease. The conductive hearing loss can be differentiated from ossicular abnormalities by acoustic reflex testing. The possibility of dehiscence other than the SSC must be considered if symptoms and/or testing suggest SSCD but SSCD is not seen on the CAT scan. Most commonly the posterior canal is affected and is dehiscent with the jugular bulb.

Superior Semicircular Canal Dehiscence Treatment

Treatment options for SSCD usually include the extremes of observation and surgery. Not all patients choose surgery. Once the diagnosis is established, many patients report that either the symptoms are nonlimiting or that they do not warrant surgery. An occasional situation allows symptomatic intervention such as a hearing aid for the hearing loss or hearing protection for the sound-induced symptoms.

Surgical intervention is carried out through either a transmastoid or middle cranial fossa approach. The dehiscence is either resurfaced or occluded once identified. In a look at the results, Ward et al.[51] reviewed 43 cases of SCCD plugging via the middle cranial fossa approach. In those with a preoperative low-frequency air-bone gap >10 dB, 63% improved to <10 dB 1 month postoperatively. Bone conduction pure tone averages declined in 25% of patients, hyperacusis was generally improved and there was no significant change in speech discrimination 1 month postoperatively. In a retrospective review of 19 cases, Crane et al.[52] showed significant patient reported symptom improvement after middle cranial fossa plugging using the Dizziness Handicap Index. As with many other dizziness treatments, they found that those scoring higher (worse symptoms) preoperatively were more likely to experience an improvement after repair. They also noted normalization of cervical vestibular evoked myogenic potentials (cVEMP) thresholds in 10 of 11 patients. Of interest is that preoperative cVEMP thresholds did not correlate significantly with preoperative DHI scores.

Patients are counseled preoperatively about the risks that include hearing loss, tinnitus, dizziness, and cerebrospinal fluid leak. Dizziness/disequilibrium postoperatively is more common with plugging than resurfacing and is usually temporary. Cerebrospinal fluid leak is a greater risk in the middle cranial fossa (MCF) approach and can occur related to the SSCD repair or be related to the multiple tegmen dehiscences that are usually present separate from the SSCD. Stroke and intracranial bleeding are unusual but possible complications with MCF approaches.

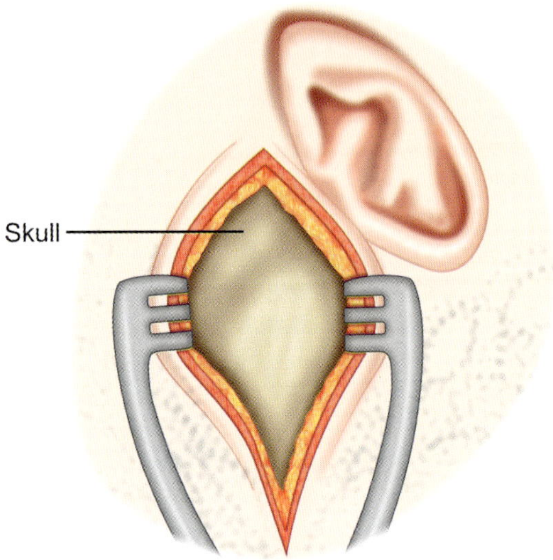

Fig. 9.51: Middle cranial fossa incision.

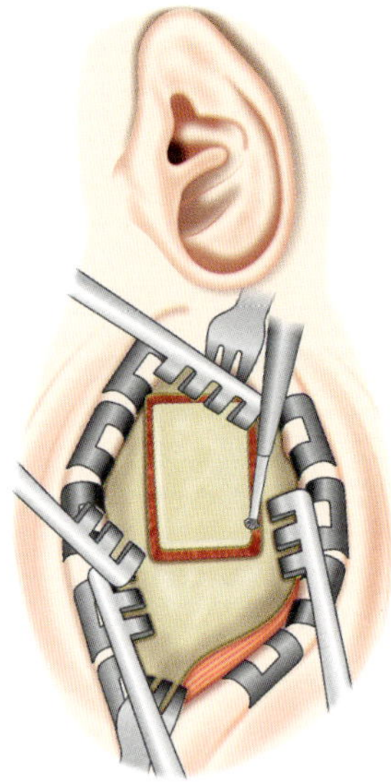

Fig. 9.52: Middle cranial fossa craniotomy for superior semicircular canal dehiscence.

Middle Cranial Fossa Repair of Superior Semicircular Canal Dehiscence Procedure

After adequate anesthesia, the patient is placed in the supine position with the head turned with the affected ear up. Perioperative antibiotics are given. Dexamethasone is given preoperatively for nausea. Facial nerve and ABR monitoring electrodes are placed. Mannitol is given and the patient is hyperventilated to a $Paco_2$ of 26 to reduce intracranial pressure.

Step 1

An approximately 6 cm vertical incision originating in the immediate preauricular area just above the tragus is made (Fig. 9.51). It is carried down to the temporalis fascia. A piece of temporalis fascia is usually harvested depending on the intent with the SSCD. The incision is then carried down to the bone.

Step 2

A 5 × 5 cm craniotomy is created centered on the external auditory canal (Fig. 9.52).

Step 3

The dura is widely elevated and the temporal lobe is retracted superiorly. A middle fossa retractor is placed (Fig. 9.53). Commonly there are multiple bony dehiscences, if not frank encephaloceles, lateral to the SSCD. More medially, the pneumatized bone transitions to the solid labyrinthine bone as the superior canal are approached. The dura is very gently elevated in this area to least disrupt the intralabyrinthine fluid and structures.

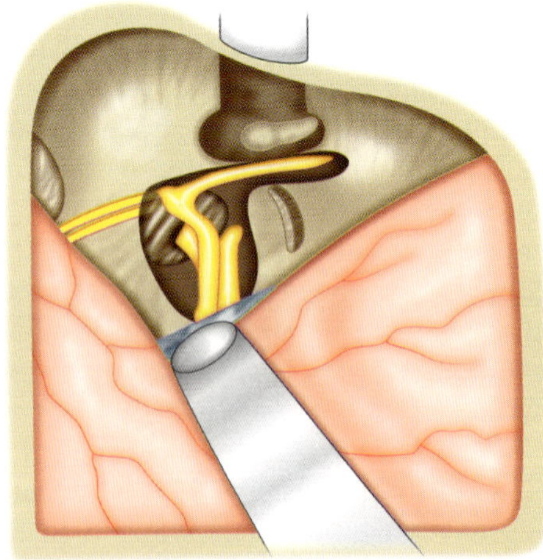

Fig. 9.53: Middle cranial fossa retractor in position exposing the floor of the middle cranial fossa.

Step 4

Once exposed, the SSCD (Fig. 9.54) can be definitively repaired. It can be occluded with bone wax, bone pate, or fascia. Bone cement can also be used. A layer of fascia is usually placed over this. For resurfacing, a layer of fascia is usually placed over the dehiscence. Bone cement,

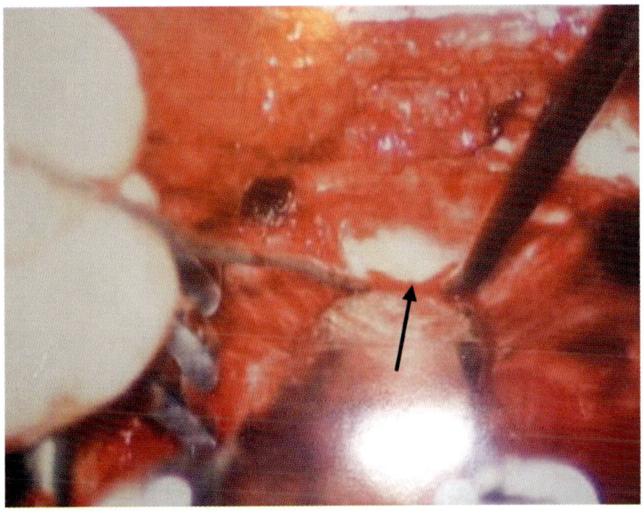

Fig. 9.54: Intraoperative photo showing the large superior semicircular canal dehiscence (arrow).

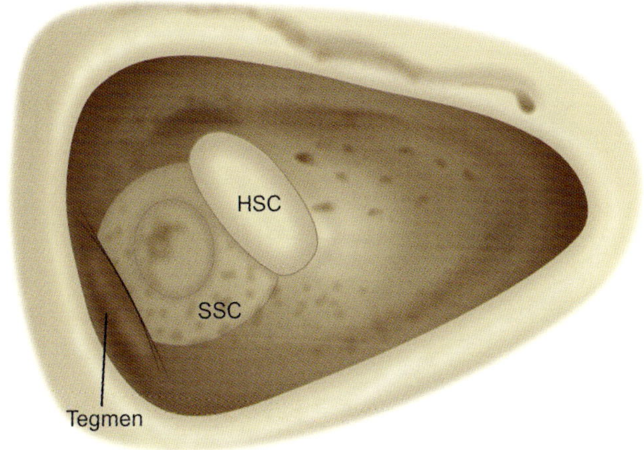

Fig. 9.55: Transmastoid exposure of the superior semicircular canal.
(SSC: Superior semicircular canal; HSC: Horizontal semicircular canal).

a hydroxylapatite plate, calvarial bone, or even Silastic[53] can be placed to support the dura and separate it from the repair.

Step 5

The retractor is removed being careful not to disrupt the repair. The calvarial bone is plated back in position. The wound is carefully closed in layers.

A pressure dressing is placed. The patient is observed in the intensive care unit overnight. If stable, discharge is possible the first morning. Patients are instructed to avoid strenuous activity for 3 weeks. The level of postoperative disequilibrium varies and is an important factor in length of hospital stay and total recovery. For those with disequilibrium, there is immediate instruction in vestibular therapy exercises. The sutures are removed 10 days postoperatively.

Transmastoid Repair of Semicircular Canal Procedure

After adequate anesthesia, the patient is placed in the supine position with the head turned with the affected ear up. Perioperative antibiotics are given. Dexamethasone is given preoperatively for nausea. Facial nerve monitoring is performed.

Step 1

A standard postauricular incision is made and a cortical mastoidectomy is completed as in ELS surgery (Figs. 9.1 to 9.4) carefully identifying the horizontal semicircular canal and the tegmen. As noted above there will frequently be multiple tegmen dehiscences.

Step 2

Drilling is continued superior and medial to the horizontal canal until the outline of the SSC is identified (Fig. 9.55). The level of the dura can usually be seen cutting off some of the contour of the SSC.

Step 3

Most will approach the dehiscence over the top. For this, the dura immediately lateral to the SSC is carefully drilled away (Fig. 9.56). For resurfacing, fascia is usually placed over the dehiscence, and a bone graft, hydroxylapatite plate, piece of cartilage, or Silastic is placed over the fascia. For occlusion, placing a piece of bone wax over the dehiscence and compressing it into the SSCD will complete the repair. An alternative to directly exposing the dehiscence is to leave the dura in place and occlude the SSC anterior and posterior to the dehiscence[54] (Fig. 9.57) as in PSCD (*see* Figs. 9.45 and 9.46).

Step 4

The incisions are then closed in routine fashion for a postauricular approach and a mastoid dressing is placed.

Discharge is possible whenever the patient is medically capable. Disequilibrium is likely in plugging

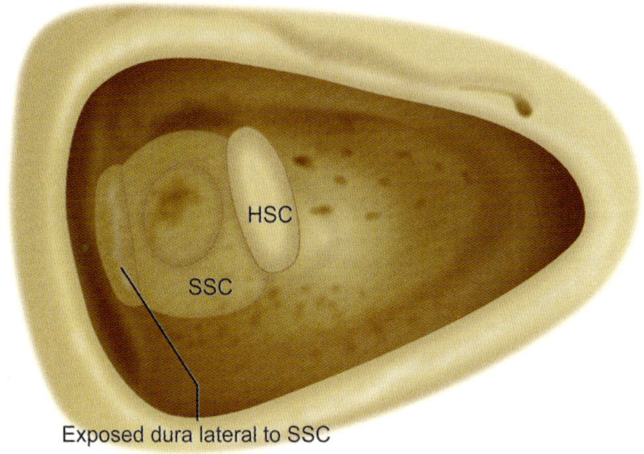

Fig. 9.56: Removal of the bony tegmen lateral to the superior semicircular canal to allow access to the dehiscence on top of the superior semicircular canal.

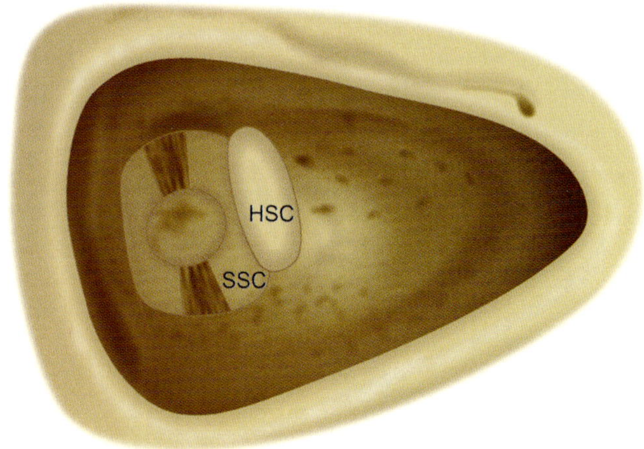

Fig. 9.57: Areas of occlusion of the superior semicircular canal when occlusion is planned.

procedures but can occur in with resurfacing techniques. The patient is instructed to avoid strenuous activity for 3 weeks. The level of postoperative disequilibrium varies and is an important factor in length of hospital stay and total recovery. There is immediate instruction in vestibular therapy exercises for those with disequilibrium.

Transcanal Surgical Treatment of Semicircular Canal Dehiscence

Although controversial, an alternative to direct repair is RW reinforcement.[55] The attractive aspect of this is the minimization of risk with little chance of hearing loss or postoperative dizziness. This is a consideration for those wanting to limit risk. It is also a consideration when the medical risk of a general anesthetic for more formal repair is unacceptably high.

PERILYMPHATIC FISTULA SURGERY

Introduction

A perilymphatic fistula (PLF) is an abnormal direct connection of the inner ear with any area outside the labyrinth. For this chapter, the term will specifically refer to an abnormal connection from the perilymphatic space of the inner ear to the pneumatized space of the middle ear with leakage of perilymph fluid. An extensive review of the topic was presented by Friedland and Wacky.[56]

The most likely sites for PLF are the oval window and round window membranes. There are a variety of possible microfissures in and around the windows where leakage is possible. The most identifiable of these sites is the fissula ante fenestram, which lies anterior to the oval window and posterior to the cochleariform process.

PLFs can be broadly classified into iatrogenic and noniatrogenic. Surgery, most frequently stapedectomy, is the most common cause of iatrogenic fistulae. It is considered primary if the fistula occurs immediately after the procedure without evidence of ever completely healing. They are classified as secondary fistulas if there is apparently a period of time where the inner ear has sealed.

Noniatrogenic PLFs can be divided into traumatic, erosive, congenital, and spontaneous/idiopathic. Traumatic PLF can result from blunt or penetrating traumas that can disrupt the otic capsule. Implosive injury can occur from significant external pressure transmitted through the ear canal such as a fall on water or a slap to the ear. Aggressive nose blowing may also potentially generate enough pressure to disrupt a membrane. Explosive trauma resulting from increase CSF pressure, such as a cough or weight lifting, can be causative. If powerful enough, acoustic trauma such as a blast or loud noise can create a disruption.

Erosive PLF can be the result of cholesteatoma, chronic otitis media, neoplasm, or luetic otitis. Congenital PLFs result from a malformation of the temporal bone, resulting in an anatomic defect or weakness or an abnormal connection with the intracranial space. These can predispose to meningitis.[57] Spontaneous/idiopathic PLFs are those without any identified etiology. Kohut et al.[58] argue against the use of spontaneous and feel that idiopathic is the appropriate term for PLFs without identified etiology.

The symptoms of PLF are quite variable. Hearing loss is frequently, but not always, present and can be progressive, sudden, or fluctuant. Dizziness can be persistent or episodic with symptoms being spontaneous or positional. Although not always present, one looks for the presence of exertion-related symptoms as a possible indicator. PLF can unfortunately mimic other disorders such as Meniere's disease.

On physical examination, one looks for Tullio's phenomenon (sound-induced nystagmus) and Hennebert's sign (dizziness, nystagmus with pressure changes in ear canal). Although this would be suspected to be a more reliable finding, Hennebert's is found in less than half of patients with PLF.

Audiometry is routinely performed, but there is no characteristic finding. VNG with pressure testing ("fistula test") can be supportive but like Hennebert's sign it can be unreliable. A unilateral weakness will increase suspicion but is by no means pathognomonic. ECoG has been reportedly positive in half of PLF patients with the theory being than it can be abnormal because a PLF would create a relative hydrops with the perilymph pressure being reduced instead of the endolymph pressure being elevated.

The diagnosis of PLF rests primarily on clinical suspicion and elimination of other clinical possibilities. Some situations are more straightforward than others. Postsurgical and post-traumatic forms are easier to identify because of the history. Idiopathic forms are controversial in their existence to begin with and particularly difficult to make decisions on without a convincing history, examination, or tests.

Perilymphatic Fistula Treatment

Once the diagnosis is suspected, treatment recommendations are straightforward. In all but extremely acute situations, an initial period of inactivity is recommended. The recommendation includes bed rest, head elevation, and avoidance of Valsalva including nose blowing, lifting, straining, and bending. Stool softeners are recommended for those prone to constipation. The length of restrictions varies from days to weeks. There has been no real analysis of success of conservative therapy. One slight issue that can be encountered is that many patients will be symptomatically improved with the restrictions without true improvement of the PLF.

For those who do not recover with conservative therapy, surgical repair is recommended. Theoretically, middle ear exploration is the only way to truly verify the diagnosis. This concept is muddied by several facts. The rate of fluid accumulation in the middle ear at the time of surgery is quite variable, and not all patients with positive explorations improve with repair though. Additionally, a moderate percentage of suspected PLF patients with negative middle ear explorations improve with surgical repair. The final point may simply be lack of improvement is due to unsuccessful repair, which leads to a final complicated question—if a suspected PLF patient does not improve with surgery, is it because of a wrong diagnosis or failure of technique?

Various materials have been used for repair. Fascia, areolar tissue, perichondrium, and adipose are the most common. There has been some criticism of use of fat in that some early reports site higher failure rates. Blood and fibrin glue have also been utilized with the initial patching materials to assist in the seal. In one of the larger single series, Black et al.[4] reported the use of fat, tragal perichondrium, or fascia early but then altering the technique and using areolar tissue with a mixture of autologous cryoprecipitated fibrinogen, reconstituted microfibrillar bovine collagen (Avitene), and thrombin.

In idiopathic situations, the rate of fistula identification at the time of surgery ranges from 0% up to near 100%. Most surgeons will complete an oval and round window repair even if no fistula is seen intraoperatively. In general, success rates are reportedly higher when a PLF is seen, but reasonable improvement rates are noted even in negative explorations. Postsurgical fistulas are generally considered differently, with higher rates of identification of PLF and higher rates of success.

Perilymphatic Fistula Repair Surgical Procedure

The procedure is preferably performed under local anesthesia with sedation, although general anesthesia is possible. Intravenous dexamethasone is given for postanesthesia nausea prevention.

Step 1

The patient is placed in the supine position with the affected ear up. A circumferential auricular block with

1% lidocaine with 1:100,000 epinephrine is competed. The external meatus is also injected. The periauricular area is prepared and draped in the usual sterile manner.

Step 2

The external canal is inspected under the operating microscope. The external auditory canal is injected with a minimal amount of local anesthesia to minimize the possibility of unwanted fluid entering the middle ear.

Step 3

Standard tympanomeatal incisions are made and the flap is elevated as in transcanal labyrinthectomy (Figs. 9.23 and 9.24). The flap is elevated and the middle is entered as bloodlessly as possible. Typically, a portion of the posterior-superior annulus needs to be removed to allow complete visualization of the round and oval window areas.

Step 4

In some procedures, such as poststapedectomy PLF, the middle ear exploration can be focused. In most other situations, careful exposure and more complete examination of the middle ear are critical. The middle ear windows and adjacent fissures are carefully assessed. Although it can be helpful to remove some of the bone of the round window niche, this will frequently induce some bleeding and make assessment more difficult.

Step 5

The mucosa adjacent to the area of repair is gently abraded—generally with a small rasp.

Step 6

Fascia or areolar tissue can be harvested from an incision in the superior postauricular area. If utilized, adipose can be harvested from either the posterior auricle or the lobule.

Step 7

Appropriate sized pieces of tissue are trimmed. In most surgeries, the tissue is carefully placed over the stapes footplate and in the round window niche. In more specific situations, such as poststapedectomy, the tissue is packed in a more directed manner.

Step 8

Gelfoam is generally placed lateral to the repair to support the tissue in its intended position and support the tympanic membrane laterally. The tympanomeatal flap is returned to its initial position. A strip of moist Gelfoam is placed along the posterior external auditory canal. The remainder of the canal is filled with bacitracin ointment.

Postsurgical activity restriction is an important part of the treatment. Activity recommendations vary but generally include at least 3 weeks for significant Valsalva and lifting restriction, head elevation, and avoidance of nose blowing. Stool softeners are frequently recommended unless opposed by the patient.

REFERENCES

1. Portmann G. Surgical treatment by opening saccus endolymphaticus. Arch Otolaryngol. 1927;6:309-19.
2. Telischi FF, Luxford WM. Long-term efficacy of endolymphatic sac surgery for vertigo in Meniere's disease. Otolaryngol Head Neck Surg. 1993;109:83-7.
3. Brackmann DE, Nissen RL. Meniere's disease: results of treatment with the endolymphatic subarachnoid shunt compared with the endolymphatic mastoid shunt. Am J Otol. 1987;8:275-82.
4. Gianoli GJ, LaRouere MJ, Kartush JM, et al. Sac-vein decompression for intractable Meniere's disease: two year treatment results. Otolaryngol Head Neck Surg. 1998; 118(1):22-9.
5. Thomsen J, Bretlau P, Tos M, et al. Placebo effect in surgery for Meniere's disease. Arch Otolaryngol. 1981;107:230-36.
6. Pillsbury HC 3rd, Arenberg IK, Ferraro J, et al. Endolymphatic sac surgery. The Danish sham surgery study: an alternative analysis. Otolaryngol Clin North Am. 1983;16(1):123-7.
7. Wilson WR, Byl FM, Laird N. The efficacy of steroids in the treatment of idiopathic sudden hearing loss. Arch Otolaryngol. 1980;106:772-6.
8. Rauch SD, Babu S, Carey JP, et al. Oral vs. intratympanic corticosteroid therapy for idiopathic sudden sensorineural hearing loss. A randomized trial. JAMA. 2011;305(20):2071-79.
9. Roebuck J, Chang CYJ. Efficacy of steroid injection on idiopathic sudden sensorineural hearing loss. Otolaryngol Head Neck Surg. 2006;135:276-9.
10. Kakehata S, Saski A, Oji K, et al. Comparison of intratympanic and intravenous dexamethasone treatment on sudden sensorineural hearing loss with diabetes. Otol Neurotol. 2006;27:604-8.
11. Plontke S, Lowenheim H, Preyer S, et al. Outcomes research analysis of continuous intratympanic glucocorticoid delivery in patients with acute severe to profound hearing loss: basis for planning randomized controlled trials. Acta Otolaryngol. 2005;125:830-9.

12. Parnes LS, Sun AH, Freeman DJ. Corticosteroids pharmacokinetics in the inner ear fluids: An animal study followed by clinical application. Laryngoscope. 1999;109:1-17.
13. Fowler EP Jr, Seligman E. Otic complications of streptomycin therapy. Preliminary report. JAMA. 1947;133:87.
14. Fowler EP Jr. Streptomycin treatment of vertigo. Trans Am Acad Ophthalmol Otolaryngol. 1948;52:293-301.
15. Schuknecht H. Ablation therapy for relief of Meniere's disease. Laryngoscope. 1956;60:859-70.
16. Schuknecht H. Ablation therapy in the management of Meniere's disease. Acta Oto-Laryngologica Suppl. 1957; 132: 1-42.
17. Beck C, Schmidt CL. 10 years of experience with intratympanically applied streptomycin (gentamicin) in the therapy of Morbus Meniere. Arch Otorhinolaryngol. 1978; 221:149-52.
18. Nedzelski JM, Chiong CM, Fradet G, et al. Intratympanic gentamicin instillation as treatment of unilateral Meniere's disease: Update of an ongoing study. Am J Otol. 1993;14(3): 278-82.
19. Driscoll CW, Kasperbauer JL, Facer GW, et al. Low-dose intratympanic gentamicin and the treatment of Meniere's disease: Preliminary results. Laryngoscope. 1997;107:83-9.
20. Magnusson M, Padoan S, Larlberg M, et al. Delayed onset of ototoxic effects of gentamicin in patients with Meniere's disease. Acta Otolaryngol (Stockh). 1991;Suppl 485:120-2.
21. Soderman ACH, Ahlner K, Bagger-Sjoback D, et al. Surgical treatment of vertigo—the Karolinska hospital policy. Am J Otol. 1996;16:93-8.
22. Hirsch BE, Kamerer DB. Intratympanic gentamicin therapy for Ménière's disease. Am J Otol. 1997;18(1):44-51.
23. Lake R. Removal of the semicircular canals in a case of unilateral aural vertigo. Lancet. 1904;1:1567-8.
24. Diaz RC, LaRouere MJ, Bojrab DI, et al. Quality-of-life assessment of Meniere's disease patients after surgical labyrinthectomy. Otol Neurotol. 2007;28(1):74-86.
25. Jackler RK, Whinney D. A century of eighth nerve surgery. Otol Neurotol. 2001;22:401-16.
26. McKenzie KG. Intracranial division of the vestibular portion of the auditory nerve for Meniere's disease. CMAJ. 1936;34:369-381.
27. Thedinger BS, Thedinger BA. Analysis of patients with persistent dizziness after vestibular nerve section. Ear Nose Throat J. 1998;77:290-2.
28. Nedzelski JM, Barber HO, McIlmoyl L. Diagnosis in a dizziness unit. J Otolaryngol. 1986;15(2):101-4.
29. Oghalai JS, Manolidis S, Barth JL, et al. Unrecognized benign positional vertigo in elderly patients. Otolaryngol Head Neck Surg. 2000;122(5):630-4.
30. Schuknecht HF. Cupulolithiasis. Arch Otolaryngol. 1969;90: 765-78.
31. Moriarity B, Rutka J, Hawke M. The incidence and distribution of cupular deposits in the labyrinth. Laryngoscope. 1992;102(1):56-9.
32. Hall SF, Ruby RRF, McClure JA. The mechanics of benign paroxysmal positional vertigo. J Otolaryngol. 1979;8(2):151-8.
33. Kveton JF, Kashgarian M. Particulate matter within the membranous labyrinth: pathologic or normal? Am J Otol. 1994;15(2):173-6.
34. Fife TD, Iverson DJ, Lempert T, et al. Practice parameter: therapies for benign paroxysmal positional vertigo. Neurology. 2008;70(22):2067-74.
35. Gacek RR. Transection of the posterior ampullary nerve for the relief of benign paroxysmal positional vertigo. Ann Otol Rhinol Laryngol. 1974;83:596-605.
36. Gacek RR. Singular neurectomy update. II. Review of 102 cases. Laryngoscope. 1991;101:855-62.
37. Gacek RR, Gacek MR. Results of singular neurectomy in the posterior ampullary recess. ORL J Otorhinolaryngol Relat Spec. 2002;64:397-402.
38. Silverstein H, White DW. Wide surgical exposure for singular neurectomy in the treatment of benign positional vertigo. Laryngoscope. 1990;100:701-6.
39. Epley JM. Singular neurectomy: hypotympanotomy approach. Otolaryngol Head Neck Surg. 1980;88:304-9.
40. Parnes LS, McClure JA. Posterior semicircular canal occlusion for intractable benign paroxysmal positional vertigo. Ann Otol Rhinol Laryngol. 1990;99:330-4.
41. Zappia JJ. Posterior semicircular canal occlusion for benign paroxysmal positional vertigo. Am J Otol. 1996;17(5):749-54.
42. Shaia WT, Zappia JJ, Bojrab DI, et al. Success of posterior semicircular canal occlusion and application of the dizziness handicap inventory. Otolaryngol Head Neck Surg. 2006;134(3):424-30.
43. Leveque M, Labrousse M, Seidermann L, et al. Surgical therapy in intractable benign paroxysmal positional vertigo. Otolaryngol Head Neck Surg. 2007;136:693-8.
44. Walsh RM, Bath AP, Cullen JR, et al. Long-term results of posterior semicircular canal occlusion for intractable benign paroxysmal positional vertigo. Clin Otolaryngol Allied Sci. 1999;24(4):316-32.
45. Minor LB, Solomon D, Zaiteich JS, et al. Sound- and pressure-induced vertigo due to bone dehiscence of the superior semicircular canal. Arch Otolaryngol Head Neck Surg. 1998;124:249-58.
46. Carey JP, Minor LB, Nager GT. Dehiscence or thinning of bone overlying the superior semicircular canal in a temporal bone survey. Arch Otolaryngol Head Neck Surg. 2000;126(2):137-47.
47. Williamson RA, Vrabec JT, Coker NJ, et al. Coronal computed tomography prevalence of superior semicircular canal dehiscence. Otolaryngol Head Neck Surg. 2003;129(5):481-9.
48. Chien W, Ravicz ME, Rosowski JJ, et al. Measurements of Human Middle- and Inner-Ear Mechanics with Dehiscence of the Superior Semicircular Canal. Otol Neurotol. 2007;28(2):250-57.
49. Minor LB. Clinical manifestations of superior semicircular canal dehiscence. Laryngoscope. 2005;115:1717-27.
50. Cloutier JF, Belair M, Saliba I. Superior semicircular canal dehiscence: positive predictive value of high resolution CT scanning. Eur Arch Otorhinolaryngol. 2008;265:1455-60.

51. Ward BK, Agerwal Y, Nguyen E, et al. Hearing outcomes following surgical plugging of the superior semicircular canal by middle cranial fossa approach. Otol Neurotol. 2012;33(8):1386-91.
52. Crane BT, Minor LB, Carey JP. Superior canal dehiscence plugging reduces dizziness handicap. Laryngoscope. 2008; 118:1809-13.
53. Hahn Y, Zappia J. Modified resurfacing repair for superior semicircular canal dehiscence. Otolaryngol Head Neck Surg. 2010;142(5):763-4.
54. Agrawal SK, Parnes LS. Transmastoid superior semicircular canal occlusion. Tool Neurotol. 2008;29:363-7.
55. Silverstein H, Van Less MJ. Complete round window niche occlusion for superior semicircular canal dehiscence syndrome: a minimally invasive approach. Ear Nose Throat J. 2009;88(8):1042-56.
56. Friedland DR, Wacky PA. A critical appraisal of spontaneous perilymphatic fistulas of the inner ear. Am J Otol. 1999;20:261-79.
57. Rope V, Agarwal I, Rajshekhar V. Congenital perilymph fistula causing recurrent meningitis: Lessons learnt from a single-institution case series. Otolaryngol Head Neck Surg. 2014;150(2):285-91.
58. Kohut RI, Hinojosa R, Ryu JH. Update on idiopathic perilymphatic fistulas. Otolaryngol Clin N Am. 1996;29(2): 343-52.

CHAPTER

10 Cochlear Implantation

Robert S Hong

INTRODUCTION

Cochlear implants are devices that have revolutionized the treatment of severe to profound deafness. Prior to cochlear implants, the most common treatment for those with significant hearing loss was conventional hearing aids. However, as hearing worsened to severe to profound levels, the effectiveness of hearing aids decreased. Repeated adjustment of hearing aids would lead to speech sounding louder but not any clearer, leaving these patients isolated from the hearing world. With the advent of cochlear implants, we are now able to provide useful hearing to deaf individuals. Such individuals can go from having no speech understanding at all to obtaining excellent results on tests assessing the understanding of sentences in quiet after cochlear implantation.

The cochlear implant is a device that provides electrical stimulation to the cochlea to restore the sensation of hearing to deaf individuals (Fig. 10.1). It consists of an external component that sits behind the ear and an internal component that is surgically implanted into the cochlea (Figs 10.2 and 10.3). When sound is presented to the implanted ear, it is picked up by the microphone and converted by the sound processor into a digital signal. This signal is then transmitted wirelessly across the skin to the internal device, where the information is presented by the electrode array as electric pulses to different regions of the cochlea to allow patients to hear. Patients who have cochlear implants do not have normal hearing, as the implant itself provides a relatively crude representation of the acoustic signal. However, over time, patients are able to adapt to the electric stimulation and obtain useful hearing.

Cochlear implants are considered mainstream technology and have been available to the general public since the 1980s for treating hearing loss. The US Food and Drug Administration (FDA) estimates that as of December 2012, over 320,000 people have received a cochlear

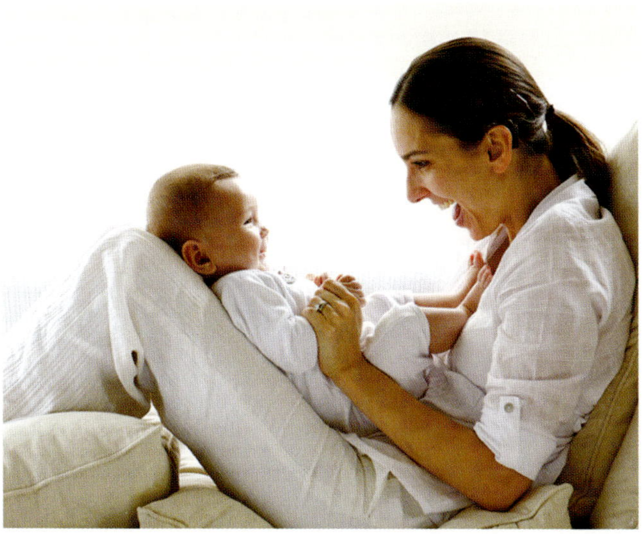

Fig. 10.1: Cochlear implant. A cochlear implant recipient is shown, wearing her sound processor behind her left ear.
Courtesy: Cochlear Americas, ©2014 Cochlear Americas

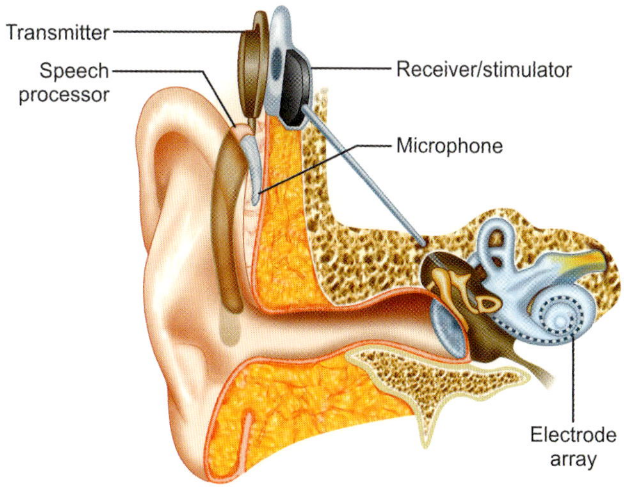

Fig. 10.2: Cochlear implant. A right ear is shown with the external and internal components of the cochlear implant. The external part consists of a speech processor, microphone, and transmitter located behind the auricle. The internal part consists of the receiver/stimulator under the skin and the electrode array within the cochlea.

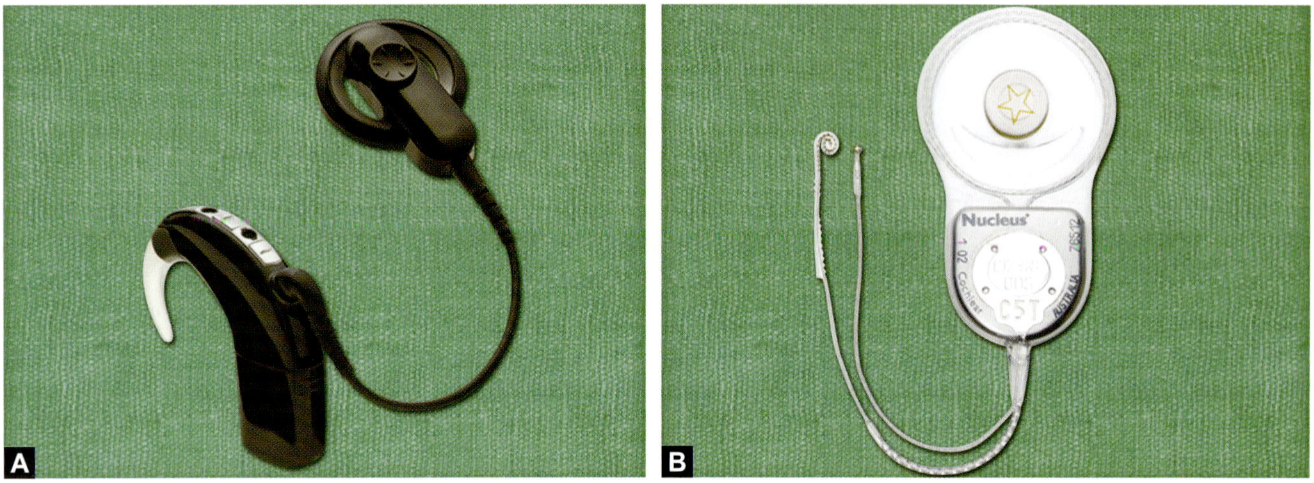

Figs. 10.3A and B: Cochlear implant. Close-up of the (A) external and (B) internal components of the cochlear implant. The implant shown is an example of a Nucleus cochlear implant (Cochlear Limited, Australia).
Courtesy: Cochlear Americas, ©2014 Cochlear Americas

implant worldwide. Currently, there are three major manufacturers of cochlear implants: (1) Advanced Bionics Corporation (Valencia, CA), (2) Cochlear Limited (New South Wales, Australia), and (3) MED-EL Corporation (Innsbruck, Austria). Each company is well respected within the otolaryngology community and has produced implants of comparable quality and performance over the years.

PATIENT SELECTION

Adults

Cochlear implants are intended for patients with significant bilateral hearing loss who receive little to no benefit from conventional hearing aids. Current audiologic criteria for cochlear implantation in adults include (1) bilateral moderate to profound sensorineural hearing loss and (2) open-set sentence recognition in the best-aided condition <50% in the ear to be implanted and <60% in the contralateral ear. It is preferable that adults have a postlingual onset of deafness (occurring after acquisition of speech and language), though adults with prelingual deafness can be implanted so long as they are aware that their benefit may be more limited.[1] It is also important to note that health insurances may use different criteria for coverage of cochlear implants than those mentioned above; for example, Medicare criteria are currently more restrictive than FDA guidelines.

CHILDREN

For children, the rule of thumb is that the younger a child is implanted, the better the child will perform with respect to speech, language, and auditory development.[2-4] Thus, it is imperative that children who are identified with hearing loss during newborn hearing screening have close follow-up throughout infancy. This allows those with severe hearing loss and poor auditory development despite appropriate hearing amplification to proceed to cochlear implantation at the earliest reasonable date. In the United States, the FDA has approved cochlear implantation for children as young as 1 year of age. However, children have been implanted younger than this, particularly if the hearing loss is secondary to meningitis, where intracochlear ossification preventing favorable cochlear implantation can occur if surgery is not performed expediently. Specific audiologic criteria for implantation in children include (1) bilateral profound hearing loss (12–24 months old) or bilateral severe to profound hearing loss (25 months to <18 years old), (2) open-set word recognition <30% in best-aided condition, and (3) lack of progress in development of auditory skills. Additionally, a supportive family and educational environment are critical to the success of the child after implantation.

Contraindications

Cochlear nerve aplasia and complete agenesis of the cochlea are considered absolute contraindications. However, a number of recent studies have shown that some patients can still perform well with a cochlear implant despite imaging consistent with these contraindications, suggesting that residual cochlear fibers are present near the implanted device, but just not detectable on imaging.[5-7] Relative contraindications include prelingual onset of deafness in adults, intracochlear ossification or fibrosis, congenital malformations of the inner ear, and active chronic otitis media. Patients who have significant medical comorbidities preventing safe administration of general anesthesia or those with psychiatric conditions inhibiting use and maintenance of the implant are also considered poor implant candidates. Notably, there is no upper age limit for cochlear implantation, so motivated adults of any age may be considered.

PREOPERATIVE EVALUATION

It is important to obtain a thorough medical history to assess for factors that may influence the success of cochlear implantation. The cause of hearing loss should be explored. Patients with a history of radiation therapy involving the temporal bone, meningitis, or post-traumatic sensorineural hearing loss are at a greater risk for ossification/fibrosis of the cochlea, which may impact the ability to perform implantation. Those who have had prior acoustic neuroma surgery are not candidates for cochlear implantation if the cochlear nerve was sacrificed intraoperatively. Patients should also be asked if they are pre- or postlingually deafened, as adults with prelingual deafness have poorer outcomes following cochlear implantation. The duration of deafness and consistency of hearing aid use should be assessed. This can affect the side selected for implantation, as patients with similarly poor hearing in both ears will often have the side with a shorter duration of deafness chosen based on theoretically better nerve survival in that ear. The duration of deafness is the only reliable predictor of cochlear implant performance, with a shorter duration correlated to better performance.[8] The utility of a patient's aided hearing in each ear should also be determined. A patient who believes that they have more useful (albeit limited) acoustic hearing in one ear will often be implanted on the contralateral side, to provide the opportunity to combine aided acoustic hearing in one ear with a cochlear implant in the other. Additionally, those who have useful residual hearing may be considered for cochlear implantation via a soft technique that can preserve this hearing and allow for the use of both a hearing aid and cochlear implant in the implanted ear. Finally, the presence of recent or ongoing ear infections should be elicited. Active chronic otitis media needs to be addressed first before implantation can proceed, as implantation in an infected field may lead to a higher risk of postoperative infections including meningitis.

On physical examination, the patient's facial nerve function should be documented. Hearing loss should be confirmed with Weber and Rinne tuning fork examinations. Otomicroscopic examination of the ear should be performed, including assessment for an ear infection or tympanic membrane perforation. Patients should also be evaluated for the presence of craniofacial abnormalities, which may correspond to an increased likelihood for abnormalities in the course of the facial nerve.

Audiometric evaluation in adults should include a complete audiogram and a test of sentence recognition (e.g. AzBio sentence test) in the best-aided condition. All patients should have a trial of appropriately fit hearing aids for at least 3 months prior to implantation. Children should have age appropriate audiometric testing and tympanometry. Open-set word recognition [using the Multisyllabic Lexical Neighborhood Test (MLNT) or Lexical Neighborhood Test (LNT)] may be assessed in children >2 years old. Objective testing including otoacoustic emissions (OAE), auditory brainstem response (ABR), and auditory steady state response (ASSR) is also useful to assess hearing loss, particularly in infants where behavioral audiometry may be unreliable. Parents should also be asked for their observations of their child's (lack of) response to sound stimuli at home and in other environments to further confirm suspected deafness prior to cochlear implantation.

Vestibular testing may be considered preoperatively in adults with a suspected history of vestibular injury or those being considered for bilateral cochlear implantation. The insertion of a cochlear implant into the inner ear may occasionally cause injury to the vestibular system, leading to postoperative imbalance. This imbalance is usually temporary, so long as the patient has a contralateral ear with good vestibular function. However, patients who already have a preoperative unilateral vestibular hypofunction are at a higher risk for developing debilitating bilateral hypofunction. Thus, caloric testing may influence the choice of ear that is implanted or influence the surgeon to be more cautious in pursuing bilateral implantation if a preoperative injury is found.

Radiological examination should be performed in all patients prior to cochlear implantation. In adults, high-resolution computed tomography (CT) imaging without contrast of the temporal bone is performed to assess for patency of the cochlea. Additionally, the CT scan provides useful information for surgical planning. A contracted mastoid cavity, abnormal course of the facial nerve, or presence of inner ear malformations may lead to modifications in surgical technique. In patients in whom a suspicion of cochlear fibrosis exists (such as those with meningitis, radiation, or otic capsule fracture), a high-resolution magnetic resonance imaging (MRI) scan without contrast of the temporal bone is useful. In particular, the T2 (CISS or FIESTA) sequence is helpful for determining the presence of fluid within the cochlea, a finding consistent with cochlear patency. In contrast, CT imaging can detect lack of patency secondary to cochlear ossification but not cochlear fibrosis.

In children with congenital deafness, MRI is the preferred modality for preoperative imaging. It is advantageous over CT imaging because it can evaluate for the presence of the cochlear nerve and avoids delivering radiation to the developing child. A high resolution T2-weighted three-dimensional fast spin echo MRI sequence should be included, with oblique cuts perpendicular to the internal auditory canal, to look for the cochlear nerve. The presence of middle ear fluid and congenital inner ear malformations including the patency of the cochlea should also be assessed.

All patients should receive vaccination against *Streptococcus pneumoniae* prior to cochlear implantation to protect against meningitis. The current recommendations for vaccination from the Centers for Disease Control (CDC) are summarized by the American Academy of Otolaryngology at: http://www.entnet.org/HealthInformation/Cochlear-Meningitis-Vaccination.cfm. Children who are candidates for cochlear implants should receive the 13-valent pneumococcal conjugate vaccine (PCV13 = Prevnar 13) according to the age-related dosing schedule released by the CDC, which can take up to 8 weeks to complete (http://www.cdc.gov/mmwr/preview/mmwrhtml/mm5909a2.htm). Adults who are candidates for cochlear implants should receive a single dose of PCV13, followed by a single dose of the 23-valent pneumococcal polysaccharide vaccine (PPSV23 = Pneumovax 23) 8 weeks later. The vaccination schedule for both children and adults should be completed at least 2 weeks prior to surgery. A revaccination dose with PPSV23 should be given to children older than 2 years of age after completing the PCV13 series. A revaccination dose (5 years later) of the PPSV23 is recommended for adults 65 years and older. Additionally, the guidelines are different for those who may have received prior dosages of different pneumococcal vaccines.

Informed consent should include a thorough discussion of the benefits, alternatives, and risks of cochlear implantation. Patients may expect to receive improvement in hearing with a cochlear implant, as most can obtain good open-set speech recognition in quiet following implantation. However, they need to have realistic expectations and know that this can take months if not years of consistent use of the cochlear implant to achieve. The most viable alternative to cochlear implantation is communication via sign language or with other assistive devices. However, most hearing parents will not elect this option for their deaf child, as they want their child to be part of their hearing world. Most postlingually deafened adults will not elect this option, as they have had hearing most of their life, so the concept of learning a new (sign) language if often foreign and unappealing.

Risks of cochlear implantation include bleeding, infection, numbness, facial paralysis, taste changes, tinnitus, dizziness, cerebrospinal fluid leak, and meningitis, along with the usual risks of general anesthesia. Complications related to the device itself include device failure, device migration, facial nerve stimulation, and need for explantation or revision surgery. Patients who have residual acoustic hearing should be counseled to expect to lose all acoustic hearing in the implanted ear. On occasion, some hearing can be saved with hearing preservation techniques, but this is unpredictable. Finally, candidates should be warned that special precautions must be undertaken if they have a MRI scan in the future with their cochlear implant.[9] This may include needing to have the internal magnet of the implant surgically removed prior to MRI, and replaced after imaging is finished. Alternatively, placement of a tightly fit head bandage over the implant may be sufficient to prevent migration, though this has only been FDA approved for a select group of MED-EL cochlear implants in 1.5 Tesla MR systems.

SURGICAL TECHNIQUES

General Considerations

One important issue to consider is whether a patient should receive one or two cochlear implants. Bilateral cochlear implantation has been demonstrated to result in improved speech perception in noise, sound localization, and language development (in children) compared to unilateral cochlear implantation.[10,11] However, the cost-effectiveness of adding a second cochlear implant is controversial,[12] and thus some insurance companies are reluctant to provide coverage for a second implant. If bilateral cochlear implantation is considered, it is most often done in children.[13] For such children, bilateral cochlear implantation can be performed either simultaneously or sequentially. Simultaneous cochlear implantation may be preferable as it has the allure of requiring

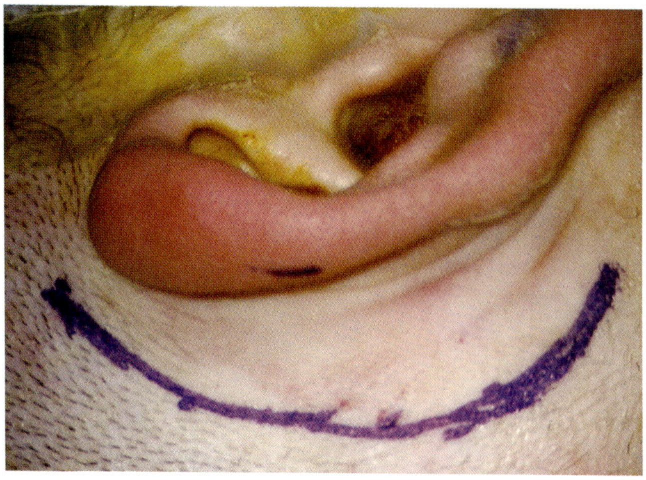

Fig. 10.4: Incision. A curvilinear postauricular incision is shown.

only one general anesthetic, leading to decreased risk from anesthesia exposure and decreased cost compared to sequential implantation.[14] It also has been shown to result in earlier speech and language development, as patients receive earlier stimulation of the bilateral auditory system and avoid central processing mismatch between the two sides.[11] However, parental concerns such as lack of acceptance that their child is deaf, not wanting to give up the hearing aid in the opposite ear, or wanting to save the other ear for potential future technologies may influence a child to have a single implant first.[15]

Another consideration in surgical preparation is the patient with active chronic otitis media. Patients should not have an active middle ear infection at the time of cochlear implantation, as this may lead to a higher risk of postoperative infections including meningitis. Those who continue to have infections despite multiple courses of antibiotics may require pressure equalization tubes, which may be left in place for cochlear implant surgery so long as the ear is dry.[16,17] Patients with persistent otorrhea despite these measures may be candidates for a two-stage procedure in which a subtotal petrosectomy (radical mastoidectomy with overclosure of the ear canal, plugging of the Eustachian tube and mastoid obliteration) is performed in the first stage, with cochlear implantation performed weeks to months later.[18]

Anesthesia

Cochlear implantation is performed under general anesthesia. Instruction should be given to the anesthesia team to avoid any long-acting muscle relaxants during anesthesia induction, to avoid hindering intraoperative facial nerve monitoring.

Surgical Technique

Step 1

The patient is placed in a supine position with the head turned away from the operative side while supported by a headrest. The operating table is turned 180° away from the anesthesia team.

Step 2

Preoperative antibiotics and steroids are administered. Steroids are particularly important if hearing preservation is to be attempted intraoperatively.

Step 3

Facial nerve monitoring is set up and used continuously throughout the case. Intraoperative ABR may be used if hearing preservation is to be attempted.

Step 4

Plan the incision: A curvilinear postauricular incision near the hairline is created (Fig. 10.4). The superior aspect of the incision can be extended posterosuperiorly as needed. Hair is shaved as needed.

Step 5

Incision: A #15 blade is used to make the incision through the skin and soft tissue, down to the level of the temporalis fascia. This plane is carried inferiorly toward the mastoid tip and the auricle is retracted forward. An anteriorly based Palva flap is then created incorporating the underlying fascia, muscle, and periosteum to expose the mastoid bone (Fig. 10.5). The superior border of this flap should be at the linea temporalis, and the posterior border should be offset posteriorly from the skin incision.

Step 6

Mastoidectomy: A limited cortical mastoidectomy is performed under the operating microscope using a high-speed drill with cutting and diamond burrs. The tegmen and sigmoid sinus are identified first. Deepening of the dissection through Koerner's septum leads to identification of the lateral semicircular canal, antrum, and incus (Fig. 10.6).

Step 7

Facial recess: The facial recess is opened and entered, with preservation of the facial nerve posteriorly, the chorda tympani anteriorly, and the incus buttress superiorly

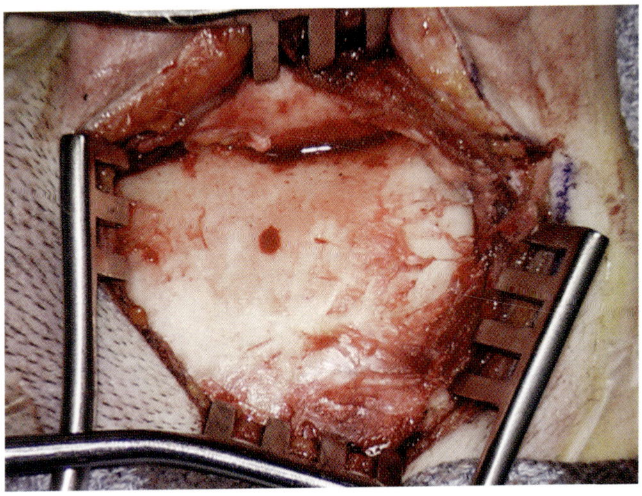

Fig. 10.5: Mastoid exposure. The soft tissues are elevated to expose the underlying mastoid bone, in preparation for drilling.

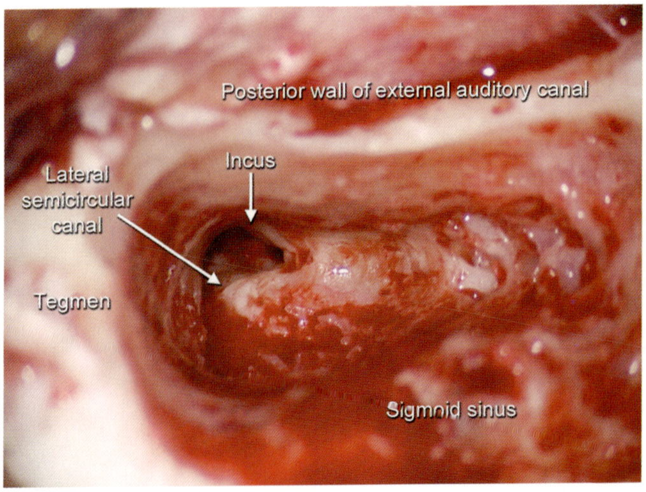

Fig. 10.6: Cortical mastoidectomy. A limited cortical mastoidectomy is performed with the borders defined by the tegmen superiorly, sigmoid sinus posteriorly, and posterior wall of the external auditory canal anteriorly. The antrum has been opened with identification of the lateral semicircular canal and incus.

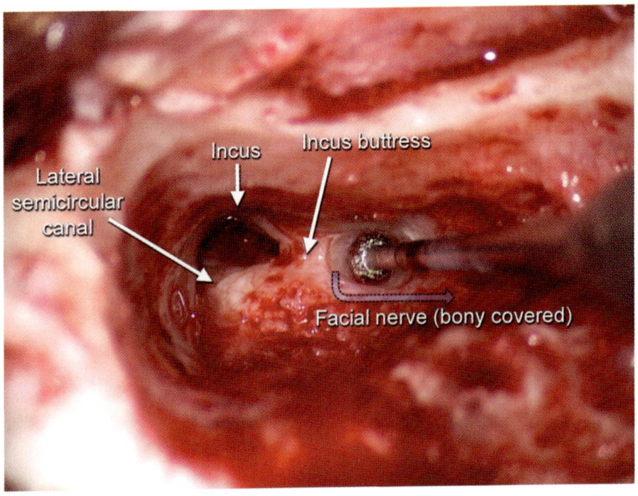

Fig. 10.7: Facial recess. The facial recess is opened with a small diamond drill, with care taken to preserve the facial nerve posteriorly and incus buttress superiorly.

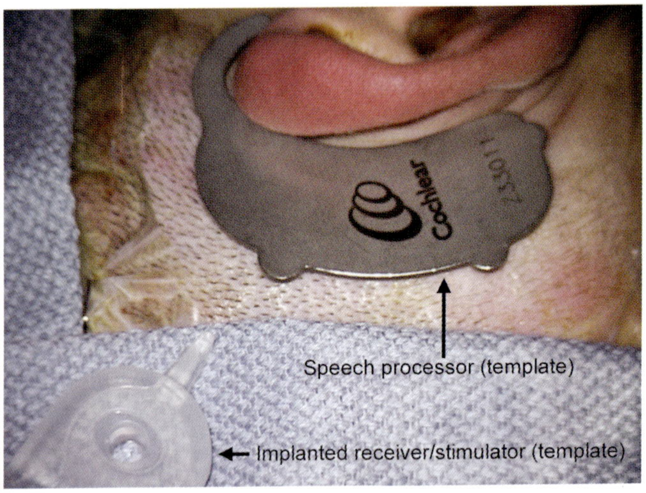

Fig. 10.8: Location of implanted receiver/stimulator. It is important to place the well for the receiver/stimulator far enough posteriorly and superiorly to the auricle, so that it will not overlap with the speech processor placed behind the ear after completion of surgery.

(Fig. 10.7). The recess is widened until the entire round window niche is visible. The short process of the incus points toward the facial recess and is a useful landmark for its identification. Occasionally, the chorda tympani is sacrificed to create enough room within the facial recess for cochlear implantation. If hearing preservation is not to be attempted, the incus buttress can be taken down and the incus removed to create additional exposure and to provide another landmark for identification of facial nerve (by tracing it from the readily visible tympanic segment to the descending segment).

Step 8

Drill the well: The periosteum is elevated posterior-superiorly from the sinodural angle to create a subperiosteal pocket for the well. It is important to place the well far enough posteriorly so that there will be room for the external transmitter to sit over the implanted receiver/stimulator when the speech processor is placed behind the ear (Fig. 10.8). The dummy templates for the speech processor and the implant can be used as a guide. A drill is used to create a bony well for the implant to prevent device migration, with a channel created from

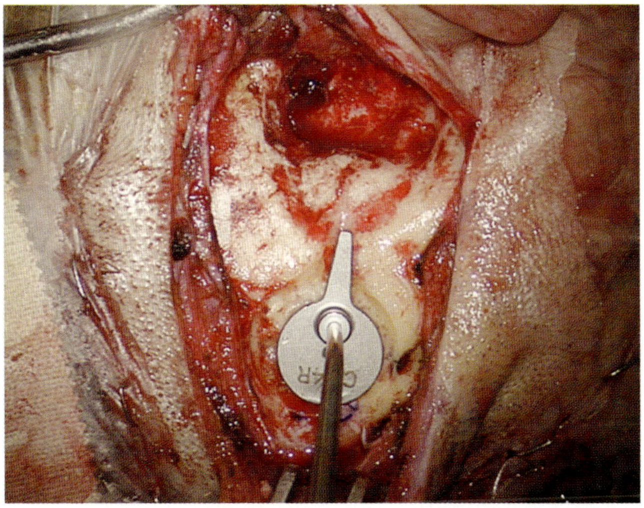

Fig. 10.9: The well. A well has been drilled into the bone behind the mastoid cavity. The template for both the receiver/stimulator and the channel extending anteriorly from it toward the mastoid cavity is shown in the figure.

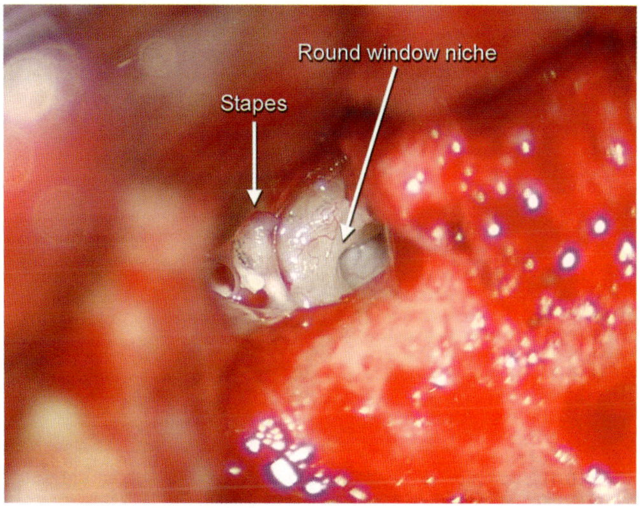

Fig. 10.10: The middle ear. Identification of the stapes (superiorly) and the round window niche (inferiorly) is shown. The view shown is similar to what would be seen through the facial recess. However, in this specific case, the posterior canal wall has been removed for improved visualization of the structures within the facial recess (Incidentally, note that the stapes is shown without its articulation to the incus).

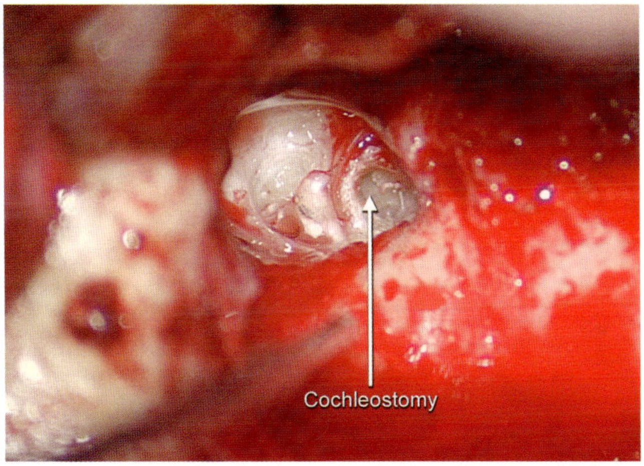

Fig. 10.11: Cochleostomy. After the round window niche has been drilled off, the cochleostomy is created extending anteriorly and inferiorly from the round window.

the well to the mastoid cavity for the electrode array (Fig. 10.9). In young children, it may be necessary to thin the bone of the well to the level of the dura for the implant to sit securely within it.

Step 9

Cochleostomy: Two general approaches through the facial recess may be considered for placement of the cochlear implant into the cochlea. The implant may be inserted directly through the round window, or a separate cochleostomy may be created in the basal turn of the cochlea. We prefer the cochleostomy approach, as this allows the implant to avoid having to take an initial sharp turn (at the hook region) within the cochlea. For the cochleostomy, a small diamond burr (1 mm) is used to remove the round window niche to allow for definitive identification of the round window (Fig. 10.10). The cochleostomy is then created anterior and inferior from the round window (Fig. 10.11).

The receiver/stimulator of the implant is placed into the well. The electrode array is then inserted into the cochlea (with the specific technique of insertion varying from manufacturer to manufacturer) using a two-handed technique, with a claw in one hand used to guide the tip into the cochlea and a forceps in the other used to advance the electrodes into the scala tympani. Ideally, a full insertion of the electrode array should be performed (Fig. 10.12). Several small pieces of fascia/muscle are placed around the array at the cochleostomy to secure the implant in place and seal the cochlea (Fig. 10.13). Any excess length of the electrode array is curled underneath bony ledges created superiorly and posteriorly within the lateral mastoid cavity to minimize the risk of device extrusion. If a separate ground electrode is present, it is placed into the zygomatic root, deep to the temporalis muscle.

In cases where hearing preservation is desired, a soft technique is used to perform the cochleostomy. Care is

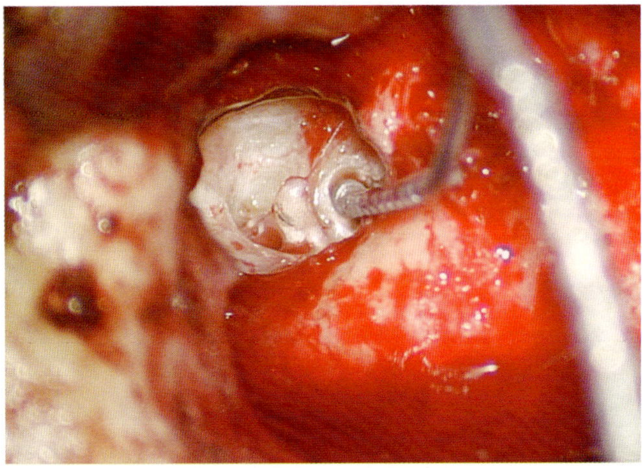

Fig. 10.12: Insertion of electrode array. A full insertion of the cochlear implant has been performed, with all electrodes placed within the cochlea.

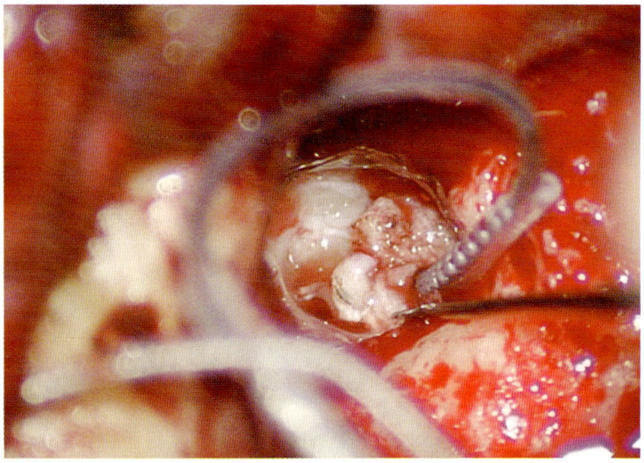

Fig. 10.13: Securing the array. A fascia/muscle plug is used to at the cochleostomy site to secure the electrode array in place.

taken to blue line the cochlea and avoid entry into the cochlea with the drill. A small rasp is used to enter the membranous cochlea and the electrodes are slowly inserted. ABR monitoring may be helpful for providing feedback to the surgeon about impending cochlear trauma during electrode insertion. Fascia is placed around the electrode array at the cochleostomy to seal the site in an expedient manner, and care is taken to avoid suctioning the perilymph.

Occasionally, intracochlear ossification may be encountered. This can be addressed by performing a drill out of the cochlea, past the site(s) of ossification. To facilitate the drill out, the posterior canal wall is taken down, and at the end of the case, the external auditory canal is closed off. It may be necessary to drill two separate cochleostomies, one at the basal turn and one at the apical turn, in which case a cochlear implant with a split electrode array is inserted. Additionally, intraoperative fluoroscopy may be helpful for confirmation of the correct electrode placement.

Intraoperative electrical testing of the implant can also be performed. This is especially important in children as the function of the implant can be confirmed and programming levels can be predetermined.

Step 10

Closure: Sutures placed in the soft tissue are generally used to secure the body of the implant against the bone. The Palva flap is then closed over the implant. The overlying soft tissue is sutured together in a separate layer and finally the skin is closed. If electrocautery is needed for hemostasis, it is important to use only bipolar cautery after the cochlear implantation has been performed, to avoid damage to the implant from monopolar cautery. A mastoid dressing is placed.

POSTOPERATIVE CARE

Cochlear implant surgery is performed on an outpatient basis. Postoperatively, patients receive a 1-week course of prophylactic oral antibiotics. Routine wound care instructions are given and sutures are removed 1 week after surgery.

The cochlear implant is turned on 1 month after surgery. Typically, multiple sessions are required over the first few months to adjust the settings on the implant. Patients typically experience improvement in their hearing over the course of months to years, with children continuing to improve throughout childhood.

COMPLICATIONS

Complications include all of the routine complications that can occur after surgery, including bleeding, infection, and wound breakdown. With respect to postoperative infections, these should be treated aggressively with antibiotics, to try to avoid colonization of the implant with bacteria and the need for explantation. Other complications specific to the ear include dizziness (usually transient), tinnitus (usually improved with the cochlear implant turned on), and facial weakness (rare).

A couple additional complications specifically related to the cochlear implant merit mentioning. The first is device failure. The internal components of cochlear implants are designed to last a lifetime, and overall, rates of device failure have been very low. However, over the years, there have been specific batches of cochlear implants that have been found to have defects that predispose to device failure. If device failure is suspected, reprogramming of the implant by the audiologist should first be performed before considering surgical removal of the implant. Also, if the cochlear implant fails to work from the initial hookup, CT imaging should be performed to confirm that the electrode array is in the right location. There have been reports of the implant being placed into the hypotympanic air cells, semicircular canals, or internal auditory canal, all of which result in device malfunction.

Another important complication is meningitis. Meningitis is a rare complication following cochlear implantation. Vaccination against *S. pneumoniae* is an important preventative measure, though it does not protect against meningitis from other strains of bacteria. In the past, there was one technique of cochlear electrode implantation, using a positioner with the electrode array, that led to a higher than expected rate of postoperative meningitis. This technique is no longer used and no current cochlear implants have such a positioner available for use during surgery.

FUTURE DEVELOPMENTS IN COCHLEAR IMPLANTS

One emerging area of research in cochlear implants is related to the benefits of residual hearing preservation in the implanted ear. While this residual hearing is generally quite poor, as patients who qualify for an implant are effectively deaf, research has nevertheless shown that when residual acoustic hearing (with a hearing aid) can be combined with electric hearing, patients have improved speech perception.[19] Numerous different types of electrode arrays have been designed with the goal of creating less trauma to the cochlea during surgical insertion, including arrays of different lengths, thicknesses, and contours. It is unclear at this time whether one array is better than another for hearing preservation, and results of hearing preservation are variable.

As bilateral cochlear implantation has become more widely accepted, attention has turned to other potential indications for cochlear implantation. These include cochlear implantation for the treatment of single-sided deafness and intractable tinnitus. (It is important to note that neither of these are currently a FDA approved indication for cochlear implantation). First, the use of a cochlear implant has the potential to restore true binaural hearing to patients with single-sided deafness. This is in contrast to the bone conduction devices or CROS hearing aids currently used for unilateral deafness, which only route sound from the deaf ear to the contralateral good cochlea. A number of small studies have demonstrated improvements in speech understanding in noise and sound localization from cochlear implants used to treat single-sided deafness, though more research is needed to substantiate these findings.[20] Second, cochlear implantation has also been advocated to treat severe, intractable unilateral tinnitus. Many patients who receive cochlear implants experience a decrease in their tinnitus from having the implant turned on.[21] However, the benefit is unpredictable and more research is needed to obtain a better understanding of what types of electrical stimulation may be most effective for the suppression of tinnitus.

REFERENCES

1. Waltzman SB, Cohen NL. Implantation of patients with prelingual long-term deafness. Ann Otol Rhinol Laryngol Suppl. 1999;177:84-7.
2. Geers AE, Nicholas JG. Enduring advantages of early cochlear implantation for spoken language development. J Speech Lang Hear Res. 2013;56:643-55.
3. Manrique M, Cervera-Paz FJ, Huarte A, et al. Advantages of cochlear implantation in prelingual deaf children before 2 years of age when compared with later implantation. Laryngoscope. 2004;114:1462-9.
4. Niparko JK, Tobey EA, Thal DJ, et al. Spoken language development in children following cochlear implantation. JAMA. 2010;303:1498-506.
5. Kontorinis G, Goetz F, Giourgas A, et al. Aplasia of the cochlea: radiologic assessment and options for hearing rehabilitation. Otol Neurotol. 2013;34:1253-60.
6. Kutz JW, Jr, Lee KH, Isaacson B, et al. Cochlear implantation in children with cochlear nerve absence or deficiency. Otol Neurotol. 2011;32:956-61.
7. Zanetti D, Guida M, Barezzani MG, et al. Favorable outcome of cochlear implant in VIIIth nerve deficiency. Otol Neurotol. 2006;27:815-23.
8. Friedland DR, Venick HS, Niparko JK. Choice of ear for cochlear implantation: the effect of history and residual hearing on predicted postoperative performance. Otol Neurotol. 2003;24:582-9.
9. Azadarmaki R, Tubbs R, Chen DA, et al. MRI information for commonly used otologic implants: review and update. Otolaryngol Head Neck Surg. 2014;150(4):512-9.
10. Basura GJ, Eapen R, Buchman CA. Bilateral cochlear implantation: current concepts, indications, and results. Laryngoscope. 2009;119:2395-401.

11. Lammers MJ, Venekamp RP, Grolman W, et al. Bilateral cochlear implantation in children and the impact of the inter-implant interval. Laryngoscope. 2014;124(4)993-9.
12. Lammers MJ, Grolman W, Smulders YE, et al. The cost-utility of bilateral cochlear implantation: a systematic review. Laryngoscope. 2011;121:2604-9.
13. Peters BR, Wyss J, Manrique M. Worldwide trends in bilateral cochlear implantation. Laryngoscope. 2010;120 (Suppl 2): S17-44.
14. Merdad M, Wolter N, Cushing S, et al. Surgical efficiency in bilateral cochlear implantation: a cost analysis. Cochlear Implants Int. 2014;15(1):43-7.
15. Ramsden JD, Papaioannou V, Gordon KA, et al. Parental and program's decision making in paediatric simultaneous bilateral cochlear implantation: who says no and why? Int J Pediatr Otorhinolaryngol. 2009;73:1325-8.
16. Baranano CF, Sweitzer RS, Mahalak ML, et al. The management of myringotomy tubes in pediatric cochlear implant recipients. Arch Otolaryngol Head Neck Surg. 2010;136: 557-60.
17. Kennedy RJ, Shelton C. Ventilation tubes and cochlear implants: what do we do? Otol Neurotol. 2005;26:438-41.
18. Baranano CF, Kopelovich JC, Dunn CC, et al. Subtotal petrosectomy and mastoid obliteration in adult and pediatric cochlear implant recipients. Otol Neurotol. 2013;34: 1656-9.
19. Incerti PV, Ching TY, Cowan R. A systematic review of electric-acoustic stimulation: device fitting ranges, outcomes, and clinical fitting practices. Trends Amplif. 2013;17:3-26.
20. Hansen MR, Gantz BJ, Dunn C. Outcomes after cochlear implantation for patients with single-sided deafness, including those with recalcitrant Meniere's disease. Otol Neurotol. 2013;34:1681-7.
21. Arts RA, George EL, Stokroos RJ, et al. Review: cochlear implants as a treatment of tinnitus in single-sided deafness. Curr Opin Otolaryngol Head Neck Surg. 2012;20: 398-403.

CHAPTER

11 Surgery for Neoplasms of the Posterior Fossa and Skull Base

Michael J LaRouere, Brent J Benscoter

INTRODUCTION

The most common lesions encountered in the posterior fossa include acoustic neuromas (90%), meningiomas (3%), epidermoids (3%), and facial nerve neuromas (1%). Other rare lesions make up the remaining 3% including arachnoid cysts, hemangiomas, paragangliomas, ependymomas, choroid plexus tumors, and primary nerve sheath tumors.[1]

Acoustic neuromas occur in about 1/100,000 individuals, are slow growing at a rate of 1–2 mm per year and are almost always benign. Over 95% are unilateral. Type II neurofibromatosis, a rare disorder localized to a gene on chromosome 22, is characterized by bilateral acoustic neuromas in 96–97% of cases.[2]

The most common symptoms of acoustic neuromas in order of occurrence are sensorineural hearing loss, tinnitus, imbalance, and facial numbness. Ironically, about 5% of patients have normal hearing irrespective of tumor size.[3]

Magnetic resonance imaging (MRI) with gadolinium is the gold standard diagnostic study for acoustic neuromas. ABR testing, although helpful in diagnosing acoustic neuromas, has been shown to have a false negative rate of 20–30% for small tumors and a false positive rate of 10%.[4]

Meningioma, the second most common cerebellopontine angle (CPA) tumor, can usually be diagnosed by its imaging characteristics. These include, on MRI scanning, (1) a dural tail and (2) localized to the porous with minimal to no internal auditory canal extension (although full extension can occur). On CT scanning, meningiomas can be calcified and show hyperostotic bone adjacent to the tumor.[5] Meningiomas and acoustic neuromas cannot be differentiated from each other based on audiologic and vestibular testing.

Epidermoids are primary cholesteatomas of the cerebellopontine angle. They cause neural deficits due to pressure on adjacent cranial nerves. Facial twitching or paralysis is much more common with epidermoids compared to acoustic neuromas or meningiomas. MRI scans are the most accurate diagnostic test. T1 images show the lesion to be hypointense and T2 images show hyperintensity. Diffusion weighted images show restricted diffusion (the epidermoid is bright) as opposed to an arachnoid cyst which is dark.[5]

Glomus tumors are the most common secondary tumor involving the posterior fossa. The most common symptoms of glomus tumors include pulsatile tinnitus and conductive hearing loss.[6] Late symptoms of cranial nerve dysfunction can occur. Cranial nerves IX, X, XI, and XII as well as cranial nerve VII can all be affected.

Again, imaging can best diagnose glomus tumors. MRI scans show a typical salt and pepper appearance due to flow voids in the lesion. CT scans are of paramount importance, showing disruption of the jugular fossa (as opposed to glomus tympanicum tumors). Irregular borders are the norm as opposed to jugular foramen schwannomas which demonstrate smooth borders. CT angiograms have become a very useful tool in diagnosing glomus tumors giving both bony and vascular information. Angiography is useful in diagnosing and managing these tumors especially when preoperative embolization is desired.[7]

SURGERY FOR CPA TUMORS

There are multiple approaches used in removing tumors of the cerebellopontine angle and internal auditory canal (IAC). Each has specific indications and risks associated with their selection. Approaches include translabyrinthine, retrosigmoid, middle cranial fossa, and extended middle cranial fossa. Other less often used but versatile approaches include retrolabyrinthine, transpetrosal, transcochlear, and transotic approaches.

The translabyrinthine approach is the workhorse approach for neurotologists in removing cerebellopontine angle tumors. Although loss of hearing is a given, the approach offers the best chance of facial nerve preservation and the least amount of cerebellar retraction. It is an excellent approach for medium to large tumors as well as smaller tumors with poor hearing.[8]

The retrosigmoid approach is used for tumors of the cerebellopontine angle that do not go into the internal auditory canal or have limited extension into the IAC with serviceable hearing.[9] In addition to the ability to preserve hearing, the retrosigmoid approach offers a wide view from the tentorium to the foramen magnum. The disadvantages include more cerebellar retraction than the translabyrinthine approach and postoperative headaches.

The middle cranial fossa approach is utilized for patients with good hearing whose tumors are confined to the internal auditory canal or fill the internal auditory canal with slight (<1 cm) cerebellopontine angle extension. Because of the presence of the facial nerve superiorly, there is a greater risk of facial nerve dysfunction both short and long term with this approach. There is also temporal lobe retraction that can lead to aphasia or seizures. This procedure is not usually performed on patients older than 65.[10] The extended middle cranial fossa approach involves removing bone over the internal auditory canal and anteriorly up to the foramen lacerum and cavernous sinus. It is best suited for lesions of the petroclival region in patients with useful hearing.

The retrolabyrinthine approach involves a wide mastoidectomy with exposure of the posterior fossa dura between the sigmoid sinus and the posterior semicircular canal. Hearing preservation is a goal of this procedure. It can be used for vestibular nerve section or microvascular decompression and can also be used for nonacoustic lesions affecting the posterior fossa.

Other approaches to the cerebellopontine angle include the transpetrosal approaches. These approaches involve combining a middle cranial fossa approach with either a retrolabyrinthine or retrosigmoid approach. The transpetrosal approaches are most often used for patients with petroclival lesions who have serviceable hearing. The superior petrosal vein is ligated. Care must be taken to preserve the vein of Labbé so as to avoid a temporal lobe venous infarct. Also damage to the IVth cranial nerve can occur when dividing the tentorium.[11]

The transcochlear approach is an extension of the translabyrinthine approach with displacement of the facial nerve posteriorly and removal of the cochlea. The external auditory canal is over sewn. This approach is most often used for petroclival meningiomas, extensive epidermoids and squamous cell carcinomas of the temporal bone.[12] The transotic approach is similar to the transcochlear approach but the facial nerve is not transposed. This approach is used for lesions extending to the clivus and for large acoustic neuromas associated with a high jugular bulb.[12]

The infratemporal fossa (type A) approach is the most utilized procedure for removing glomus jugulare tumors.[3] It involves an upper neck dissection identifying the lower cranial nerves as they enter the jugular foramen and ligating the internal jugular vein. A canal wall down mastoidectomy is performed with overclosure of the ear canal. The facial nerve can be transposed anteriorly or can be kept in the fallopian canal and tumor removed around it with stimulus dissectors. The sigmoid sinus is usually externally compressed prior to opening the jugular bulb. Intradural tumor extension is generally handled by a second-stage surgery.

SURGICAL TECHNIQUE

Translabyrinthine Approach

Exposure

Step 1: A wide postauricular incision is made in a curvilinear manner approximately two finger breadths behind the postauricular crease and carried down to the mastoid cortex and temporalis fascia. Soft tissue is reflected to the posterior ear canal and periosteum over the mastoid is harvested to pack the middle ear and eustachian tube. A large piece of temporalis fascia is harvested for later graft use (Fig. 11.1).

Step 2: A simple mastoidectomy is performed with wide beveling. The epitympanum is opened and the incus and malleus head are removed. A simple maneuver with a small hook placed between the body of the incus and the head of the malleus and pulling up and back removes

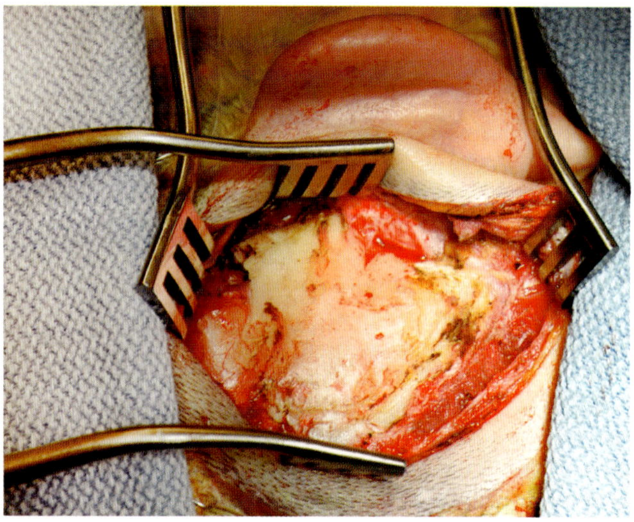

Fig. 11.1: Right postauricular incision carried down to mastoid cortex with soft tissue reflected to the external auditory canal.

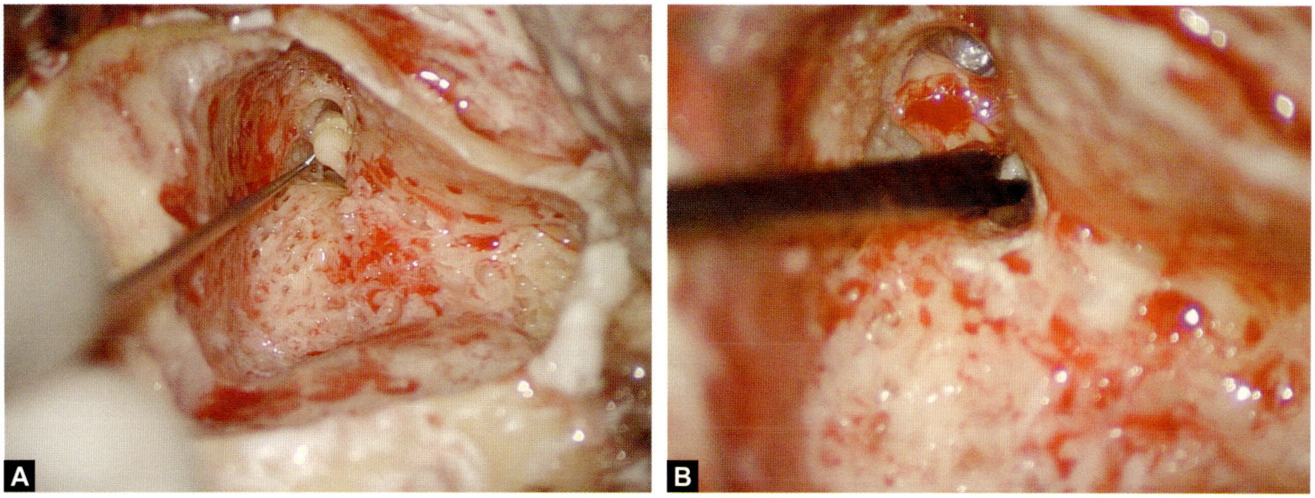

Figs. 11.2A and B: (A) Right mastoidectomy performed. A medium hook is used to remove the incus. (B) The tensor tendon is cut with scissors exposing the middle ear.

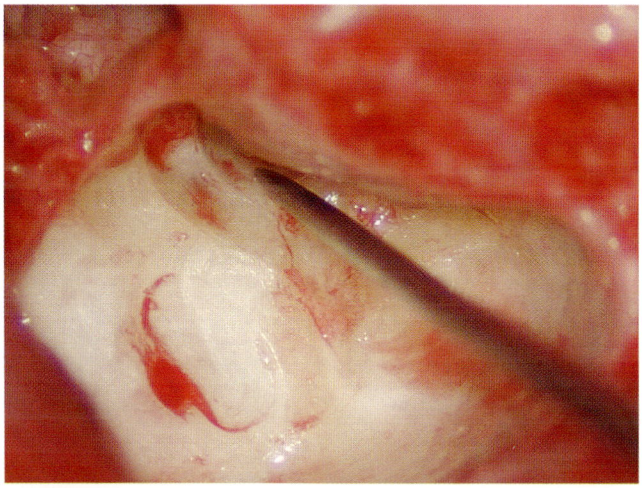

Fig. 11.3: A complete labyrinthectomy is performed. The pointer is in the spherical recess of the saccule.

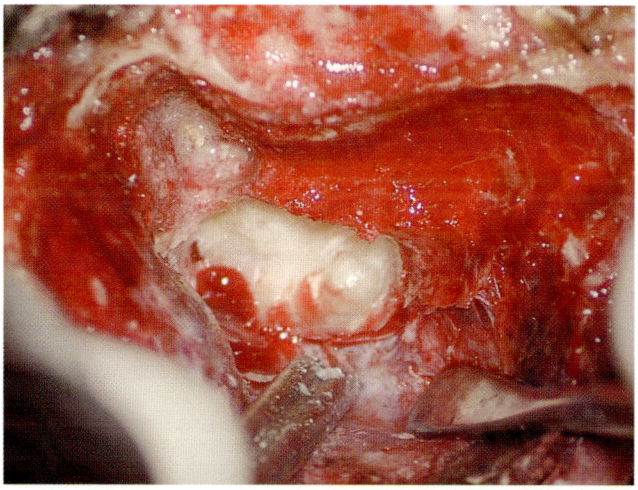

Fig. 11.4: Bone is removed over the middle and posterior fossa dura including the sigmoid sinus with diamond burrs.

the incus without dislocating the stapes. The neck of the malleus is exposed and cut with a malleus nipper. The tensor tendon is cut (Figs. 11.2A and B).

Step 3: A complete labyrinthectomy is performed exposing all three semicircular canals and the vestibule. Care is taken to achieve good exposure of the spherical recess of the saccule to allow for more lateral exposure of the internal auditory canal (Fig. 11.3).

Step 4: Bone is removed from over the middle cranial fossa and posterior cranial fossa dura and sigmoid sinus. Bipolar cautery over the sigmoid sinus and dura can shrink these structures to allow broader visualization for drilling. Care is taken to preserve the superior petrosal sinus (Fig. 11.4).

Step 5: Skeletonization of the internal auditory canal is the last step in drilling. Bone is removed approximately 270° around the internal auditory canal. The falciform crest, the bone between the superior and inferior vestibular nerves, is preserved. Due to the steep incline of the IAC, much more bone is removed near the porous than near the fundus of the IAC. We generally leave an eggshell of bone over the IAC until the IAC is fully exposed and then the thin bone is removed with a small hook (Fig. 11.5). The facial nerve can be identified just deep to Bills Bar in the superior lateral portion of the fundus. This is generally done with a stimulating microhook set at 0.05 m amps. We have also been decompressing the facial nerve in its labyrinthine segment allowing for better identification

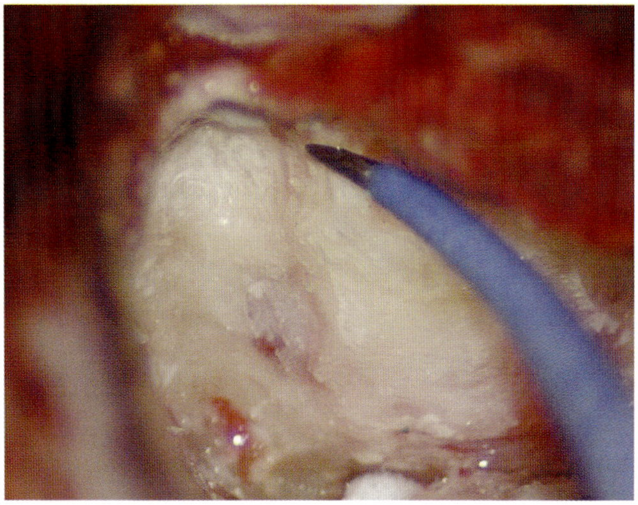

Fig. 11.5: Bone is removed over the internal auditory canal. A thin eggshell of bone is left over the internal auditory canal and is removed last.

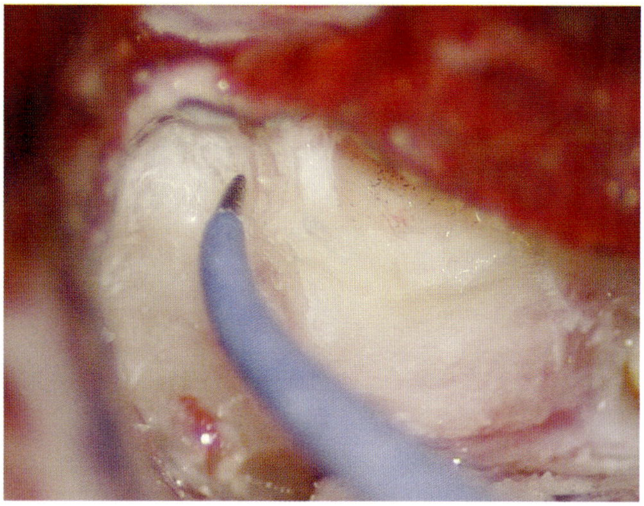

Fig. 11.6: The facial nerve is decompressed at the meatal foramen. This allows for identification of the nerve and may allow for a lower incidence of delayed facial paralysis.

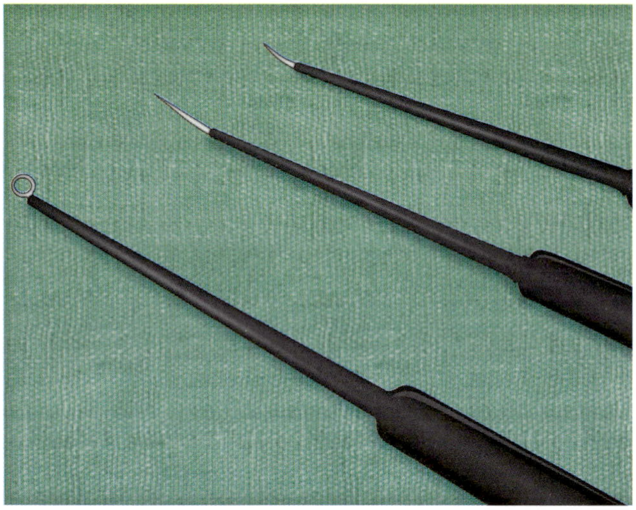

Fig. 11.7: Kartush stimulus dissectors, insulated to the tip, allow for simultaneous dissection and stimulation.

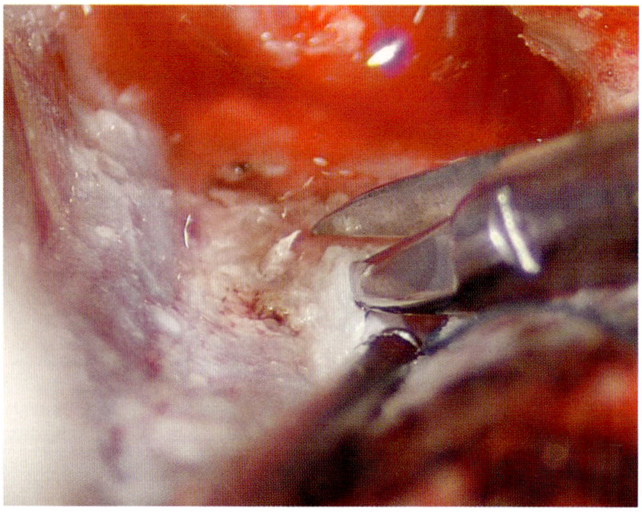

Fig. 11.8: Opening the posterior fossa dura from the sigmoid sinus to the internal auditory canal.

of the nerve and possibly reducing the incidence of postoperative delayed facial paresis secondary to swelling of the facial nerve in the area of the meatal foramen (Fig. 11.6).

Tumor Removal

Tumor removal is performed in several stages in order to maximize tumor removal as well as facial nerve preservation. In our practice, Kartush-stimulating dissectors (Fig. 11.7) are routinely used. These instruments are insulated except at their tip, allowing continuous facial nerve monitoring while dissecting.

Step 1: The dura over the posterior fossa is incised and cerebrospinal fluid is suctioned, allowing for decompression of the contents of the posterior fossa. Care is taken to incise the dura over the IAC with stimulus dissectors (Fig. 11.8).

Step 2: The tumor is stimulated on its posterior surface and an incision is made in its capsule. The tumor is debulked while maintaining the integrity of the tumor capsule. This allows the tumor to collapse on itself (Fig. 11.9).

Step 3: Tumor capsule is removed from the brainstem. Small vessels entering the tumor are coagulated with bipolar cautery. The cochleovestibular nerve is identified.

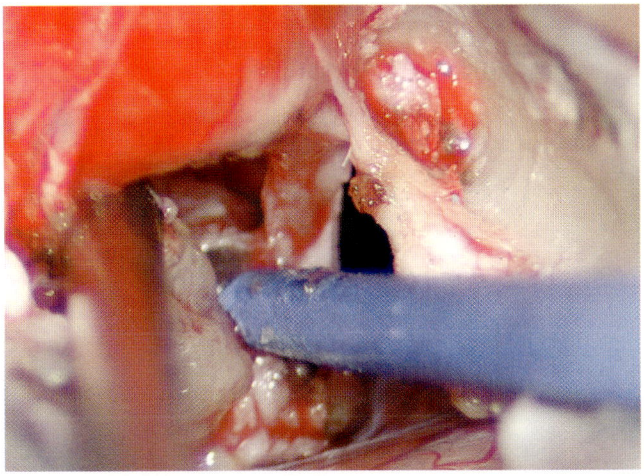

Fig. 11.9: The tumor capsule is opened on its posterior surface and the inside is gutted with stimulus dissectors with care to preserve the capsule.

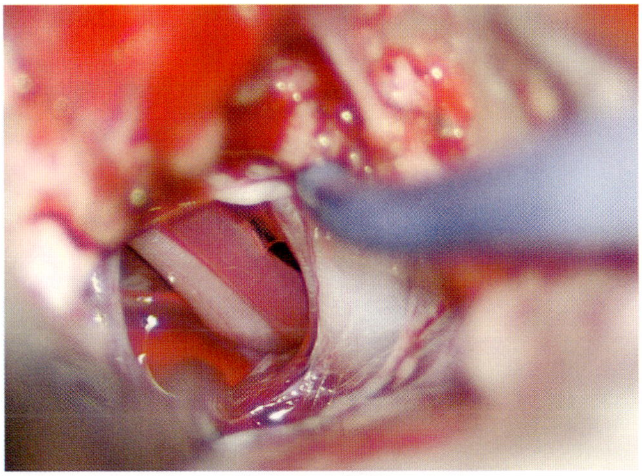

Fig. 11.10: The cochlear nerve (foreground) and the facial nerve (deep) are often separated by a loop of the AICA at the root entry zone.

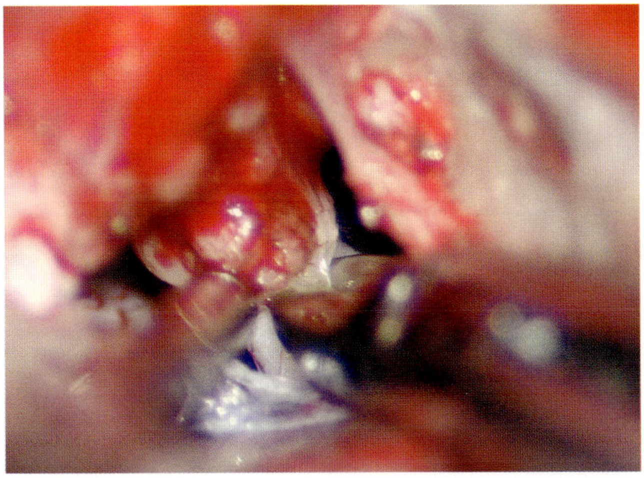

Fig. 11.11: The cochleovestibular nerve is sectioned at the brainstem.

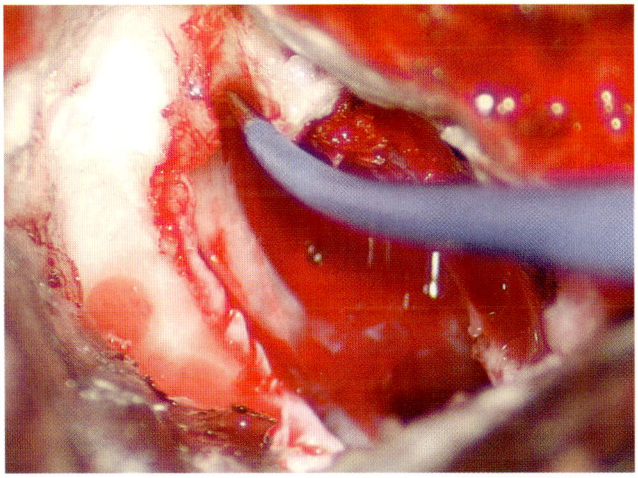

Fig. 11.12: The facial nerve is located laterally with the use of stimulus dissectors and the anatomical landmark of Bills Bar.

The facial nerve is located deep to the cochleovestibular nerve. Many times a branch of the anterior inferior cerebellar artery (AICA) is found between the two nerves (Fig. 11.10). The cochleovestibular nerve is then sectioned (Fig. 11.11). Tumor is then removed off the facial nerve from a medial to lateral direction with stimulus dissectors.

Step 4: The superior vestibular nerve is sectioned at the fundus and the facial nerve is isolated beneath it using Bill's Bar as an anatomical dividing landmark (Fig. 11.12). The tumor is gently reflected medially exposing the intracanalicular portion of the facial nerve.

Step 5: Tumor is finally removed from around the facial nerve at the porous using stimulus dissectors with the ability to follow the facial nerve from both a medial and lateral direction. The tumor/facial nerve plane is most obscure at the porous. It is in this region that facial nerve injury could occur (Fig. 11.13).

Closure

Step 1: The middle ear and eustachian tube are packed with fascia. A large fascia graft is placed over the antrum and bone wax is used to occlude any remaining mastoid air cells (Fig. 11.14).

Step 2: Hemostasis is checked by having anesthesia hold positive pressure and the CPA examined. An abdominal fat graft is then placed in the mastoid cavity and secured in place with 2-0 Vicryl sutures in a hammock technique (Fig. 11.15).

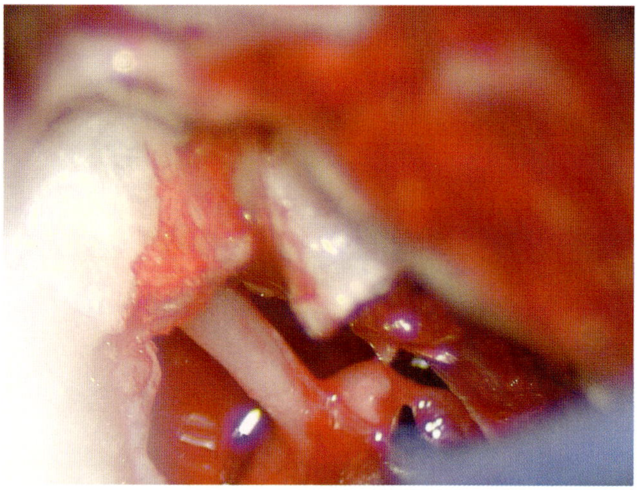

Fig. 11.13: The last portion of tumor is removed off the facial nerve at the porus acusticus, where the facial nerve is often splayed. A benefit of the translabyrinthine approach is that the facial nerve can be isolated both medially and laterally and tumor removed in between.

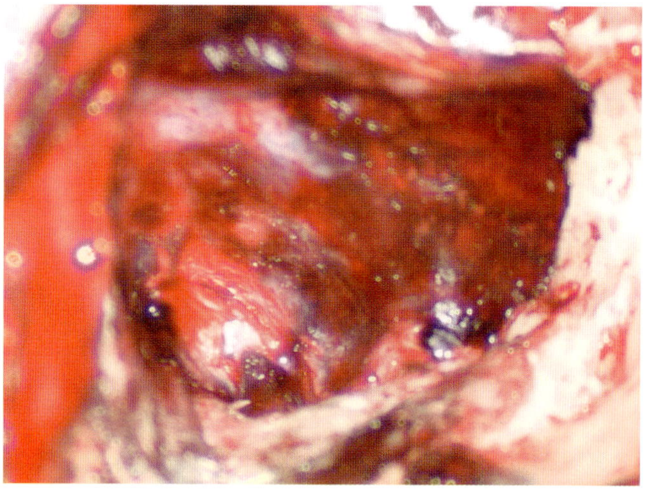

Fig. 11.14: A large fascia graft is placed over the antrum after the middle ear is packed with fascia.

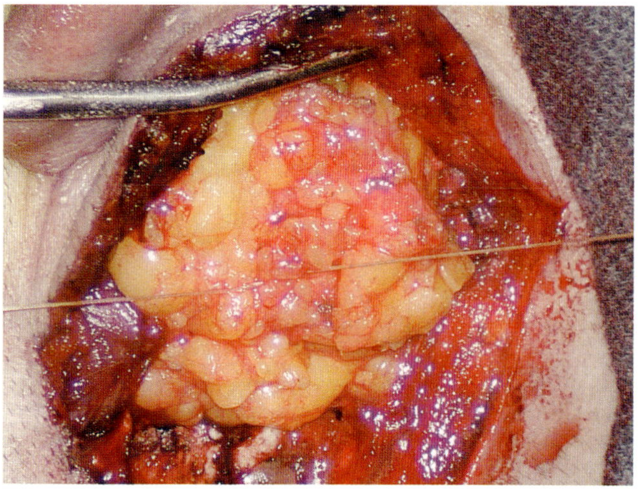

Fig. 11.15: An abdominal fat graft is placed in the mastoid cavity and sutured in place.

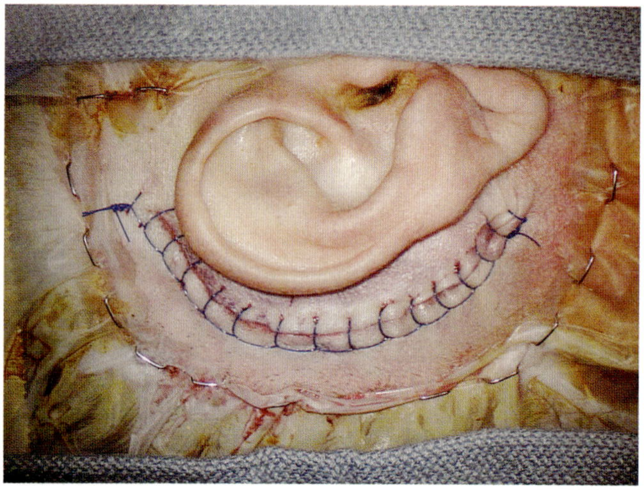

Fig. 11.16: Skin is closed with a running interlocking stitch of 2-0 Prolene.

Step 3: The wound is then closed in layers with 2-0 Vicryl in the subcutaneous tissue and 2-0 Prolene interlocking in the skin (Fig. 11.16). A pressure dressing is then applied.

Retrosigmoid Craniotomy

Exposure

Step 1: A wide postauricular C-shaped incision is made approximately three to four finger breadths behind the postauricular crease (Fig. 11.17). A fascia/muscle flap that is based inferiorly is created over the mastoid region.

Step 2: Bone is removed over the sigmoid sinus and lateral sinus. Bone is removed further posterior to the sigmoid sinus and inferior to lateral sinus exposing the posterior fossa dura (Fig. 11.18). Currently, we do not save a bone plug for later use.

Step 3: A curvilinear incision is made in the dura inferior to lateral sinus and posterior to the sigmoid sinus reflecting the dura posteriorly. Care is taken to leave a cuff of dura just posterior to the sigmoid sinus for closure (Fig. 11.19). The cisterna magna is immediately identified and cerebrospinal fluid is drained to allow retraction of the cerebellum.

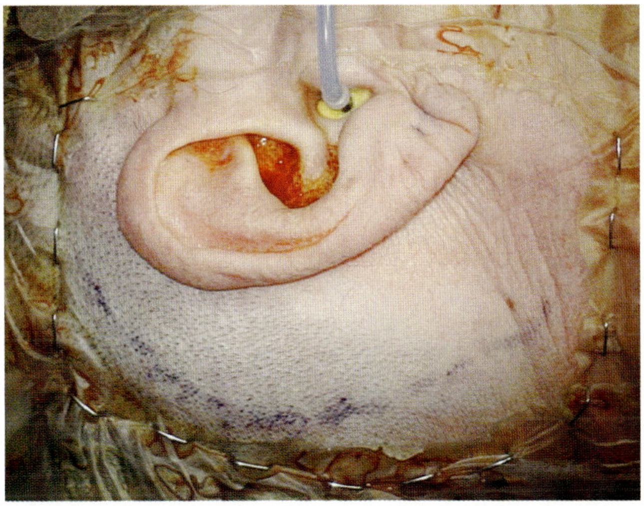

Fig. 11.17: For a retrosigmoid craniotomy a wide postauricular incision is made. Note the insert earphone for ABR monitoring.

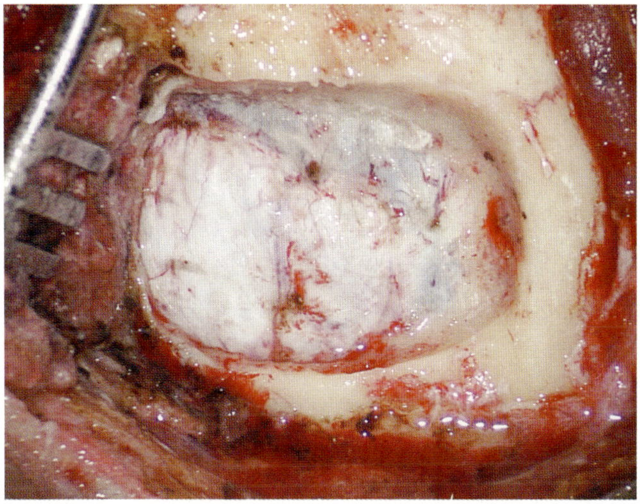

Fig. 11.18: Bone is removed over the sigmoid and lateral sinuses and inferior to the lateral sinus, posterior to the sigmoid sinus.

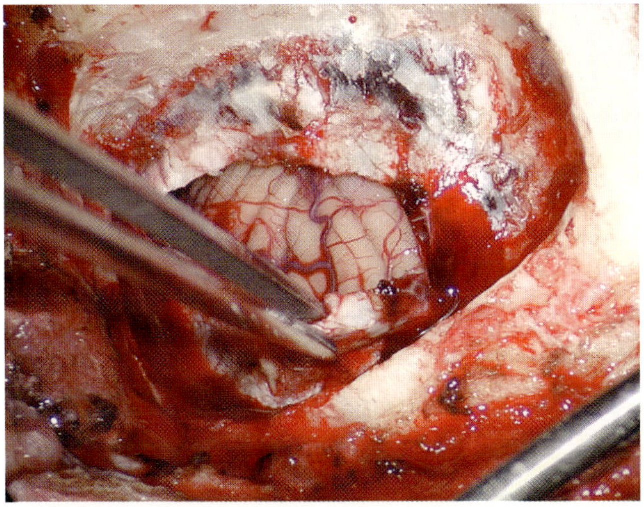

Fig. 11.19: A curvilinear incision is made in the dura and the dura is reflected posteriorly. An initial incision is made inferiorly and the cisterna magna drained to allow cerebellar relaxation.

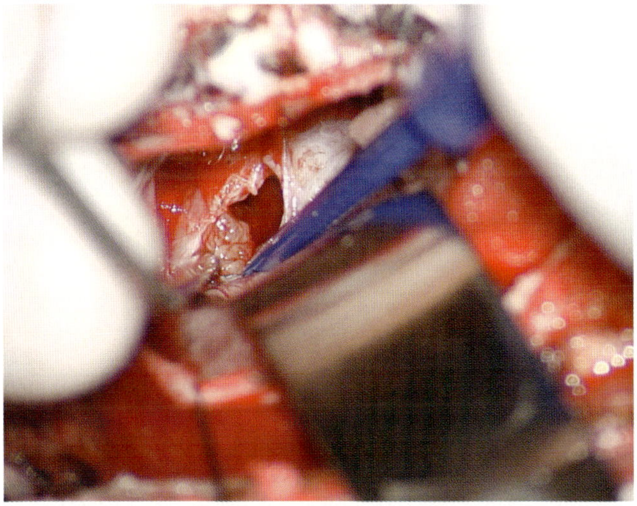

Fig. 11.20: The cerebellum is gently retracted. Bicol is placed under the retractor to protect the cerebellum.

Tumor Removal

Step 1: Tumor removal and identification of the VIIth and VIIIth cranial nerves at the brainstem are similar to that of the translabyrinthine approach. A retractor is used to gently compress the cerebellum. Bicol (a collagenous material) is placed between the retractor and cerebellum to prevent cerebellar injury (Fig. 11.20).

Step 2: Approaching the IAC from the medial direction involves creating a dural flap over the internal auditory canal based posteriorly with care taken to preserve the endolymphatic sac (Fig. 11.21). The internal auditory canal is drilled out medial to laterally exposing the tumor. The lateral extent of drilling is stopped when either the lateral extent of the tumor is identified or just as the posterior semicircular canal is blue lined (Fig. 11.22).

Step 3: Tumor is then removed from the internal auditory canal similar to the translabyrinthine approach except that the facial nerve can best be isolated with the use of stimulus dissectors going from a medial to lateral direction.

Closure

Step 1: The internal auditory canal is packed with muscle and the dural flap replaced. Any exposed air cells are closed with bone wax (Fig. 11.23).

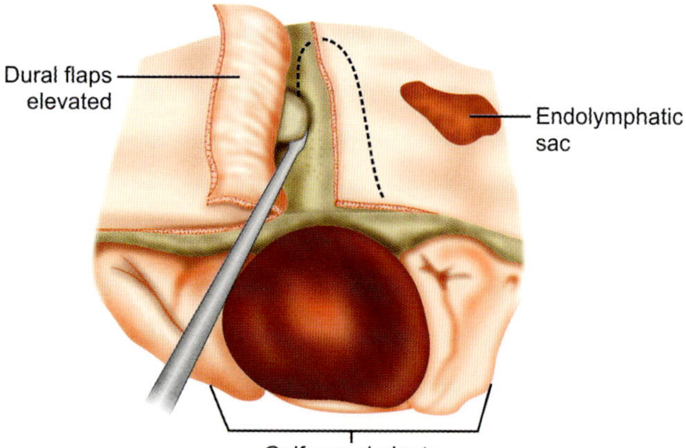

Fig. 11.21: Dural flaps are elevated over the petrous ridge protecting the endolymphatic sac.

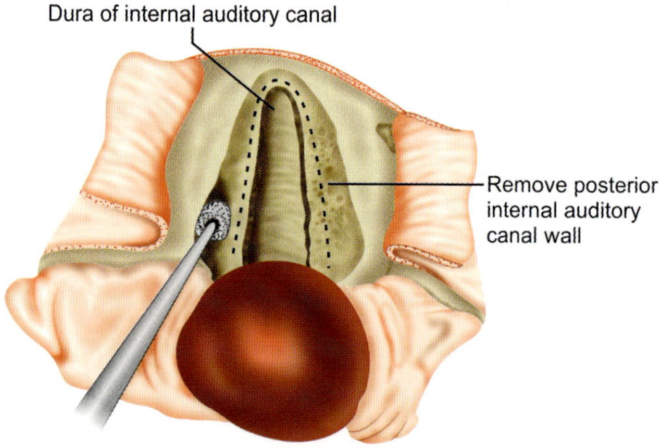

Fig. 11.22: The internal auditory canal is drilled out with small diamond burs with care to protect the endolymphatic duct and posterior semicircular canal.

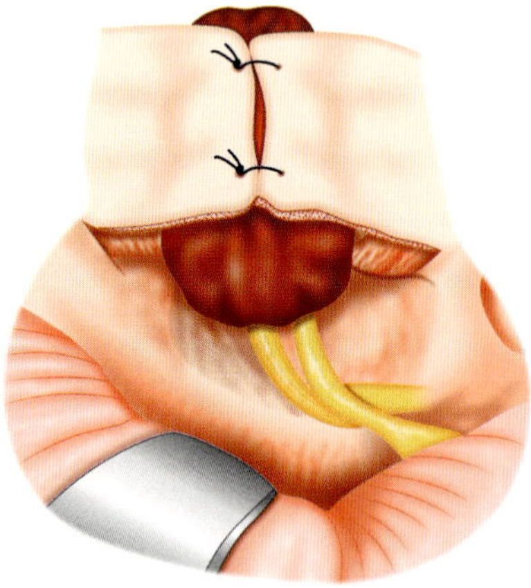

Fig. 11.23: The internal auditory canal is packed with muscle after tumor removal. The dura may or may not be able to be closed. Any exposed air cells are bone waxed.

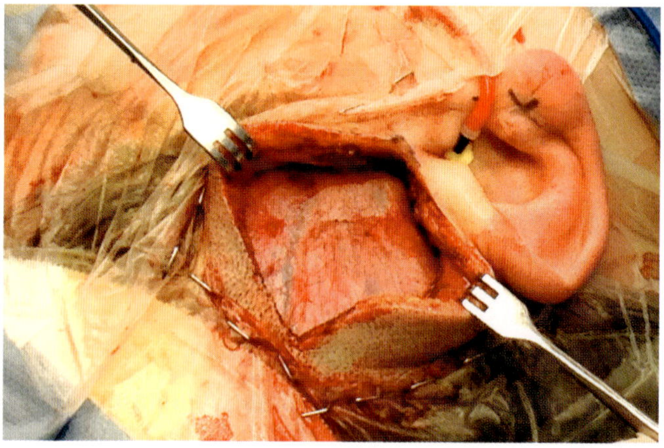

Fig. 11.24: A preauricular incision is carried up in the temporal area exposing the fascia of the temporalis muscle.

Step 2: The posterior fossa dura is closed with 4-0 Nurolon and any exposed mastoid air cells are occluded with bone wax.

Step 3: Artificial dura is placed over the dural incision and abdominal fat is placed over this. The muscle fascia flap is then reapproximated and the subcutaneous tissue and skin are closed with 2-0 Vicryl and 2-0 Prolene, respectively, using a running interlocking stitch. A pressure dressing is applied.

Middle Cranial Fossa Approach

Exposure

Step 1: A pre- or postauricular incision is made and carried upward into the temporal area of the scalp (Fig. 11.24).

Step 2: A large piece of temporalis fascia is harvested and the temporalis muscle is split (Fig. 11.25).

Step 3: A 5 × 5 cm craniotomy is made two-thirds anterior to the external ear canal and one-third posterior to the external auditory canal with small cutting and diamond burs and the bone flap is saved. Care is taken to make the inferior cut of the bone flap just above the external canal paralleling the floor of the middle cranial fossa (Fig. 11.26).

Step 4: The dura is gently retracted medially exposing the floor of the middle cranial fossa. To allow for good exposure, many times the middle meningeal artery is bipolared and divided. The foramen spinosum is packed with bone wax. The geniculate ganglion is many times exposed and should be positively identified with stimulus dissectors (Fig. 11.27).

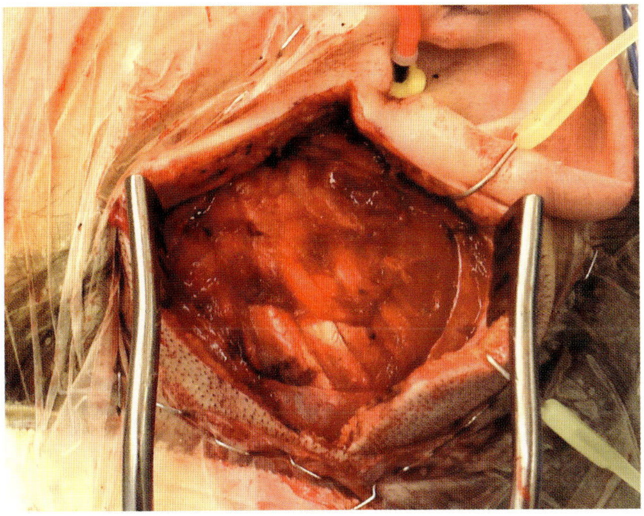

Fig. 11.25: A large piece of temporalis fascia is harvested for later use.

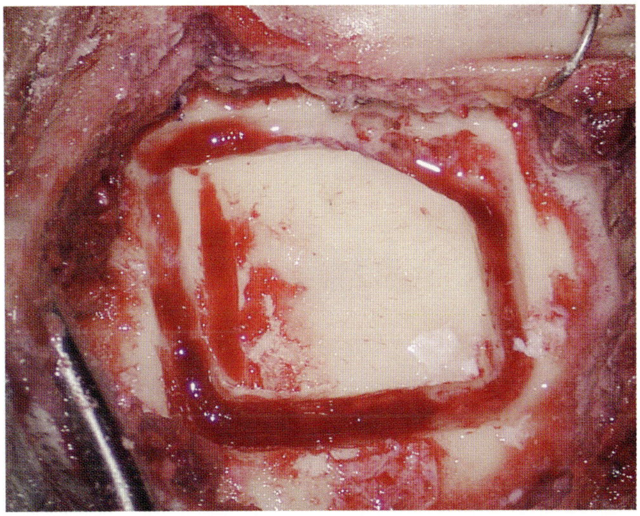

Fig. 11.26: A 5 x 5 cm bone flap is created above the external auditory canal with the anterior portion of the flap centered two-thirds anterior to the external auditory canal.

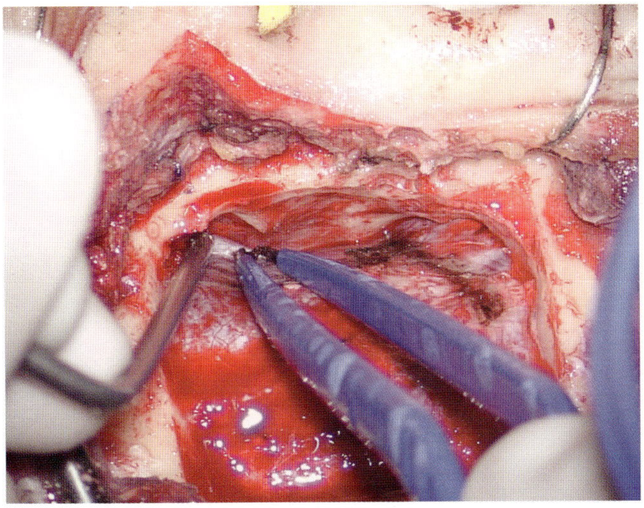

Fig. 11.27: The temporal lobe dura is retracted medially exposing the floor of the middle cranial fossa.

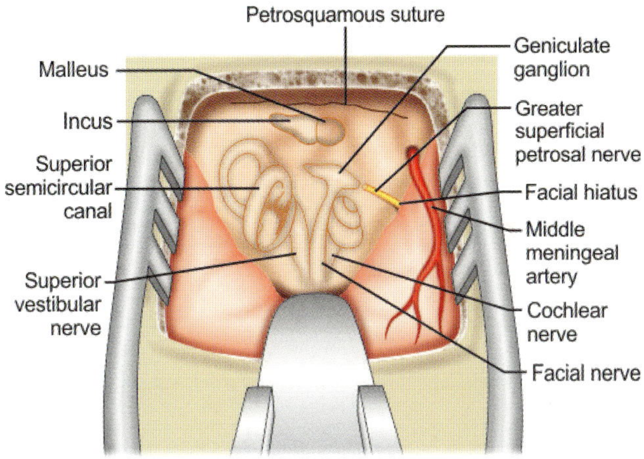

Fig. 11.28: The greater superficial petrosal nerve is identified at the facial hiatus with stimulus dissectors. The ampullated end of the superior semicircular canal is 1 cm posterior and 0.5 cm medial to the facial hiatus.

Step 5: The greater superficial petrosal nerve is isolated by stimulus dissectors and direct vision. The facial hiatus is identified. The ampullated end of the superior semicircular canal is routinely found 1 cm posterior and 0.5 cm medial to the facial hiatus. The arcuate eminence is often but not always coincidental with the superior semicircular canal (Fig. 11.28).

Step 6: The internal auditory canal is found by first blue lining the superior semicircular canal. Bone is then removed with diamond burs around the internal auditory canal from a medial to lateral direction, thereby avoiding damage to the superior semicircular canal and cochlea. Much more bone is removed medially (safe area) as opposed to laterally (Fig. 11.29).

Step 7: The labyrinthine segment of the facial nerve is usually decompressed to allow for facial nerve identification and postoperative swelling to occur. This segment of the facial nerve appears to be in a somewhat vertical plane and curves slightly anteriorly toward the geniculate ganglion (Fig. 11.30).

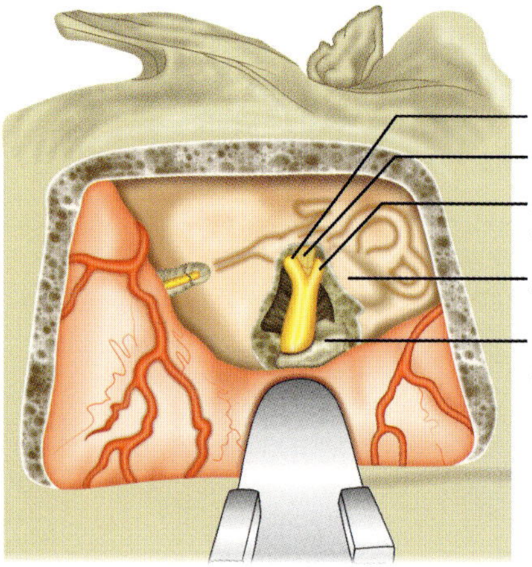

Fig. 11.29: The internal auditory canal is drilled out with diamond burs with wider exposure medially. Care is taken to preserve the superior semicircular canal and cochlea.

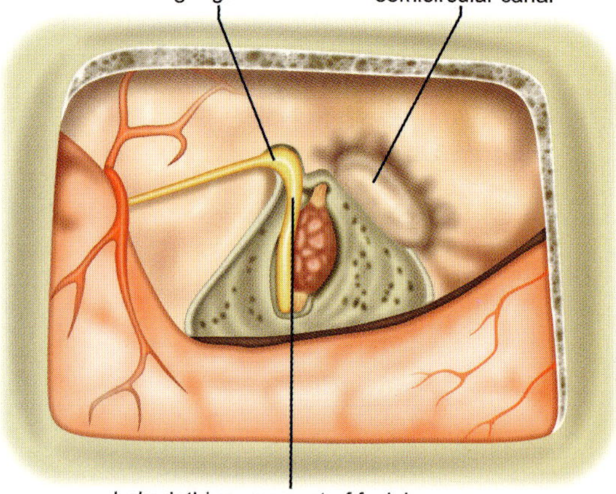

Fig. 11.30: The labyrinthine segment of the facial nerve is usually decompressed to allow for identification and postoperative swelling to occur. This may prevent postoperative facial paresis due to swelling at the meatal foramen.

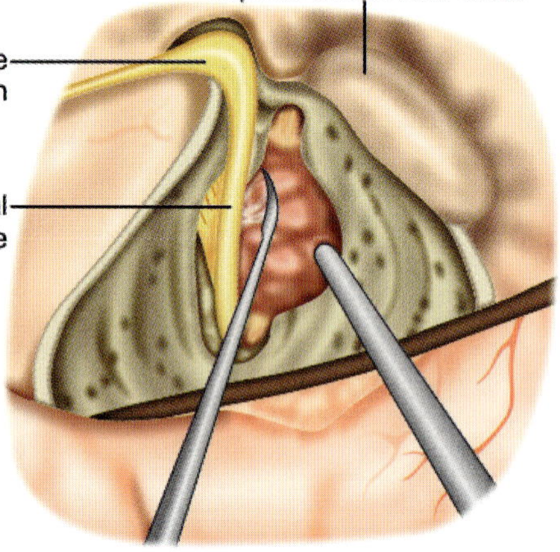

Fig. 11.31: Tumor is removed with stimulus dissectors with care to preserve the cochlear nerve and artery. The facial nerve is located superiorly.

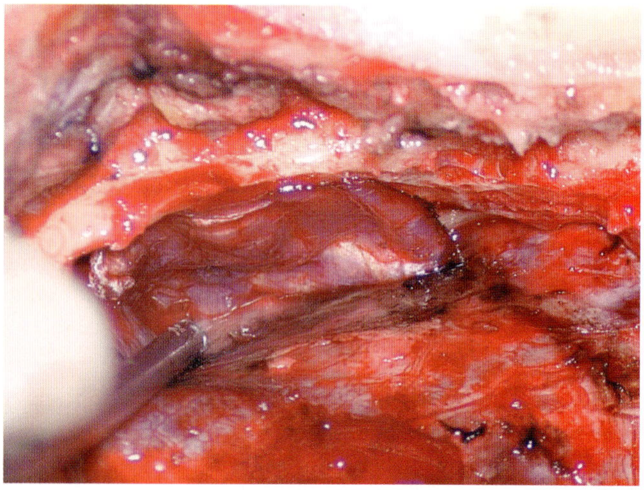

Fig. 11.32: The internal auditory canal is packed with muscle and a fascia graft is placed over the floor of the middle cranial fossa.

Tumor Removal

Step 1: The dura of the internal auditory canal is opened and the facial nerve is identified with stimulus dissectors. The facial nerve is most often just under the dura.

Step 2: The vestibular nerves are identified laterally and sectioned. The auditory nerve is identified and preserved.

Step 3: Tumor removal is best performed in a medial to lateral direction with stimulus dissectors in order to preserve both the facial and auditory nerves. Care is taken to try and preserve the internal auditory artery that runs between the facial and cochlear nerves (Fig. 11.31).

Closure

Step 1: Any opened air cells are closed with bone wax. The internal auditory canal is packed with muscle. Fat packing has been shown to have increased risk of cerebrospinal fluid leakage. Fascia is then placed over the floor of the middle cranial fossa and the brain/dura is allowed to relax (Fig. 11.32).

Step 2: The bone flap is replaced and secured to the skull with titanium plates (Fig. 11.33).

Step 3: The muscle layer and skin layer are closed with 2-0 Vicryl and 3-0 Prolene sutures in the scalp. 5-0 Prolene is used to close the pretragal skin and a pressure dressing is applied (Fig. 11.34).

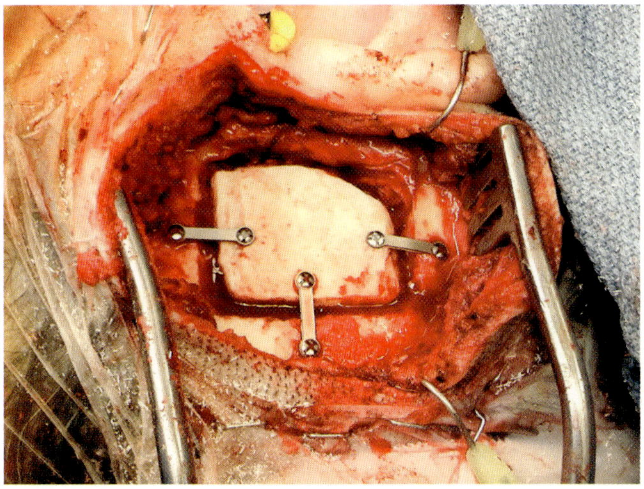

Fig. 11.33: The bone flap is secured to the skull with titanium plates.

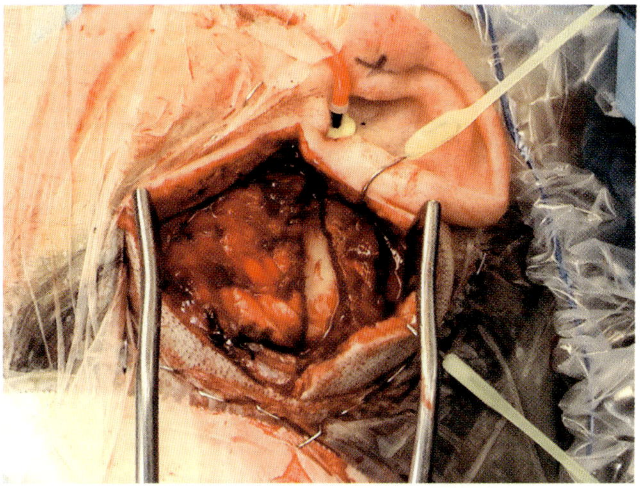

Fig. 11.34: The muscle layer and skin layer are closed separately creating a watertight closure.

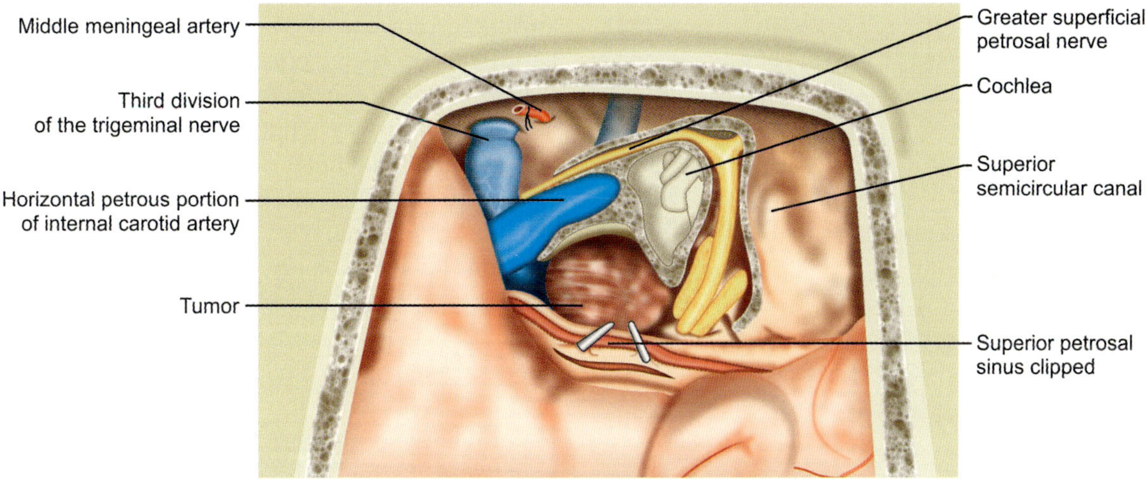

Fig. 11.35: An extended middle fossa approach exposing the carotid artery anteriorly and removing bone from the internal auditory canal to the intrapetrosal carotid artery.

Extended Middle Cranial Fossa

The extended middle cranial fossa approach is performed similar to that of the middle cranial fossa technique with the addition of the following steps.

Exposure

Step 1: A slightly wider craniotomy is made in the temporal region with more exposure anteriorly. The zygomatic arch can be reflected inferiorly to gain more exposure.

Step 2: The middle cranial fossa dura is reflected medially. The middle meningeal artery is divided. The greater superficial petrosal nerve is divided to prevent retraction of the geniculate ganglion.

Step 3: After the superior semicircular canal is blue lined and the internal auditory canal is exposed, bone is removed anteriorly up to and exposing the petrous carotid artery. This exposes the petrous apex. The third division of the trigeminal nerve should be identified and preserved unless involved by tumor. The cochlea should also be preserved (Fig. 11.35).

Step 4: Bone is removed deep to the horizontal carotid artery to the level of the inferior petrosal sinus.

Step 5: The tentorium and superior petrosal sinus can be divided to gain more superior exposure.

Step 6: The third division of the Vth cranial nerve can be mobilized or divided to provide more anterior exposure.

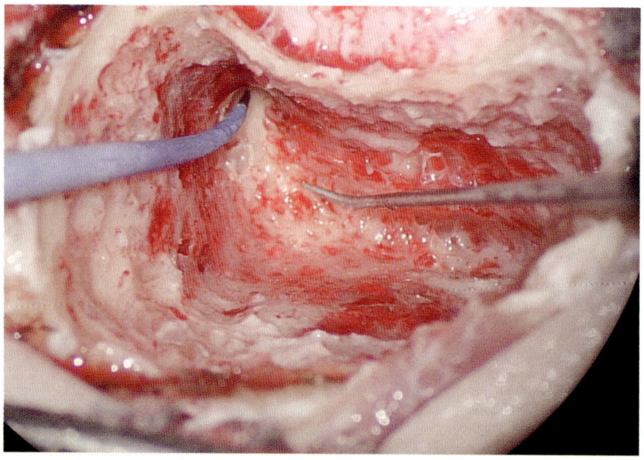

Fig. 11.36: A mastoidectomy is performed exposing the bony horizontal and posterior semicircular canals.

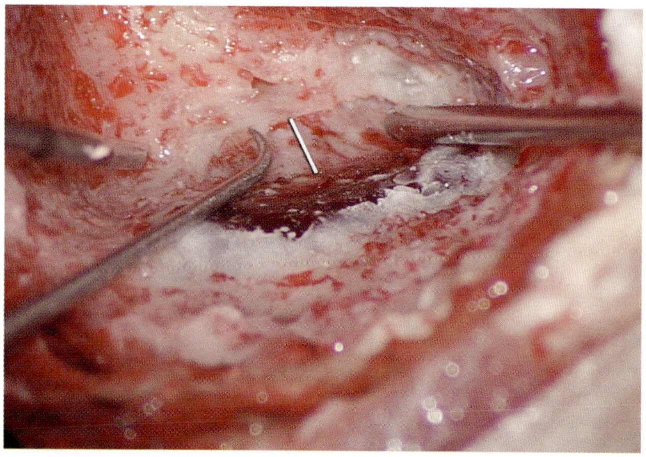

Fig. 11.37: Bone is removed over the sigmoid sinus and posterior fossa dura to the level of the posterior semicircular canal. An incision (blue line) is made in the posterior fossa dura with care to avoid the endolymphatic sac and duct.

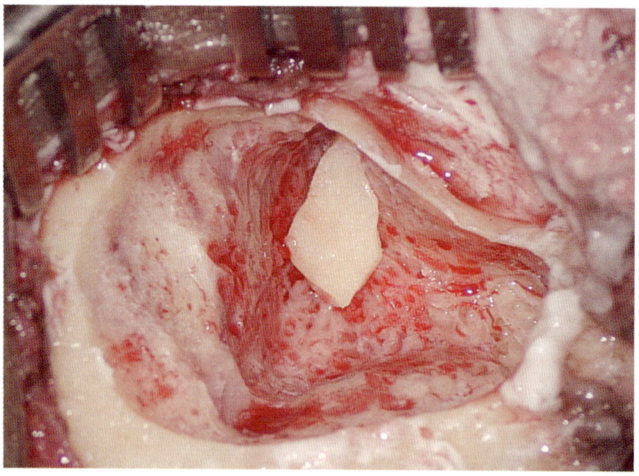

Fig. 11.38: A bone chip is used to block the antrum.

Tumor Removal

Tumor removal is similar to the previously described techniques. Stimulus dissectors are utilized.

Closure

Closure is similar to that of the middle cranial fossa technique. Occasionally, an abdominal fat graft in addition to muscle and fascia is used to obliterate the surgical defect.

Retrolabyrinthine Approach

Exposure

Step 1: A wide postauricular incision, approximately two finger breadths behind the postauricular crease is made and carried down to the periosteum/fascia layer. A muscle periosteal flap is created and based inferiorly.

Step 2: A wide mastoidectomy is performed. The epitympanum is partially opened to expose the incus keeping it intact. The bony horizontal and posterior semicircular canals are identified and preserved (Fig. 11.36).

Step 3: Bone is removed over the sigmoid sinus and posterior fossa dura to the level of the posterior semicircular canal. Bone is also removed over the middle cranial fossa dura and superior petrosal sinus depending on the intent of the surgery (Fig. 11.37).

Step 4: The posterior fossa dura is incised just inferior to the superior petrosal sinus with care to avoid the endolymphatic sac and duct (Fig. 11.37).

Step 5: Cerebrospinal fluid (CSF) is drained from the posterior fossa and its contents are exposed.

Tumor Removal

Tumor removal is accomplished similar to that in the aforementioned approaches.

Closure

Step 1: Closure is important to protect against a CSF leak and hearing loss. A bone chip is used to block the antrum without damaging the incus (Fig. 11.38).

Step 2: A large fascia graft is placed over the bone chip and the anterior portion of the mastoid cavity. Any remaining mastoid air cells are closed with bone wax (Fig. 11.39).

Step 3: An abdominal fat graft is placed in the mastoid cavity and the wound closed in layers. A pressure dressing is applied.

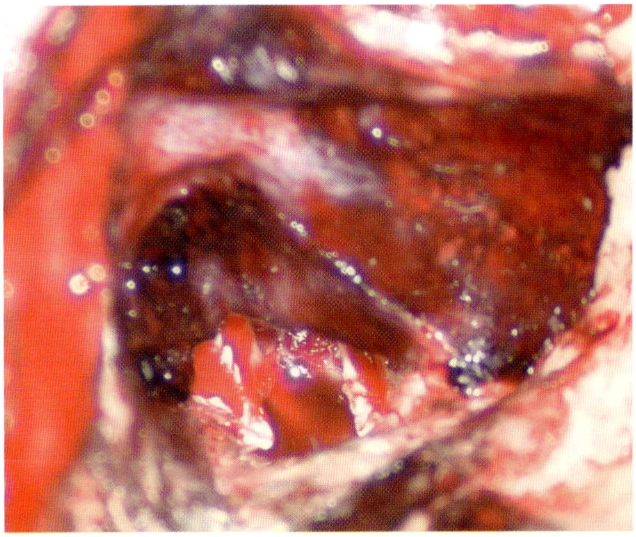

Fig. 11.39: A fascia graft is placed over the bone chip and antrum. All remaining air cells are occluded with bone wax.

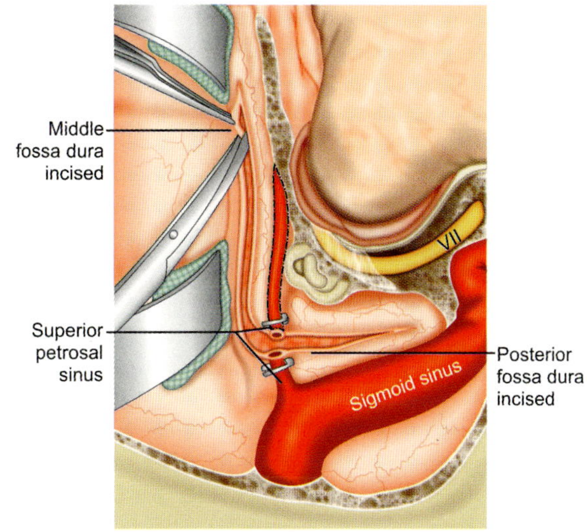

Fig. 11.40: The middle cranial fossa dura and posterior fossa dura (presigmoid) are opened and the superior petrosal vein is ligated and divided.

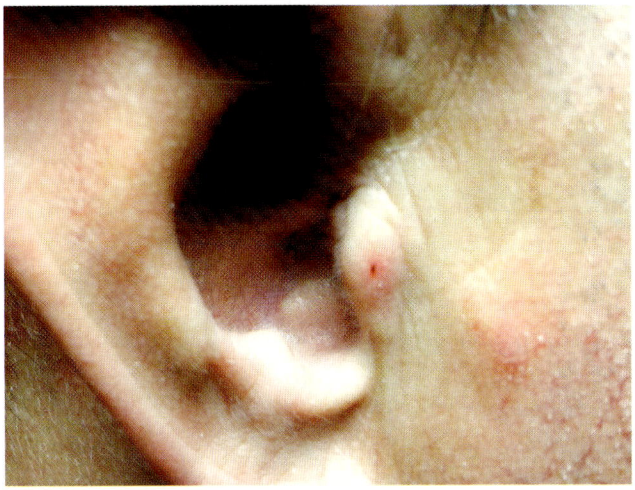

Fig. 11.41: The external auditory canal is overclosed in a two layer (soft tissue medially, skin laterally) technique.

Transpetrosal Approaches

These approaches combine a middle cranial fossa or extended middle cranial fossa approach with either a retrolabyrinthine or retrosigmoid approach. Unique features of the transpetrosal approaches include the following.

Exposure

Step 1: After completing the middle cranial fossa/retrolabyrinthine approaches described earlier, the superior petrosal vein is divided to allow for maximal exposure.

Step 2: The middle cranial fossa dura is divided to the incisura with care to preserve the IVth cranial nerve and the Vein of Labbé. Injury to the latter can result in a temporal lobe infarct. The vein arises just posterior to the sigmoid transverse sinus junction (Fig. 11.40).

Tumor Removal

Step 1: Tumor is removed similar to the previously described techniques.

Closure

Step 1: Closure is similar to that of the retrolabyrinthine approach in that a bone chip is placed over the antrum, a large fascia graft placed and abdominal fat graft packing used. The middle cranial fossa/posterior fossa bone plates are secured with titanium plates.

Transcochlear

Exposure

Step 1: Following a wide postauricular incision, the external auditory canal is divided and overclosed and all remaining external auditory canal skin, tympanic membrane, and ossicles are removed (Fig. 11.41).

Step 2: A translabyrinthine approach is then performed including a wide mastoidectomy, labyrinthectomy, and exposure of the internal auditory canal. See figures outlining the translabyrinthine approach.

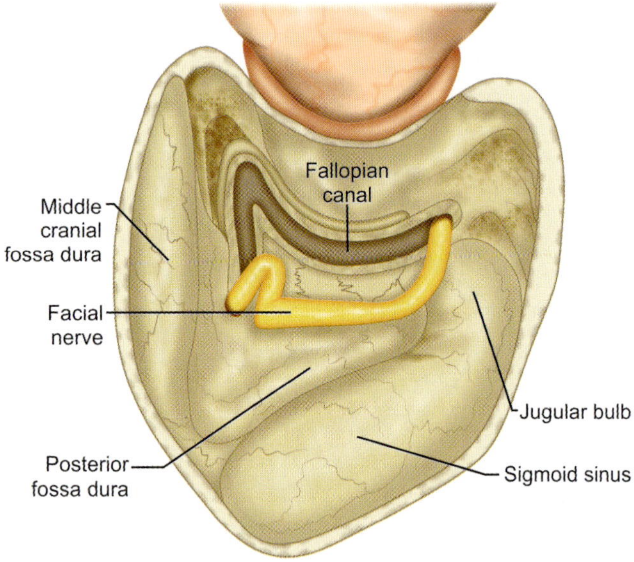

Fig. 11.42: The external auditory canal is taken down to the fallopian canal which is opened. The facial nerve is reflected posteriorly.

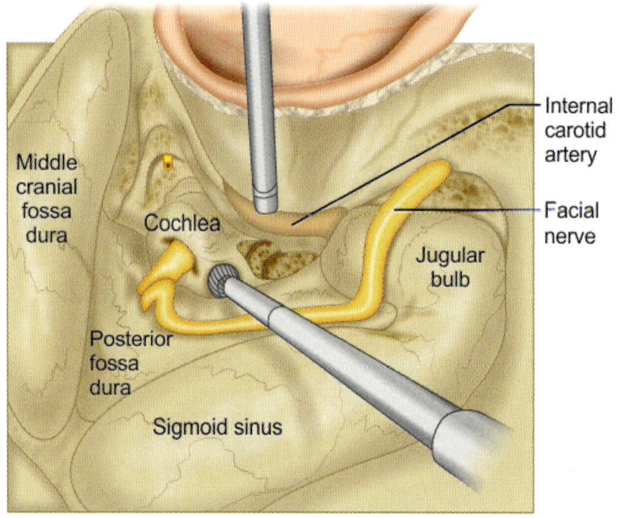

Fig. 11.43: The cochlea is drilled out exposing the internal auditory canal, carotid artery, and jugular bulb.

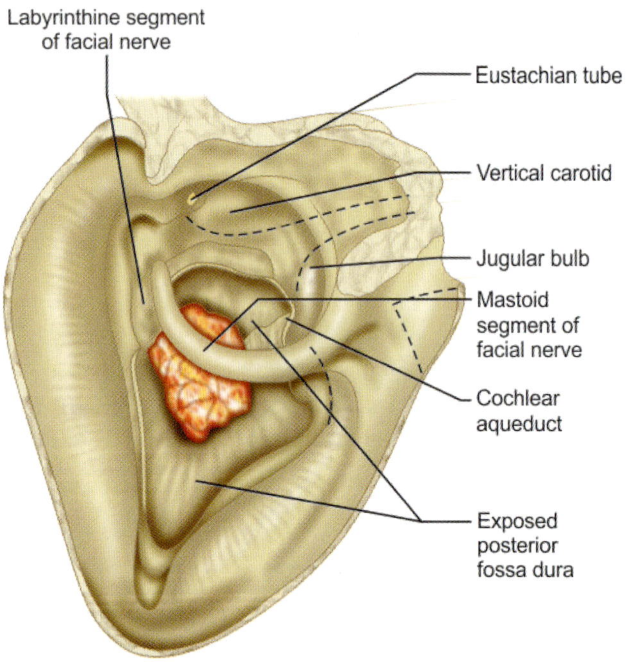

Fig. 11.44: The transotic approach involves drilling out the cochlea combined with the translabyrinthine approach while leaving the facial nerve in the fallopian canal.

Step 3: The chorda tympani nerve is sectioned as is the greater superficial petrosal nerve. The facial nerve is decompressed with diamond burs and reflected posteriorly (Fig. 11.42).

Step 4: The cochlea is then drilled out exposing the carotid artery and jugular bulb (Fig. 11.43).

Tumor Removal

Step 1: Tumor removal is similar to the translabyrinthine approach.

Closure

Step 1: Closure is similar to that of a translabyrinthine approach. Care is taken to directly pack the eustachian tube with fascia. The ear canal is tightly closed to prevent a CSF leak and an abdominal fat graft is placed in the cavity.

Transotic Approach

Exposure

Step 1: The external auditory canal is overclosed similar to the transcochlear approach. The ear canal skin, tympanic membrane, and ossicles are removed. The translabyrinthine approach is then carried out.
Step 2: The facial nerve is left in the fallopian canal, but it is skeletonized. The cochlea is drilled out (Fig. 11.44).

Tumor Removal

Tumor removal is similar to the translabyrinthine approach.

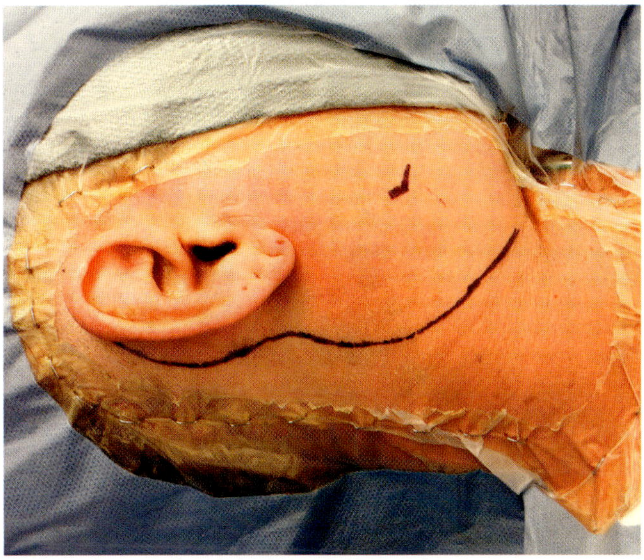

Fig. 11.45: A wide postauricular incision is made and carried down into the neck two fingerbreadths below the mandible.

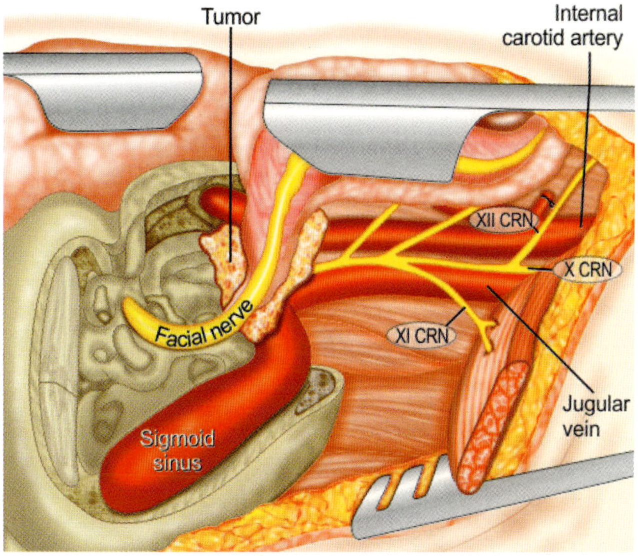

Fig. 11.46: After a mastoidectomy is performed and the external auditory canal taken down the facial nerve is decompressed (mobilized anteriorly or left in fallopian canal) and the tail of the parotid gland reflected anteriorly.

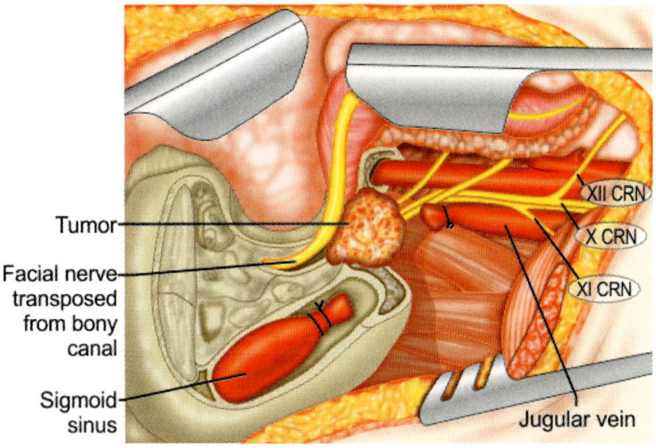

Fig. 11.47: The sigmoid sinus is divided or decompressed extraluminally with Surgicel. The jugular vein is ligated and divided then reflected under the spinal accessory nerve to the level of the jugular bulb.

Closure

Step 1: Closure is performed similar to the transcochlear approach. The eustachian tube is directly packed with fascia and a large abdominal fat graft is used.

Infratemporal Fossa Approach

Exposure

Step 1: Generally, 1–2 days following embolization, a wide postauricular incision is made at least three to four finger breadths behind the postauricular crease. This decreases the chance of devascularization of the auricle. The incision is brought down into the neck approximately two finger breadths beneath the angle of the mandible to protect the marginal mandibular branch of the facial nerve (Fig. 11.45).

Step 2: The external auditory canal is transected and overclosed, and skin is removed from the remainder of the external auditory canal. The tympanic membrane, malleus, and incus are removed (Fig. 11.41).

Step 3: The cervical portion of the neck is exposed and cranial nerves IX–XII are identified as are the internal jugular vein and carotid artery (internal, external, and common carotid arteries are identified and vascular loops applied). The internal jugular vein is then suture ligated. The posterior belly of the digastric is identified and split. Care is taken to reflect the tail of the parotid gland upward to protect the facial nerve (Fig. 11.46).

Step 4: A wide mastoidectomy is performed. The epitympanum is opened. The bony ear canal is taken down to the facial nerve. The facial nerve is skeletonized and either left in a shell of bone or totally decompressed from the geniculate ganglion to the stylomastoid foramen and reflected anteriorly (Fig. 11.46).

Step 5: The sigmoid sinus is then decompressed as is the posterior fossa dura. The sigmoid sinus is then either extraluminally compressed with Surgicel or suture ligated (Fig. 11.47).

Step 6: Bone is then removed over the jugular bulb and the posterior wall of the jugular vein. Bone is occasionally removed around the intrapetrous carotid artery (Fig. 11.48).

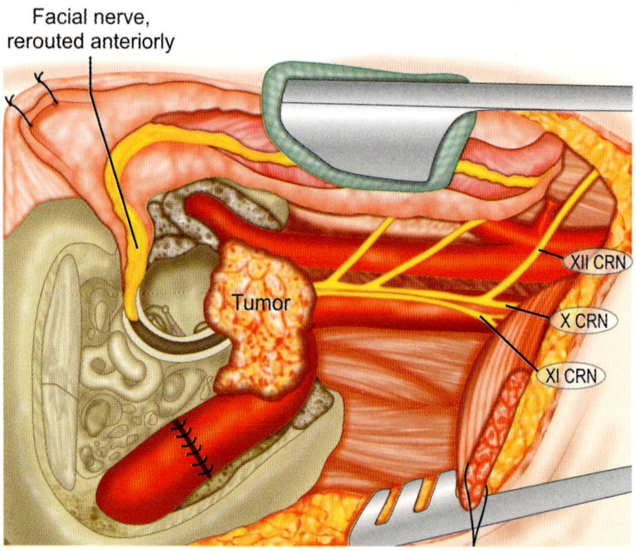

Fig. 11.48: Bone is removed from around the jugular bulb with diamond burs, etc. If the facial nerve is left in the fallopian canal, bone can be removed 360° around the nerve with diamond burs utilizing facial nerve monitoring.

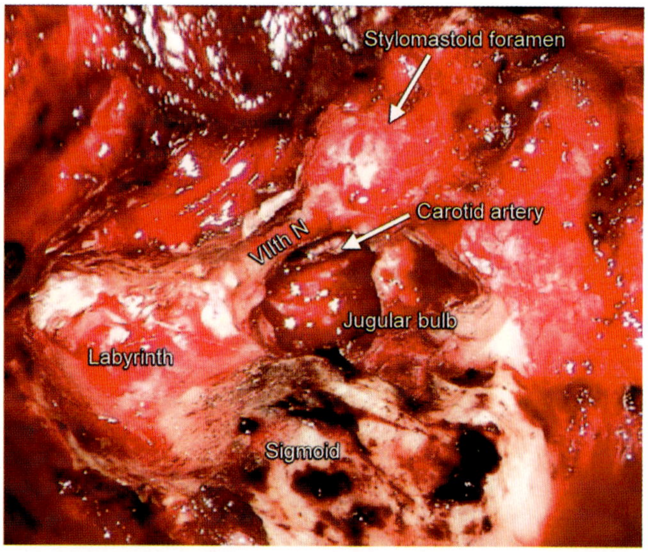

Fig. 11.49: The sigmoid sinus and jugular bulb are opened and the tumor removed. The inferior petrosal sinus openings into the jugular bulb are packed with Surgicel.

Tumor Removal

Step 1: Tumor is removed from the middle ear and mastoid. Bipolar cautery can help to shrink the tumor prior to removal.

Step 2: Tumor is removed from around the facial nerve with stimulus dissectors. One can work 360° around the facial nerve if the nerve is kept in its bony canal.

Step 3: Tumor is then removed from the jugular bulb. The inferior petrosal sinus opening(s) are packed with Surgicel. Care must be taken when packing the jugular bulb, as compression of the lower cranial nerves can occur causing weakness (Fig. 11.49).

Step 4: Intracranial tumor removal is usually performed as a second-stage procedure.

Closure

Step 1: After tumor is removed, the eustachian tube is packed with fascia and the cavity is packed with an abdominal fat graft. The wound is closed in layers. A drain can be placed in the neck unless a CSF leak is suspected. A Pressure dressing is applied.

COMPLICATIONS

The most common complications of lateral skull base surgery include injury to cranial nerves, specifically cranial verves VII and X. CSF leaks and meningitis can occur. Vascular injury, either arterial or venous, can result in stroke or death.

Injuries to the facial nerve or Xth nerve are the two most commonly seen cranial nerve palsies. Facial nerve injury has been decreased with the use of intraoperative monitoring, prophylactic facial nerve decompression, and the use of intraoperative and postoperative steroids. Postoperative use of acyclovir has been helpful in decreasing the incidence of delayed facial palsy. Treatment of facial nerve injuries including gold weight insertion and reanimation procedures can be found elsewhere in this atlas.

Vagal nerve injury has decreased with intraoperative monitoring. Both temporary and permanent procedures to medialize the vocal cord have proved beneficial in the postoperative period.

The risk of a CSF leak has been reduced in lateral skull base surgery with meticulous packing of the eustachian tube. Muscle, fascia, and abdominal fat grafts are useful in packing the surgical deficit. We have found the use of bone cements is less useful in preventing CSF leaks and rarely use bone cement to perform a cranioplasty during the primary procedure.

A lumbar drain is beneficial in treating a CSF leak. We have not used lumbar drains prophylactically in our practice. If a CSF leak occurs repacking the wound and a lumbar drain are usually employed. It is important to use a constant drainage rate (and not a dependent drainage technique) to prevent the risk of pneumocephalus.

Meningitis can complicate intradural procedures. Meningitis generally occurs 4–8 days postoperatively.

Risk factors for meningitis include increased operative time and CSF leakage. Rarely have we seen meningitis associated with a nasal CSF leak. CSF leakage through the wound is almost always associated with meningitis unless addressed immediately. Rarely does a CSF collection under the skin lead to meningitis unless a break in the wound occurs. A pressure dressing and time generally allow a CSFoma to resolve. Aggressive management including a lumbar tap and culture and prolonged intravenous antibiotics is essential in treating postoperative meningitis.

Vascular injury, either arterial or venous, can be met with serious complications. Injury to the carotid artery can cause stroke or death. The advent of endovascular intervention has reduced the morbidity of vascular injury. Injury to the AICA can result in a stroke of the lateral pons which can result in death (Atkinson's syndrome). Injury to the vein of Labbé can result in a temporal lobe infarct. This vein arises just posterior to the transverse sigmoid junction and can be damaged with retraction in this region. Generally, injury to the sigmoid and lateral sinus can be controlled with gentle pressure and Surgicel.

REFERENCES

1. Brackman DE, Arriaga MA. Neoplasms of the posterior fossa. In: Paul W Flint, Bruce H Haughey, John K Niparko, et al (Eds). Cummings Otolaryngology: Head and Neck Surgery, 5th edition. Philadelphia, PA: Elsevier Health Sciences: 2010. pp. 2514-41.
2. Guttmann DM, Wonth A, Caney JC, et al. The diagnostic evaluation and multidisciplinary management of NF1 and NF2. JAMA. 1997;278:51-7.
3. Jankins HA, Franklin DJ. Infratemporal approaches to the skull base. In: Jackson CG (Ed). Surgery of Skull Base Tumors. New York: Churchill Livingstone; 1991. p. 291.
4. Weiss MH, Kisiel DL, Bhatia P. Predictive value of brainstem evoked response. Otolaryngol Head Neck Surg. 1990;103: 583-5.
5. LoWW, Housepian MM. MRI Imaging of the cerebellopontine angle. In: Jackler RK, Brackmann DE (Eds). Neurotology, 2nd edition. New York: Mosby; 2005. pp. 349-82.
6. Rosenwasser U, Parisier SC, Edelsein DR. Glomus tumors. In: English GM (Ed). Otolaryngology, Vol 1. Philadelphia, PA: JB Lippincott; 1991. pp. 1-28.
7. Mafee MF, Raofi B, Kumar A, et al. Glomus faciale, glomus jugulare, glomus tympanicum, glomus vagale, carotid body tumors and simulating lesions. Radiol Clin North Am. 2000;38:1059-76.
8. Mamikoglu B, Wiet RJ, Esquivel CR. Translabyrinthine approach for management of large and giant vestibular schwannomas. Otol Neurotol. 2002;23:224-7.
9. Kartush JM, Telian SA, Graham MD, et al. Anatomic landmarks for labyrinthine preservation during posterior fossa acoustic tumor surgery. Laryngoscope. 1986;96:1024-8.
10. Satan B, Jackler RK, Oghalai J, et al. Risk—benefit analysis of using the middle fossa approach for acoustic neuromas with >10 mm cerebellopontine angle component. Laryngoscope. 2002;112 (pt 1):1500-6.
11. Daspit CP, Spetzler RF, Pappas CT. Combined approach for lesions involving the cerebellopontine angle and skull base, experience with 20 cases. Preliminary report. Otolaryngol Head Neck Surg. 1991;105:788-96.
12. House WF, De la Cruz A, Hitselberger WE. Surgery of the skull base: transcochlear approach to the petrous apex and clivus. Otolaryngology. 1978;86:ORL-770-9.

CHAPTER 12

Drainage Procedures of the Petrous Apex

Ilka C Naumann, Adam Folbe

INTRODUCTION

Lesions of the petrous apex may remain silent for many years and are often an incidental discovery in the workup of unrelated complaints. The petrous apex is defined as a space anteromedial to the labyrinth and lateral to the petro-occipital fissure (Fig. 12.1). If a line is drawn along the modiolus of the cochlea and the center of the internal auditory canal (IAC), the petrous apex can be divided into a larger anterior and a smaller posterior compartment. The anterior compartment is aerated in about 30% of the patients (Fig. 12.2).[1] It contains the horizontal portion of the petrous carotid canal, the foramen lacerum and the abducens nerve in Dorello's canal deep in the petrous apex. On the superior-medial surface sits the trigeminal nerve. Dense bone will frequently fill the posterior compartment and therefore it is generally not the origin of petrous apex pathologies.

CLINICAL PRESENTATION

The most common presenting symptom in patients with a diagnosed petrous apex lesion is hearing loss, found in 64% of cases. It may be conductive, in cases of eustachian tube involvement, or sensorineural if the otic capsule or the 8th nerve is affected. Vestibular dysfunction occurs in about 50% of cases, whereas headaches and tinnitus are presenting symptoms in about 40% of patients. Facial twitching is three times more common than facial paralysis. Facial paralysis, diplopia and otorrhea are uncommon and are found in about 5% of patients.[2]

DIFFERENTIAL DIAGNOSES

The most common pathologies in the petrous apex are pseudolesions (retained fluid), tumor-like lesions (encephalocele, aneurysm), benign lesions (cholesterol granuloma, cholesteatoma), and malignant lesions (often metastasis, chondrosarcoma, chordoma). A summary of these lesions can be reviewed in Table. 12.1.

IMAGING CHARACTERISTICS

Despite high-resolution magnetic resonance imaging (MRI) and computed tomography (CT), these lesions may pose a diagnostic dilemma. Both imaging modalities are complementary in most cases and are crucial for surgical planning.

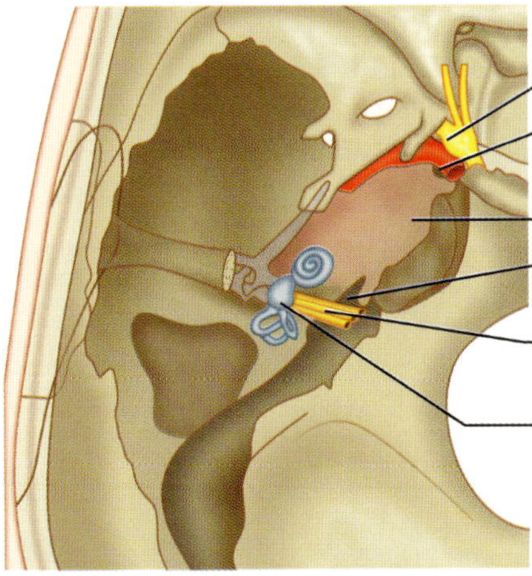

Fig. 12.1: Surgeon's view of the right petrous apex and its anatomical borders.

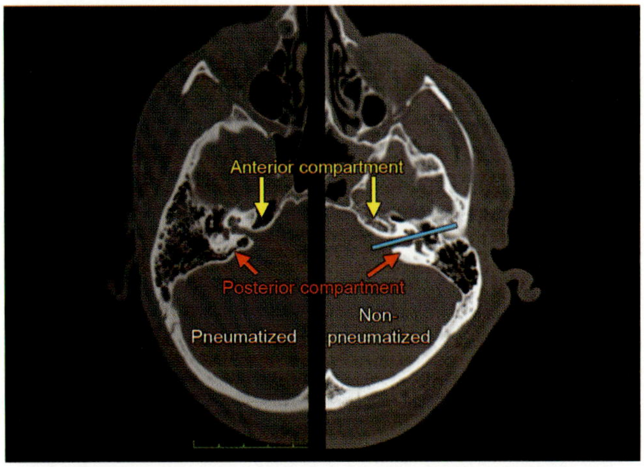

Fig. 12.2: CT scan: left, well-pneumatized petrous apex; right, no aeration of petrous apex. Line illustrates demarcation of the anterior and posterior compartments.

Table 12.1: Common petrous apex lesions

Cystic	*Solid*
Vascular: ICA aneurism, venous lake	Benign: Neurofibroma, schwannoma, meningioma, paraganglioma
Nonvascular: Cholesterol granuloma, petrous apicitis, congenital cholesteatoma	Malignant: Metastatic malignancy, eosinophilic granuloma lymphoma, plasmacytoma, chondrosarcoma

Table 12.2: Radiologic findings of petrous apex lesions on CT

		Bony erosion		
		None	Smooth	Irregular
Contrast enhancement	No	Marrow asymmetry effusion	Cholesterol granuloma cholesteatoma mucocele	
	Yes		Neurogenic tumor carotid aneurism	Petrous apicitis (rim) malig nancy meningioma

Table 12.3: Radiologic findings of petrous apex lesions on MRI

		T1	
		Hypo	Hyper
T2	Hypo		Bone marrow
	Hyper	Carotid aneurism, serous effusion, petrous apicitis, malignancy, cephalocele, epidermoid	Cholesterol granuloma

Whereas a CT scan will give a detailed evaluation of the osseous architecture (bony erosion) and determine involvement of the otic capsule, IAC or carotid canal, an MRI scan can help to differentiate different pathologies. A CT angiogram should be obtained when a vascular lesion is suspected or when CT and MRI fail to exclude an aneurysm.

An angiogram and possibly embolization of highly vascular tumors should be considered. Tables 12.2 and 12.3 help to differentiate between pathologies found in the petrous apex based on CT and MRI.

INDICATION FOR SURGERY

Most lesions found in the petrous apex do not require immediate surgery. The most common cystic lesion is a cholesterol granuloma. It is the only lesion showing hyperintensity on T1 and T2 MRI images. Unless the lesion is growing, which is confirmed by serial scans or is causing significant symptoms, these lesions should be monitored.

"Pseudolesions", such as serous fluid and asymmetric bone marrow, never need surgery. Following an acute otitis media about 1% of patients with a pneumatized petrous apex will have residual fluid deep to the otic capsule. The CT will show lack of cortical or trabecular erosion; a follow-up scan will likely show resolution. Bone marrow asymmetry is found in approximately 5% of hypopneumatized temporal bones and shows the diagnostic findings on MRI scans consisting of hyperintensity on T1 and hypointensity on T2.

PATIENT SELECTION

Treatment is highly individualized. Patient's age, health status and clinical symptomatology, suspected pathology, prognosis and location of the lesion in relation to vital structures, hearing status, and aeration patterns of the temporal bone are all taken into consideration in the discussion of possible surgical approaches. Middle cranial fossa procedures pose much higher risks, especially in the elderly patient.

The following pages describe in detail the infracochlear approach, the infralabyrinthine approach and the extended middle cranial fossa approach from the otologic perspective and the trans-sphenoid approach from the rhinological viewpoint.

Infracochlear Approach

The goal of this approach is to create a drainage passage for cystic lesions from the petrous apex into the middle

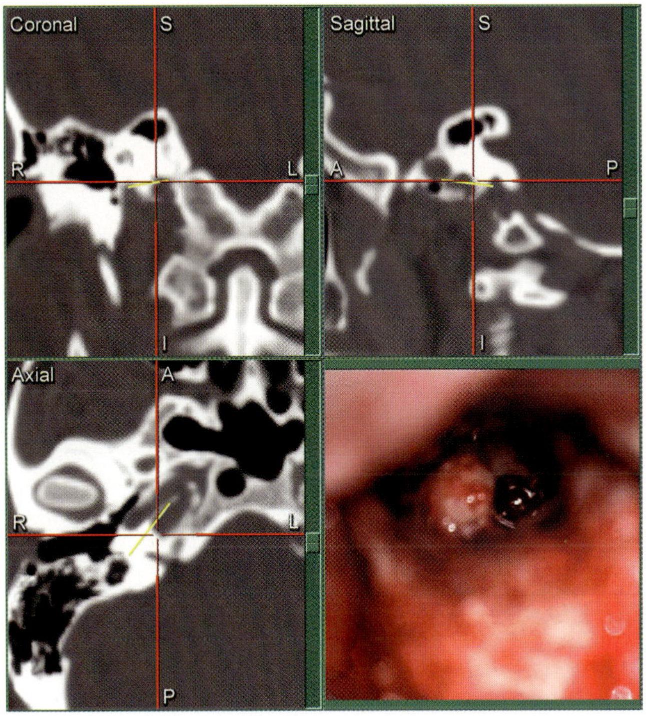

Fig. 12.3: CT guided intraoperative photograph of infracochlear approach. Rolled Silastic sheet in opened cyst lumen (right lower corner). *Courtesy*: Dr Eric Sargent, Farmington Hills, Michigan, USA

ear. Complete resection is not possible and therefore this approach is not recommended for excision of solid tumors. Stereotactic navigation can be helpful when lesions of the petrous apex are drained (Fig. 12.3).[3,4]

Surgical Steps

Step 1: The procedure is done through a transcanal approach. Through a standard postauricular incision, as used in a routine mastoidectomy, the skin and subcutaneous tissues are incised about 0.8 cm behind the postauricular crease.

Step 2: The temporalis fascia is identified and the subcutaneous tissues are separated toward the mastoid tip.

Step 3: A true temporalis fascia graft, measuring 2 × 2 cm, is harvested.

Step 4: The periosteum of the mastoid bone is incised and elevated anteriorly. The lateral canal skin is elevated, after an incision is made paralleling the annulus and release cuts are made at 6 and 12 o'clock positions. A Perkins retractor is placed.

Step 5: The ear canal is visualized. The standard incision from a tympanoplasty is modified. Special attention should be paid to the position of the inferior cut that should be as anterior as possible to allow for optimal exposure. The incision starts in the anterior ear canal skin at the 3 o'clock position and is curved to the 9 o'clock position keeping an adequate distance from the annulus. The tympanomeatal flap is then elevated (Fig. 12.4).

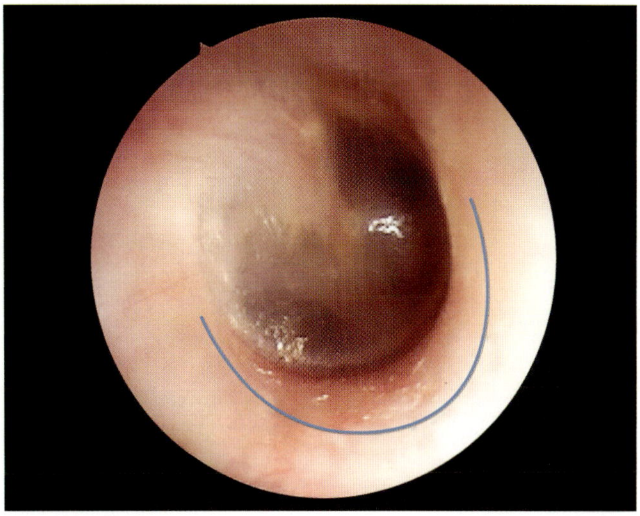

Fig. 12.4: Right ear canal. Incision outline is shown by blue line.

Step 6: A protective sheet made of a sterile foil is placed over the tympanomeatal flap. The ear canal wall is then drilled with small (2–3 mm) diamond burrs. The hypotympanum is exposed by drilling a portion of the tympanic bone inferiorly (Fig. 12.5).

Step 7: Once adequate exposure is achieved, the jugular bulb is blue-lined posteriorly inferiorly and the carotid canal is skeletonized anteriorly. Drilling inferior to the round window niche will prevent injury to the cochlea (Fig. 12.6).

Step 8: The triangular space between the carotid canal and the jugular bulb is widened with small 1–1.5 mm diamond burrs. The lumen of the cyst is entered. In the event the surgeon is in doubt, needle aspiration of the cystic fluid can be done before widening the opening. The lumen should be as large as possible to prevent bony overgrowth and scarring (Fig. 12.7).

Step 9: Generally, it is recommended to place a piece of thin Silastic (0.1 mm), as fibrous scarring can cause a recurrence of the cyst. This can be either cut into a spear-like shape to avoid extrusion or rolled and positioned into the created opening like a tubing (as visible in Figure 12.3).

Step 10: A fascia graft is often needed to cover the exposed hypotympanum. The middle ear is packed with Gelfoam. The fascia is placed under the tympanic membrane covering the hypotympanic defect and brought onto the inferior canal wall. The ear canal is packed with antibiotic-soaked Gelfoam.

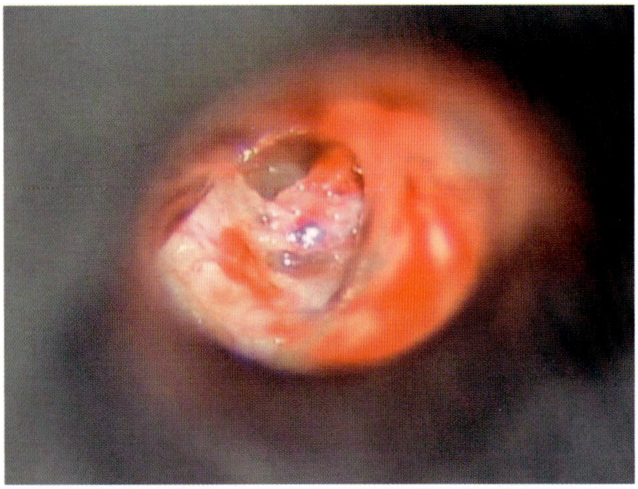

Fig. 12.5: Intraoperative photograph. Right ear transcanal infracochlear approach. Visualization of inferior ear canal wall.
Courtesy: Dr Eleanor Chan, Farmington Hills, Michigan, USA

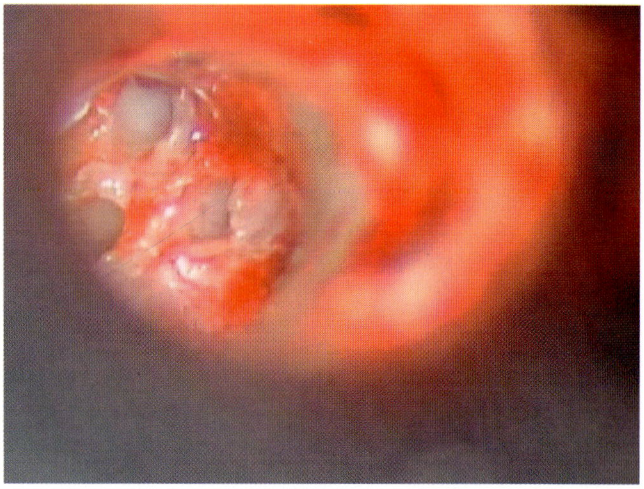

Fig. 12.6: Intraoperative photograph: right ear transcanal infracochlear approach. Hypotympanum exposed.
Courtesy: Dr Eleanor Chan, Farmington Hills, Michigan, USA

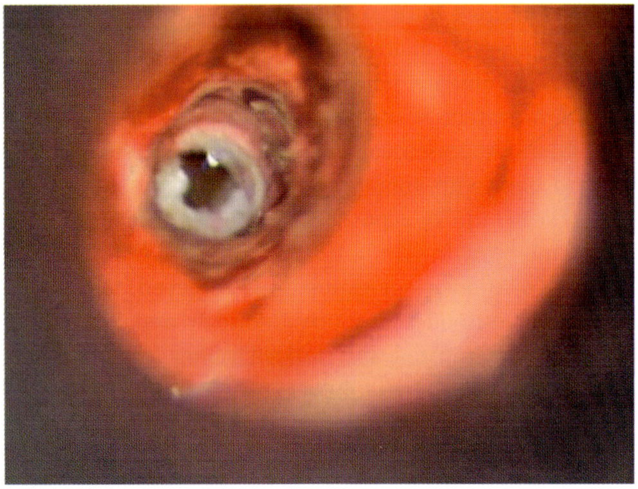

Fig. 12.7: Intraoperative photograph. Right ear transcanal infracochlear approach. Cyst entered.
Courtesy: Dr Eleanor Chan, Farmington Hills, Michigan, USA

Step 11: The periosteum is reapproximated and is closed in the postauricular area, using 3-0 and 4-0 Vicryl in a single interrupted fashion. The skin is closed with a 5-0 fast absorbing gut.

Complications

The narrow space places several structures at risk. Injury to the cochlea will lead to much greater likelihood of permanent sensorineural hearing loss compared to the semicircular canals. The intrapetrous carotid artery has a much thinner adventitia when compared to cervical portion and therefore potentially life-threatening injury can occur.

Injury to the facial nerve can occur if anatomically the nerve's position is very anterior. Using stimulating instruments for mapping can help to identify the nerves close location.

Injury to the jugular bulb can cause heavy bleeding but should be controllable by applying gentle pressure with Gelfoam and Surgicel.

Transmastoid Infralabyrinthine Approach

The infralabyrinthine approach opens into the petrous apex through a mastoidectomy approach, with the borders being the posterior semicircular canal superiorly, the posterior fossa bony plate posteriorly, the jugular bulb inferiorly and the facial nerve anteriorly. The approach allows for adequate exposure in most cases, but a high-riding jugular bulb can narrow the operating field significantly and may make it impossible to gain access to the petrous apex.

Surgical Steps

Step 1: Through a standard postauricular incision, as used in a standard mastoidectomy, the skin is incised about 0.8 cm behind the postauricular crease with a 15 blade.

The temporalis fascia is identified and the subcutaneous tissues are separated in a plane toward the mastoid tip.

A 7-shaped incision is made through the periosteum and the mastoid cortex is visualized using a Lempert elevator. Switching to freer elevator in the ear canal

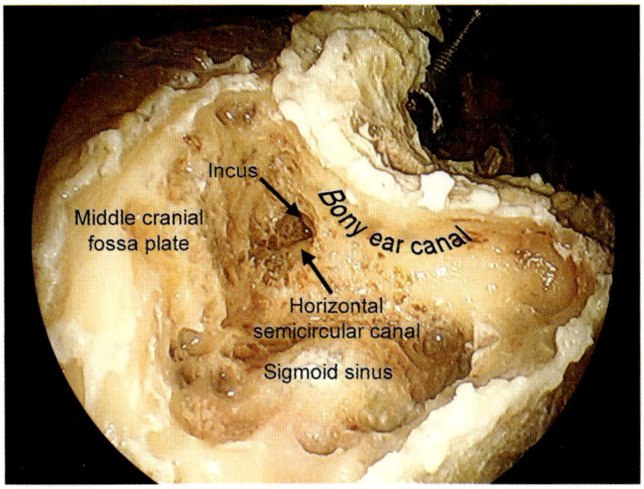

Fig. 12.8: Right ear cadaver dissection. Simple mastoidectomy.

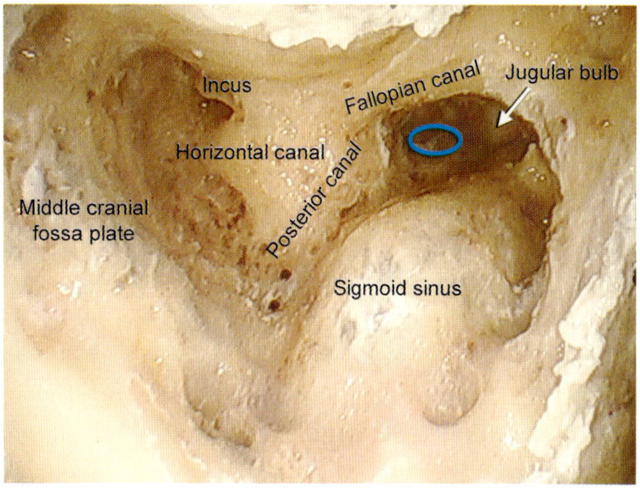

Fig. 12.9: Right ear cadaver dissection. Retrofacial air cells opened. Blue area shows location of the petrous apex.

prevents inadvertent lacerations of the ear canal skin. The spine of Henle is identified. Superiorly the temporalis muscle is elevated just above the temporal line; inferiorly and posteriorly the sternocleidomastoid muscle should be elevated widely. Weitlaner retractors are placed.

Step 2: A simple mastoidectomy is started with a 6 cutting burr, then switched to a 4 cutting burr and eventually to a 3 and 2 mm diamond burr. The sigmoid sinus, posterior fossa bony plate, tegmen, and horizontal canal are skeletonized and the ear canal is thinned. The sigmoid sinus can be decompressed to gain further space for visualization later in the case (Fig. 12.8).

Step 3: The horizontal semicircular canal is followed posteriorly and inferiorly and the posterior semicircular canal is delineated. The vertical segment of the facial canal is identified in the mastoid. The sigmoid sinus is followed inferiorly and the jugular bulb is found.

Step 4: Following the posterior fossa plate, retrofacial air cells are exenterated. The disease process is identified and drained (Fig. 12.9). The wound bed should be vigorously irrigated. A piece of thin Silastic (0.1 mm) can be placed in the opening of the cyst as fibrous scarring can cause recurrences. This can be either cut into a spear-like shape to avoid extrusion or rolled and positioned into the created opening like a tubing. Figure 12.10B shows the postoperative CT scan of the opened air cell tract (and in comparison the preoperative CT in Figure 12.10A).

Step 5: The periosteum is reapproximated and closed using 3-0 and 4-0 Vicryl in a single interrupted fashion. The skin is closed with a 5-0 fast absorbing gut. The ear canal should be inspected and suctioned.

Complications

Injury to the vertical segment of the facial nerve can be avoided by clearly identifying its location. Keeping a thin layer of bony cover over the nerve will prevent injury from the shaft "burning" the perineurium and causing paralysis.

Injury to the jugular bulb and carotid artery are possible. If in doubt if the capsule of the cholesterol granuloma is reached, an initial needle aspiration with a 27 G needle of the contents can be done.

If one of the semicircular canals (most commonly the posterior canal) is entered, sealing the opening with fascia and bone pate can potentially prevent vertigo and permanent hearing loss.

Extended Middle Cranial Fossa Approach

If the aforementioned inferior drainage procedures are prohibitive, the extended middle cranial fossa approach will evacuate the cyst at the time of surgery but no permanent and continuous drainage passage is created.

The extended middle cranial fossa approach has the widest exposure of the aforementioned drainage procedures. It is routinely used for solid lesions of the petrous apex.

Preoperative Consideration

Stereotactic navigation may be of help in this approach. Neuromonitoring should be used including CN7 and ABR. The surgeon's position is at the head of the bed.

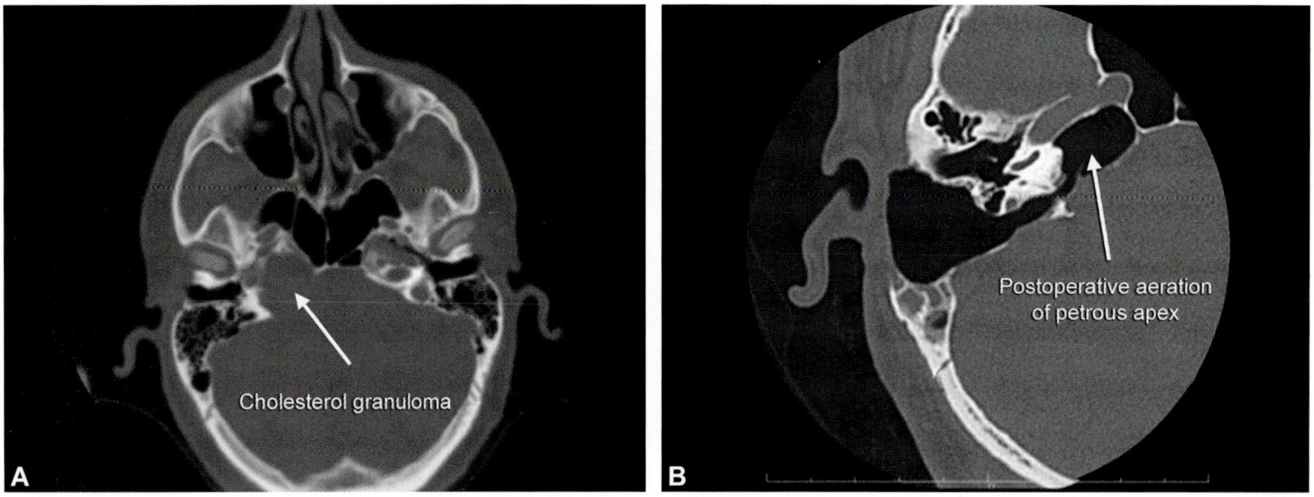

Figs. 12.10A and B: (A) CT scan. Right petrous apex cholesterol granuloma; (B) CT scan. Postoperative aerated petrous apex.

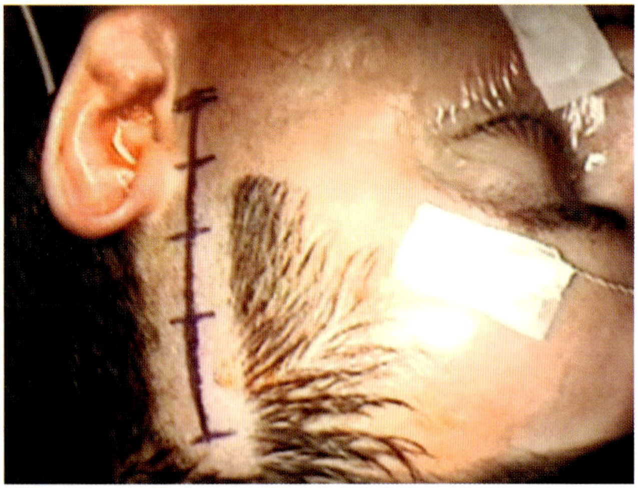

Fig. 12.11: Left middle cranial fossa incision lined out.

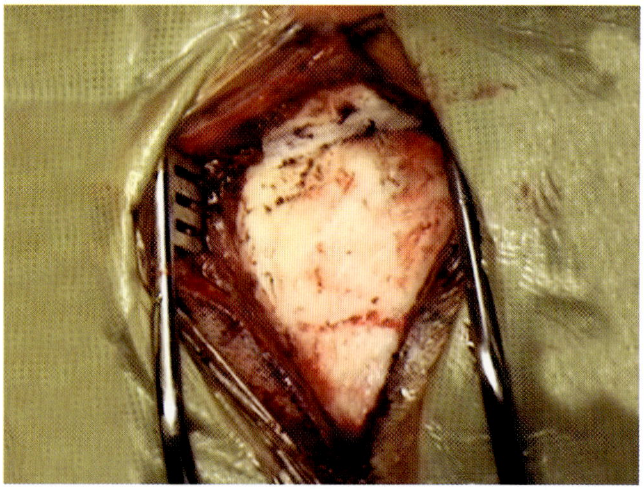

Fig. 12.12: Left middle cranial fossa exposed bone and zygomatic arch and root.

The patient is positioned with his head maximally turned so that the temple parallels the floor.

Preoperative antibiotics are given and redosed every 4–6 hours. Muscle relaxants should be avoided to guarantee accurate neuromonitoring. Mannitol, at doses of 0.5–1 mg/kg, is given about 1 hour before the dura is incised. Mild hyperventilation and additional diuretics (e.g. Lasix) should be considered if brain relaxation is insufficient.

Surgical Steps

Step 1: A preauricular incision is made from the level of the tragus extending upward. A straight incision is generally sufficient. It can be curved back and then forward for wider exposure. The temporalis fascia is identified but not transsected (Fig. 12.11).

Step 2: A temporalis fascia graft is harvested. The temporalis muscle is often incised at its attachment along the squamosa in a u-shaped fashion. The bulk it creates when retracting the muscle inferiorly has led us to use a linear incision with retraction anteriorly. Release cuts in a T-shaped fashion can be made most superiorly (Fig. 12.12).

Step 3: Positioning of the craniotomy is crucial. It is essential for the extended MCF approach to have exposure anteriorly. The ear canal and zygomatic root are clearly identified. The craniotomy should be placed two-thirds anterior to the ear canal. It should be placed close to the zygomatic root, which approximates the location of the middle cranial fossa floor.

Four mm cutting and 3 mm diamond burrs are used to make the craniotomy that measures at least 5 × 5 cm

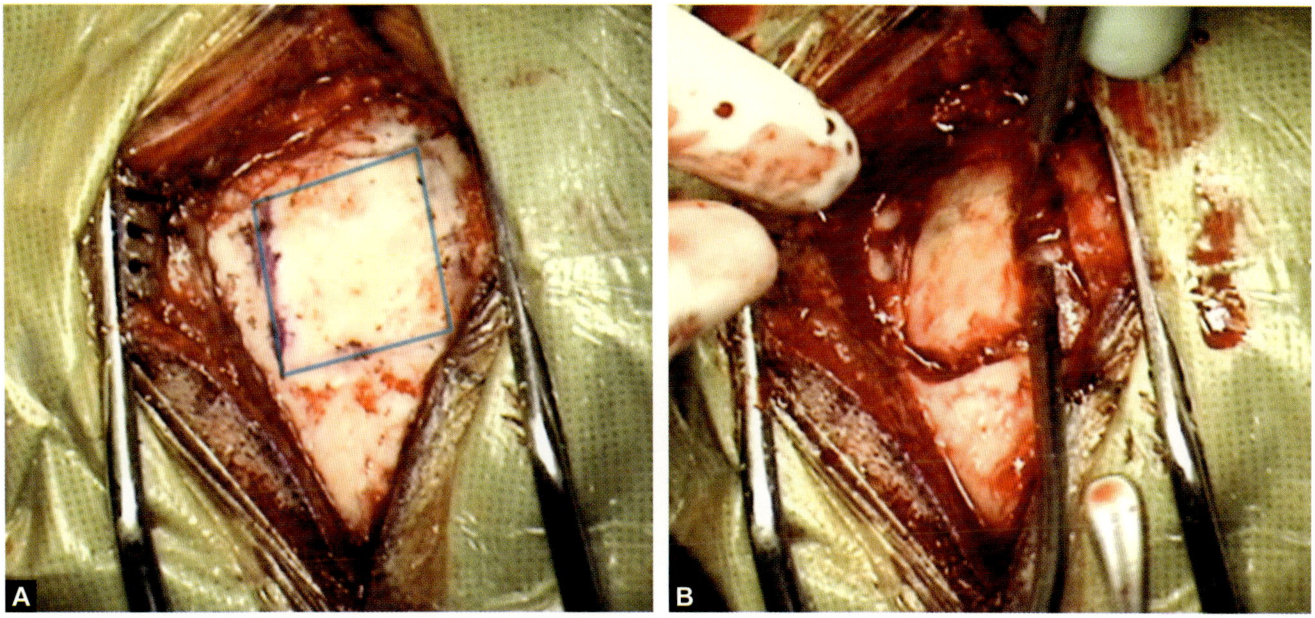

Figs. 12.13A and B: Left middle cranial fossa. (A) Craniotomy lined out. (B) Raising the bone flap.

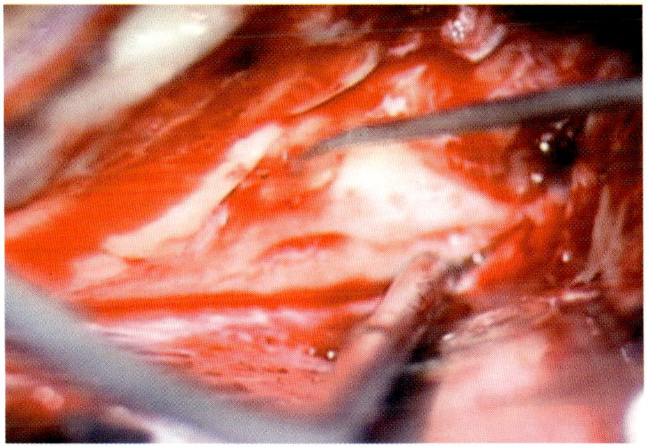

Fig. 12.14: Intraoperative photograph. Elevation of the middle cranial fossa dura and mapping the facial nerve.

(Figs. 12.13A and B). The bone flap is gently raised with a freer elevator to avoid tears in the dura or dural vessels.

Step 4: The floor of the middle cranial fossa is identified. Often it is necessary to drill the overhang from the squamosa to increase visualization. The dura is gently elevated over the arcuate eminence and meatal plane.

Dissection further anteriorly exposes the middle meningeal artery, which is then cauterized and transsected. The foramen spinosum is occluded with bone wax. The greater superficial petrosal nerve is identified and can be sharply cut from its dural attachments to avoid traction on the geniculate ganglion if needed. Bleeding should be readily controlled. Often venous oozing is encountered and controlled with thrombin or small pieces of Surgicel (Fig. 12.14).

Step 5: The House-Urban retractor is placed with its lip along the petrous ridge. Necessary care has to be taken not to tear the superior petrosal sinus. The location of the facial nerve and IAC are mapped with stimulating dissectors. The superior semicircular canal is blue lined. Its amputated end is found 1 cm posterior to the facial hiatus and 0.5 mm medially.[5] The IAC is then skeletonized. Drilling is performed anteriorly to the level of the carotid canal. The third division of the trigeminal nerve is preserved (unless involved with pathology) (Fig. 12.15).

Step 6: The cyst is readily identified and drained. Cholesterol granulomas will drain a thick yellow to brown fluid (Fig. 12.16). The cyst wall should be extentered as much as possible to avoid a recurrence. A small hand-held Doppler can be used to identify the internal carotid artery. The internal carotid artery and the cochlea are in very close proximity.

Step 7: Opened air cells are sealed with bone wax to avoid a cerebrospinal fluid (CSF) leak. A piece of fat is placed into the cavity to allow scar tissue formation (Fig. 12.17). A temporalis fascia graft and Dura-repair should be placed between the dura and the tegmen to prevent any leaks that cannot be repaired.

Step 8: The brain and dura are relaxed. Complete hemostasis should be confirmed. A positive pressure ventilation Valsalva maneuver administered by the anesthesiologist shows bleeding vessels and leaks of spinal fluid.

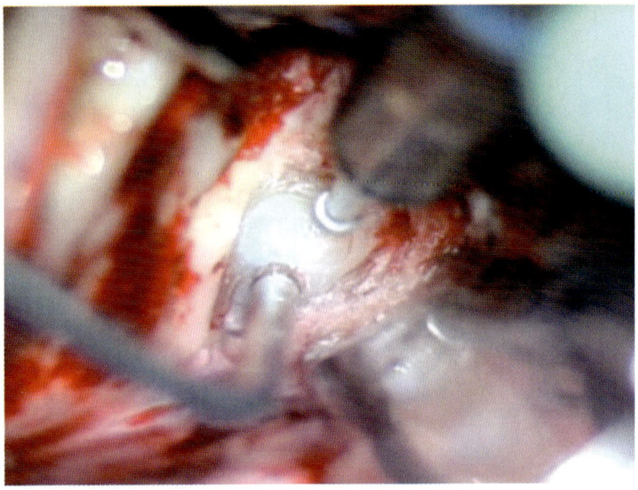

Fig. 12.15: Left middle cranial fossa drilling the bone over the cyst after retractor is placed.

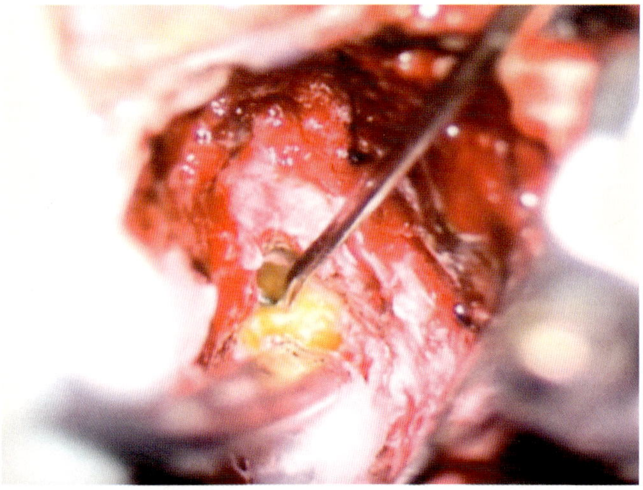

Fig. 12.16: Left middle cranial fossa opening the cyst. Yellow-brown fluid draining from the cyst lumen.

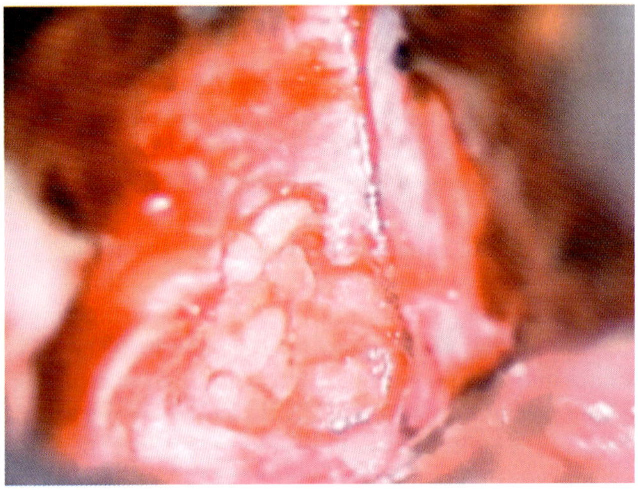

Fig. 12.17: Left middle cranial fossa. A fat graft is placed into the drained cyst cavity.

Step 9: The bone flap is secured in at least 3 points with titanium miniplates and 3 mm screws. The soft tissue layers are meticulously closed with special attention to achieve a watertight seal of the temporalis muscle. Subcutaneous tissues are approximated and the skin is closed (Fig. 12.18). A light pressure dressing is applied.

Complications

In addition to the aforementioned complications, with this approach the cochlea, superior canal, and the facial nerve are at greater risk for injury. Injury to the trigeminal nerve can cause numbness of the face. Complications from prolonged temporal lobe retraction, particularly in the elderly patient, are rare but can include seizures and stroke like symptoms. Postoperative meningitis and CSF leak are very rare, as are epidural hematomas.

Trans-sphenoid Approach

If the sphenoid sinus is well pneumatized and the cholesterol granuloma expands medial to the carotid artery an endonasal endoscopic approach could be considered (Fig. 12.19).[6] Stereotactic navigation is routinely used for this approach.

Step 1: Through a transnasal approach bilateral sphenoidotomies with a posterior nasal septectomy are performed, gaining wide exposure into the sphenoid sinus (Fig. 12.20). A binarial approach is used to access the lateral aspect of the sphenoid sinus and petrous apex.

Step 2: The sphenoid rostrum and the superior clivus are drilled to identify the medial aspect of the cholesterol granuloma if it is located medial to the first genu of the carotid artery. If more lateral access is needed the vidian nerve can be used as a landmark to identify the petrous carotid (Fig. 12.21).[7]

Step 3: The cholesterol granuloma is entered (Fig. 12.22) and the cyst is marsupialized (Fig. 12.23); often a microdebrider can be used.

Step 4: A Silastic drain can be placed into the lumen to prevent scarring of the ostium and to facilitate drainage into the nasal cavity (Fig. 12.24).

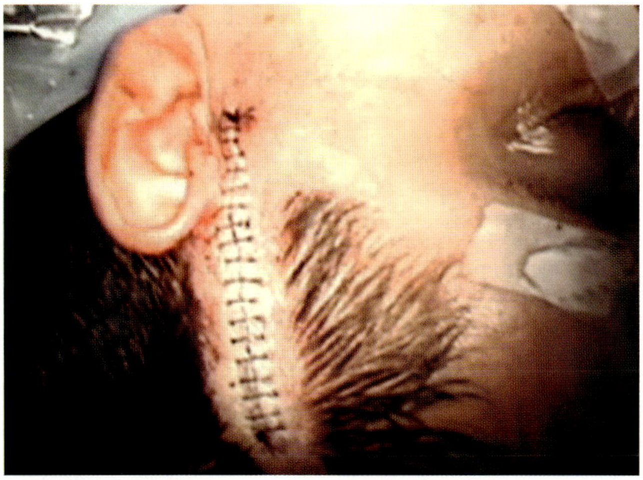

Fig. 12.18: Left middle cranial fossa closed incision.

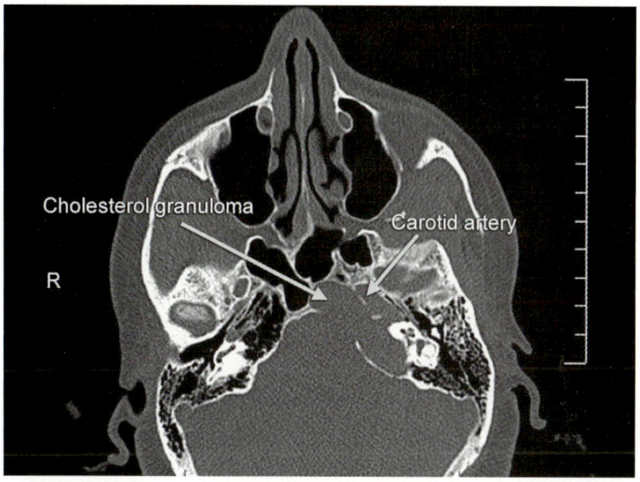

Fig. 12.19: CT scan. Left petrous apex cholesterol granuloma. Cyst extends medial to internal carotid artery.

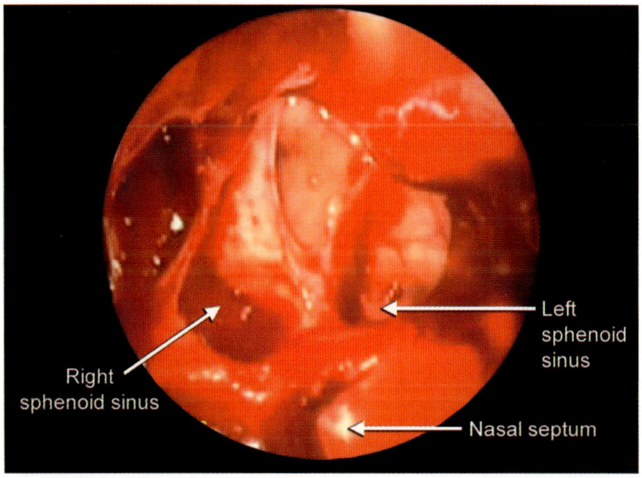

Fig. 12.20: Intraoperative endoscopic view after partial septectomy and sphenoidectomy.

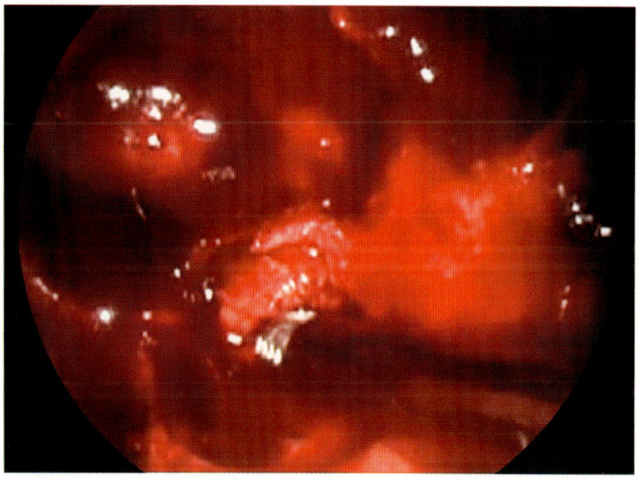

Fig. 12.21: Intraoperative endoscopic view. Drilling the bone over the cyst.

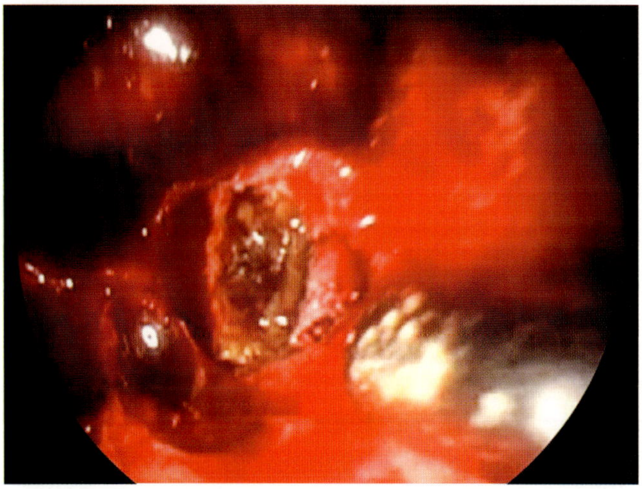

Fig. 12.22: Intraoperative endoscopic view. Opening the cyst with the microdebrider.

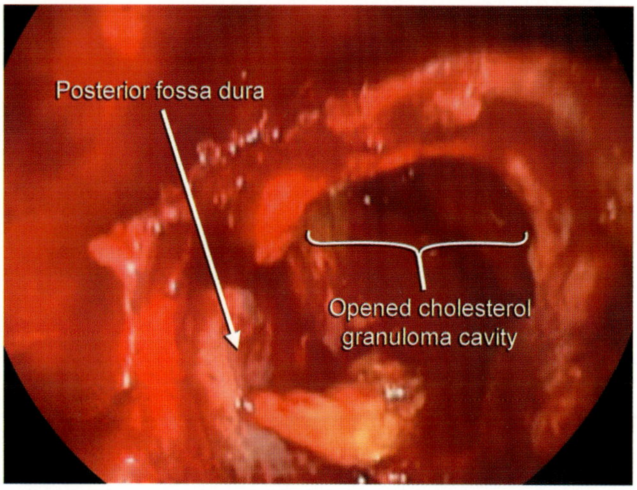

Fig. 12.23: Intraoperative endoscopic view. Opened cyst, exposed posterior fossa dura.

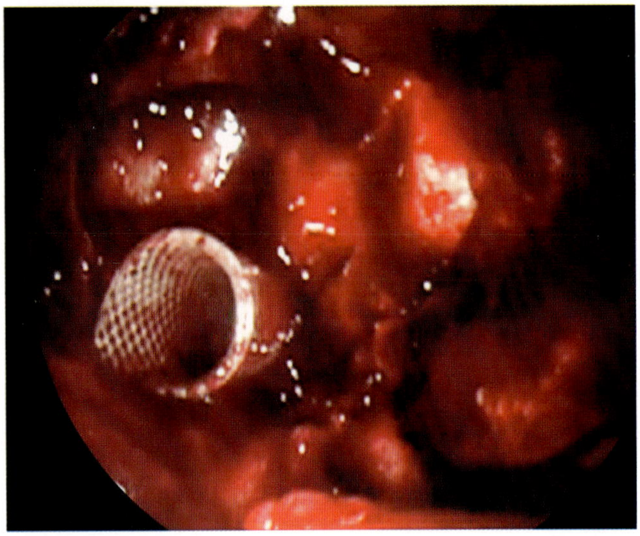

Fig. 12.24: Intraoperative endoscopic view. Silastic placed into lumen.

REFERENCES

1. Swartz JD, Harnsberger HR. Imaging of the Temporal Bone, 3rd edition. New York, NY: Thieme; 1998. p. 450.
2. Muckle RP, De la Cruz A, Lo WM. Petrous apex lesions. Am J Otol. 1998;19(2):219-25.
3. Cole RA. Petrous apicitis: surgical anatomy. Ann Otol Rhinol Laryngol. 1985;94:251-7.
4. Giddings NA, Brackmann DE, Kwartler JA. Transcanal infra cochlear approach to the petrous apex. Otolaryngol Head Neck Surg. 1991;104:29-36.
5. Kemink JL, Kartush JM, Graham MD. The arcuate eminence: topographic orientation in the middle cranial fossa surgery. Ann Otol Rhinol Laryngol. 1985;95:25-8.
6. Montgomery WW. Cystic lesions of the petrous apex: transsphenoid approach. Ann Otol Rhinol Laryngol. 1977;86 (4 Pt 1):429-35.
7. Kassam AB, Vescan AD, Carrau RL, et al. Expanded endonasal approach: vidian canal as a landmark to the petrous internal carotid artery. J Neurosurg. 2008;108:177-83.

CHAPTER 13

Facial Nerve Surgery

Eric W Sargent, Jack M Kartush

INTRODUCTION

The VIIth cranial nerve or facial nerve is a special visceral efferent nerve that innervates the stapedius muscle, branchial muscles of facial expression, and the posterior belly of the digastric muscle. The contribution of the nervus intermedius adds sensory (taste from tongue and palate and cutaneous sensation from the external auditory canal) and parasympathetic function (lacrimal, submandibular, and sublingual glands) to the nerve. The facial nerve has a long and winding course from the brainstem to the motor endplates of the facial musculature (Figs. 13.1 and 13.2). Its critical function in facial expression, maintenance of oral continence, and closure of the eyelids can make injury or pathology of the nerve socially, emotionally, and functionally devastating.

BELL'S PALSY

Bell's palsy is the most common cause of facial paralysis. It presents as acute peripheral facial weakness often associated or proceeded by upper respiratory symptoms and mild transient pain in the mastoid. Bell's palsy is not slowly progressive (although it may take 1–7 days to progress to complete paralysis), and not associated with twitching, audiovestibular symptoms, or severe otalgia. Studies have established reactivation of herpes simplex virus 1 (HSV-1) as the likely cause of most cases of Bell's palsy.[1,2] While most studies have shown that acute high-dose steroids (1 mg/kg per day for 2 weeks) initiated early in the course of the illness improve outcomes and reduce secondary defects after nerve recovery, the benefits of antiviral medication remain debated.[3,4] However, given the low cost and low risk of side effects of antivirals, it is reasonable to treat patients with both of these medications.

Patients with complete facial paralysis who present within 2 weeks of onset may be candidates for surgical treatment by decompressing the facial nerve. While most patients with typical Bell's palsy can forego imaging unless there has not been return of normal or near normal function within a reasonable amount of time, patients in whom decompression is contemplated should undergo an MRI scan.

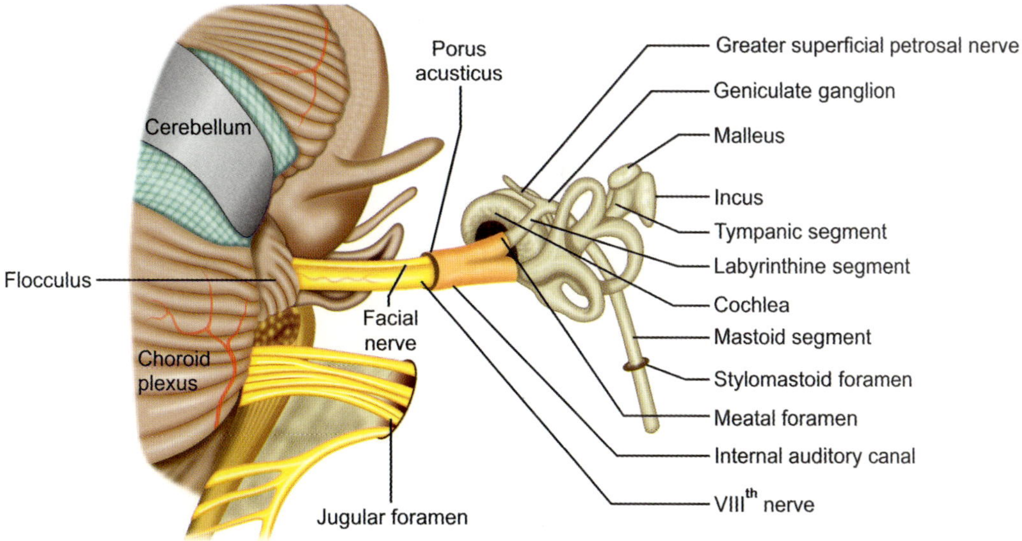

Fig. 13.1: Coronal view of the course of the facial nerve from the brainstem to the stylomastoid foramen.

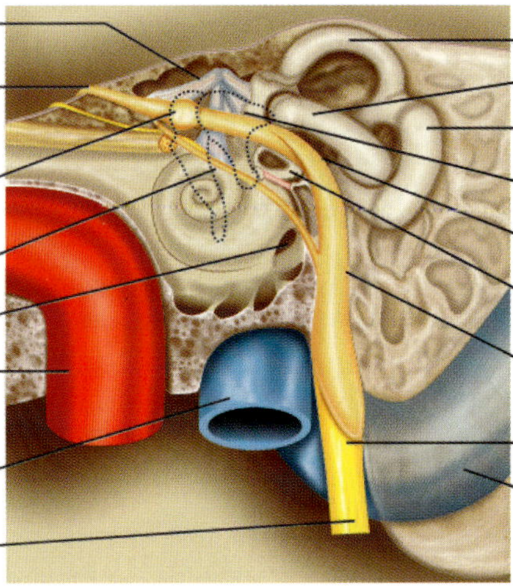

Fig. 13.2: Lateral view of the course of the facial nerve in the left temporal bone.

The constriction of the nerve at the meatal foramen, where the facial nerve enters the labyrinthine segment at the end of the internal auditory canal (IAC), is thought to be the cause of most facial nerve paralysis arising from viral cause and is probably the site of injury in delayed facial paralysis after acoustic neuroma surgery.[5] The nerve at the meatal foramen also has a dense investment of arachnoid. The meatal foramen is the narrowest part (0.61–0.68 mm diameter) of the fallopian canal and is the focus of surgical efforts in facial nerve decompression.[6,7]

TESTING

While there are several electrical tests of VIIth nerve integrity, all those in current clinical use suffer from the inability to test the nerve proximal to the stylomastoid foramen. Since, except for facial nerve disorders caused by parotid disease or penetrating facial trauma, most facial nerve pathology arises in the temporal bone or CPA, proximal facial nerve status can only in practicality be estimated indirectly from electrical testing of the distal nerve once Wallerian degeneration has extended beyond the stylomastoid foramen. Furthermore, because Wallerian degeneration takes 2–3 days to progress from a proximal intratemporal lesion to the extratemporal nerve, testing will be of no value for those first few days postinjury.

Objective data are derived from the response of the compound muscle action potential to electrical current applied with surface electrodes. This test is known as electroneurography or electroneuronography and usually abbreviated as ENoG. Using current applied at the stylomastoid foramen that causes supramaximal stimulation of the normal side of the face, the response in millivolts of the abnormal side of the face is measured and the outcome expressed as a percentage (Figs. 13.3A and B). Because the test measures the function of many fibers and relies on synchronous transmission of impulses, it is not of help in cases of demyelination or longstanding paralysis (typically a duration >3 weeks). As noted, it requires a period of 48–72 hours of complete paralysis before becoming useful to allow Wallerian degeneration to extend beyond the stylomastoid foramen. Degeneration of ENoG response that exceeds 90% within 14 days of the onset of paralysis indicates poor recovery in > 50% of patients.[8]

INDICATIONS FOR SURGERY

The current indications for decompression of the facial nerve in Bell's palsy include complete facial paralysis, ≥90% decrease in facial nerve response on ENoG within 2 weeks of onset of complete facial paralysis, and absence of voluntary action potentials on electromyography (EMG).[9] Patients should be counseled on the natural history of Bell's palsy, understanding that 70% of unselected and medically untreated patients have normal or near-normal recovery, an additional 15% may have mild or moderate asymmetric recovery and/or synkinesis, and the remaining 15% may have severely disturbed facial function.[10] Patients who meet the current criteria for decompression have a 42% chance of House-Brackmann (HB) I or II outcome if only treated medically; with decompression, their chance of HB I or II function is 91%.[9]

Like Bell's palsy, herpes zoster oticus (HZO; Ramsay Hunt syndrome), the second most common cause of facial paralysis, has a viral etiology: in the case of HZO the cause is reactivation of the varicella zoster virus.[11] Unlike Bell's palsy, HZO has a much poorer prognosis

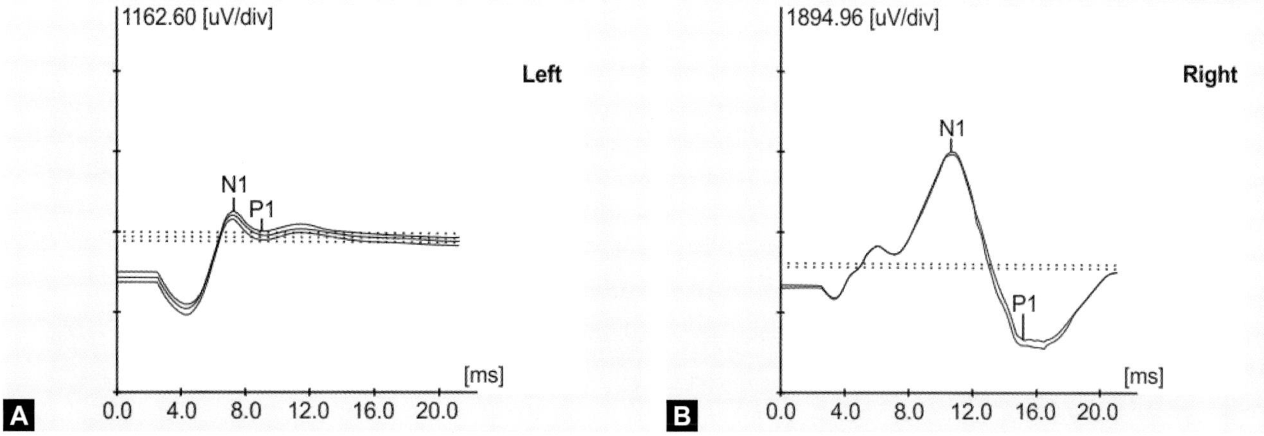

Figs. 13.3A and B: Electroneurography (ENoG) of patient after 72 hours of left facial paralysis showing >90% decrement in peak-to-peak N1/P1 left facial nerve response.

for facial nerve recovery with normal recovery observed in 49% of all untreated patient and in only 10% of patients who present with total paralysis.[12] Although the classic description of HZO is rapid onset of facial paralysis with a vesicular eruption of the auricle, hard palate or anterior two-thirds of the tongue, *zoster sine herpete*, in which patients have facial paralysis without a vesicular eruption, occurs in up to 19% of facial paralysis.[13,14] Unlike Bell's palsy, patients with HZO may have audiovestibular symptoms with partial or total loss of hearing and vestibular function. The treatment for HZO is early initiation of corticosteroid and antiviral treatment.[15] Due to the intense and diffuse inflammation of the nerve, surgery is not performed for HZO at most centers.

SURGERY—GENERAL CONSIDERATIONS

Procedures involving the facial nerve are performed under general anesthesia with the patient in supine position. Long-term paralyzing agents are avoided and facial nerve monitoring is performed if there is any chance of residual nerve function or if other nerves need to be monitored concurrently. In reanimation procedures that involve the hypoglossal nerve, electrodes can be placed in the tongue to allow positive identification of the hypoglossal nerve in the neck with a stimulating-dissecting instrument. However, because the hypoglossal nerve also innervates the geniohyoid muscle, if the surgical dissection is performed in this area, stimulation of the hypoglossal nerve near the digastric will reveal an obvious visible geniohyoid contraction, thereby confirming identification of the hypoglossal nerve and obviating the need to place needles in the tongue. This principle also applies to monitoring the spinal accessory nerve where sternocleidomastoid muscle contractions are readily apparent as long as muscle relaxants are avoided.

Procedures involving dural elevation require arterial line, urinary catheter, prophylactic antibiotics, diuretics, and hyperventilation. The patient's head is rotated away from the surgical field and taped into position with due care to avoid overextension especially in the elderly.

In all cases of facial nerve paralysis, attention must be directed to eye care to minimize the risk of secondary complications that can arise from paralytic lagophthalmos. In addition to lubricants and taping, early gold weight eyelid implantation can benefit, especially in elderly patients with early signs of ectropion, dryness, and keratitis. Because gold weight eyelid implantation is a low risk, easily reversible procedure, it should be considered early for the high-risk patients.[16]

SURGICAL STEPS—MEDIAL FACIAL NERVE DECOMPRESSION

Figures 13.4 to 13.13 show the steps in decompression of the meatal foramen and labyrinthine segment of the facial nerve in Bell's palsy or facial paralysis from temporal bone trauma. Patients should understand the risks of the surgery, which include loss of hearing and balance function in the ear from breach of the labyrinth during decompression, injury to the facial nerve, and intracranial complications such as cerebrospinal fluid leakage, intracranial bleeding, and temporal lobe injury from retraction. The operation is performed at few centers and the favorable outcomes of surgery cited in the literature are predicated on the competence and experience of the surgeon. However, even in the hands of experienced surgeons, the risks of the surgery are not insubstantial.

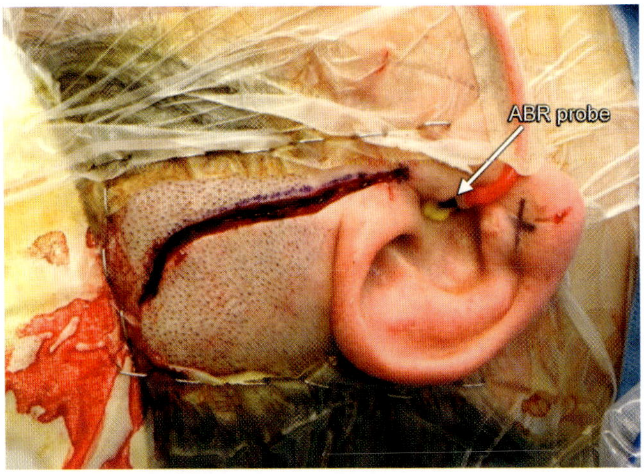

Fig. 13.4: Preauricular middle cranial fossa incision. For facial nerve decompression, the incision may start postauricularly to allow simultaneous mastoidectomy.
Source: Image used by permission from Michael J LaRouere, MD

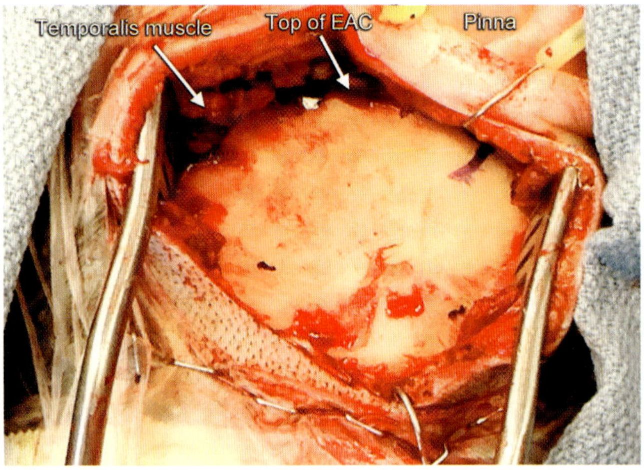

Fig. 13.5: Exposure of temporal skull before creation of bone flap craniotomy.
Source: Image used by permission from Michael J LaRouere, MD

Step 1: The hair is clipped for 5–7 cm above and behind the ear. Facial nerve monitoring electrodes are placed. A sterile probe for auditory brainstem monitoring is placed, secured, and then handed off the field to the monitorist.
Step 2: The proposed incision (which may start in the preauricular or postauricular crease depending on the preference of the surgeon) is infiltrated with lidocaine with epinephrine, taking care not to allow diffusion of the anesthetic beyond the mastoid tip where it may chemically paralyze the nerve and render monitoring useless.
Step 3: The skin incision is extended forward to create a posteriorly-based flap (Fig. 13.4).
Step 4: The temporalis muscle is reflected forward anteriorly, leaving a 1 cm cuff of muscle and fascia attached to the superior temporal line (Fig. 13.5). Leaving a cuff of muscle with fascia allows better reapproximation of the muscle at the end of the procedure.
Step 5: The surgeon typically elects to perform mastoidectomy prior to starting the middle cranial fossa (MCF) procedure to allow the tegmen above the cochleariform process to be fenestrated from below, which will aid in more rapid identification of the geniculate ganglion when later approached from the middle fossa.
Step 6: A 4–5 cm craniotomy centered over the external auditory canal is outlined and removed with an otologic drill (Fig. 13.6). Alternatively the bone flap can be made with a craniotome after drilling 5 mm holes at the corners of the bone flap. The former procedure takes a bit more time but minimizes the risk of dural injury.
Step 7: The dura is elevated from the roof of the temporal bone with a Freer elevator (Fig. 13.7). After the initial elevation is performed, elevation is the performed with stimulating-dissecting instruments (Fig. 13.8) that may allow early identification of a dehiscent nerve; however, often the nerve is not responsive to stimulation in these cases. An injured nerve will need higher current levels to achieve threshold responses. Consequently, while mapping this area seeking an injured nerve begin at 2mA and reduce current if or when a response is obtained. Elevation of dura from the floor of the MCF should proceed from posterior to anterior to reduce the risk of inadvertent avulsion of the greater superficial petrosal (GSP) and the geniculate ganglion, which in 17–20% of patients is dehiscent.[17,18] The middle meningeal artery (MMA) should be identified. If exposure of the floor of the temporal fossa is limited, the MMA should be cauterized, divided and the foramen spinosum packed with bone wax to reduce the chance of intracranial arterial bleeding.
Step 8: After placement of an articulated middle cranial fossa retractor, the critical step in middle fossa decompression is orientation, since surface landmarks are variable and can be unreliable. As mentioned before, the approximate position of the geniculate ganglion can be marked by performing mastoidectomy beforehand and making a hole in the bone of the tegmen above the cochleariform process. In the middle fossa, the surgeon may use (a) the arcuate eminence as a (fairly unreliable) proxy for the position of the underlying superior semicircular canal (SSC); (b) identification of the IAC in the "meatal plane" (measured from outer table of skull and from lip of superior petrosal sinus) on CT; (c) stereotactic

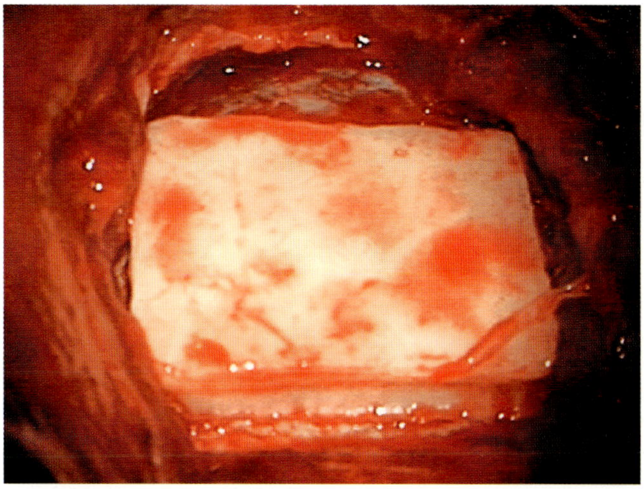

Fig. 13.6: Bone flap created for medial facial nerve decompression.
Source: Image used by permission from Michael J LaRouere, MD

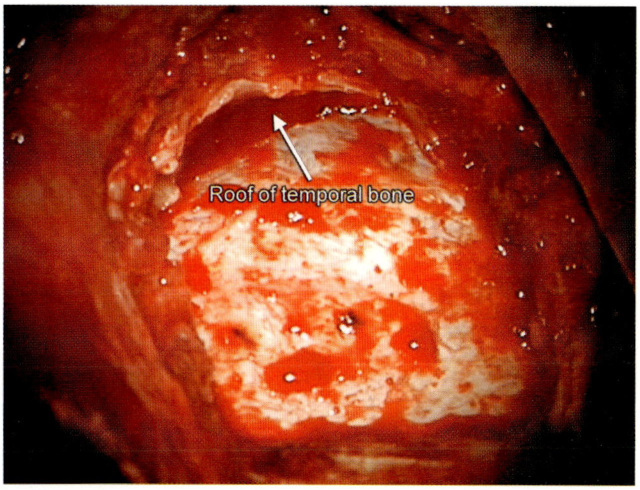

Fig. 13.7: Elevation of temporal lobe dura.
Source: Image used by permission from Michael J LaRouere, MD

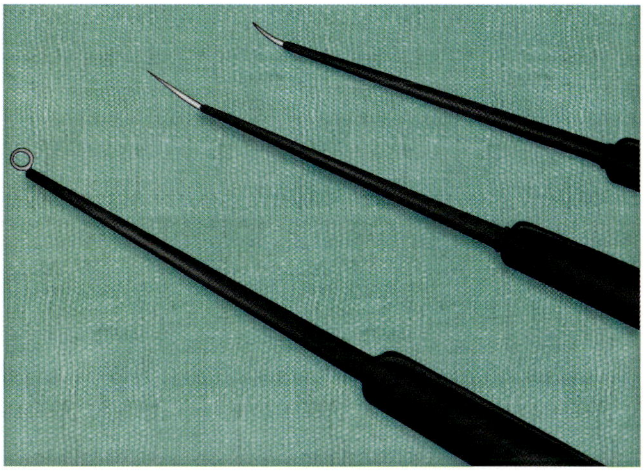

Fig. 13.8: Kartush stimulating instruments (KSIs) allow simultaneous stimulation during operative dissection (Neurosign, Wales).
Source: Image used by permission from Jack M Kartush, MD

localization; (d) identification of the facial hiatus and measurement 10 mm posteriorly and 5 mm medially from the origin of the GSP to the SSC (Kartush 10-5 rule[18]); (e) retrograde dissection via unroofing the GSP and following it posteriorly to the geniculate ganglion and labyrinthine facial nerve[19] (Fig. 13.9). The GSP nerve extends anteriorly from the geniculate ganglion and typically lies dehiscent on the middle fossa floor. Care must be taken to preserve this nerve branch to prevent a dry eye (Fig. 13.10). If it is injured in conjunction with a facial palsy, the risk of keratopathy increases dramatically.

After passing through the meatal foramen, the facial nerve is in the 4–5 mm labyrinthine segment where it becomes more rostral and arcs anteriorly. The nerve is encased in the narrowest part of the fallopian canal. It is slightly posterior and superior to the cochlea and anterior and medial to the superior semicircular canal. During middle cranial fossa dissection, this segment can be easily injured by the drill since the facial nerve is the most superior structure in the IAC, and it rises toward the surgeon as it passes from meatal foramen to the geniculate (Fig. 13.11). In surgery, more than in the temporal bone laboratory, this visual parallax issue is exacerbated because the temporal lobe dura creates an acute angle with the floor of the middle fossa.

Step 9: All bone dissection in the middle fossa is performed with a diamond bur and continuous suction-irrigation. The labyrinthine segment of the nerve is decompressed from the IAC to the geniculate ganglion (Fig. 13.12). The arachnoid investing the nerve at the meatal foramen is opened using a fine sharp ophthalmic knife. As noted, surgical decompression at the meatal foramen is made challenging by the fact that the nerve lies in a narrow 4 mm valley between basal turn of the cochlea and the superior semicircular canal's ampulla. Consequently, slight deviation of the drill may violate the labyrinth resulting in deafness, tinnitus, and dizziness. Drill burr size should be progressively reduced as the meatal foramen is approached. In addition, during the final delicate removal of bone, reducing drill speed can minimize inadvertent drill bit skipping.

Step 10: After the meatal foramen and labyrinthine segments have been decompressed, a muscle plug is typically required to prevent leakage of cerebrospinal fluid from the distal end of the IAC. The floor of the middle fossa may be covered with fascia and a part of the bone flap,

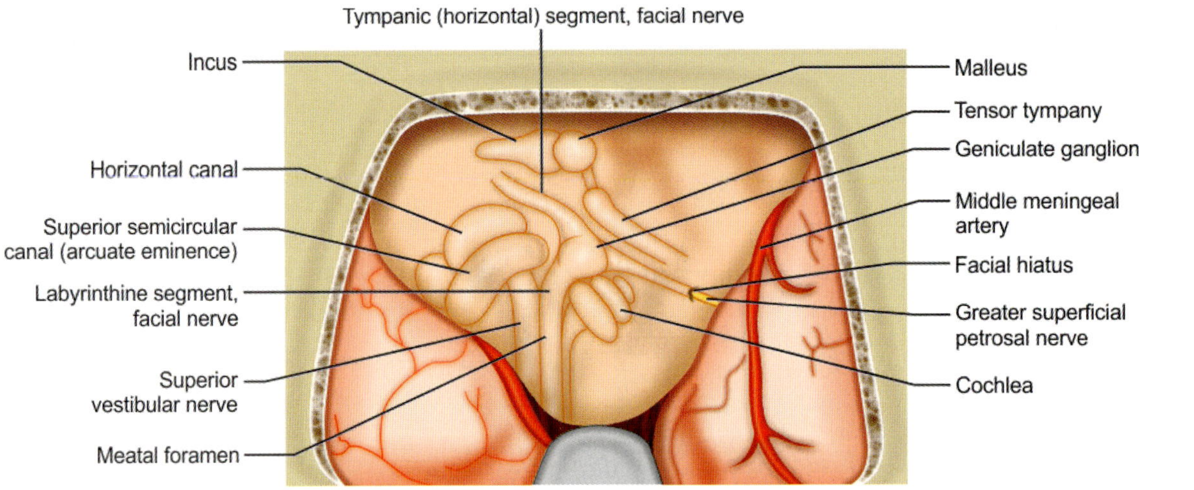

Fig. 13.9: Diagram of floor of middle cranial fossa showing key relationships important for surgical orientation during medial facial nerve decompression.

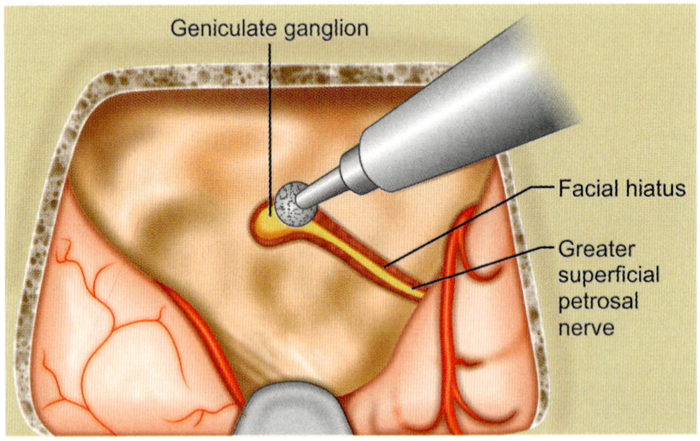

Fig. 13.10: Diagram showing orientation of middle cranial fossa dissection by following the greater superficial petrosal (GSP) nerve to the geniculate ganglion. Care should be taken to avoid injury to the nerve.

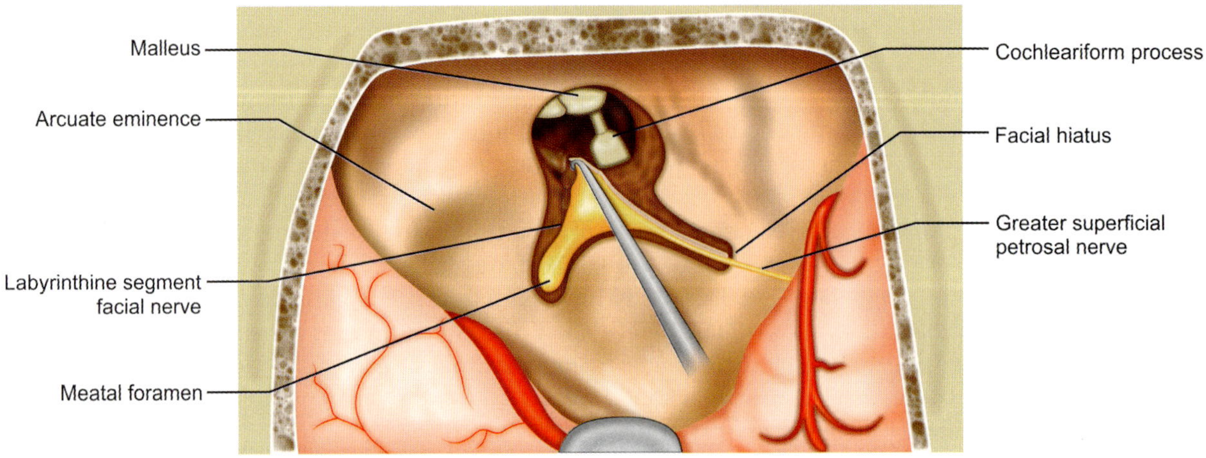

Fig. 13.11: Diagram of decompressed geniculate ganglion, labyrinthine segment and proximal horizontal segment of the facial nerve. By performing mastoidectomy before middle fossa surgery, identifying the position of the cochleariform process and heads of the ossicles can facilitate localization of the geniculate ganglion.

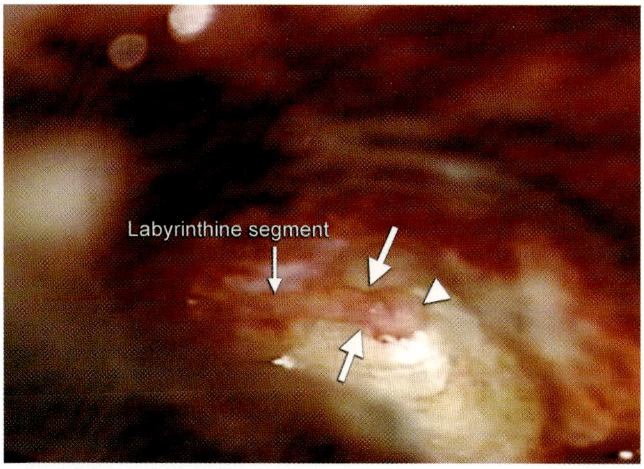

Fig. 13.12: The appearance of the labyrinthine facial nerve after decompression for Bell's palsy. The arrowhead indicates the nerve exiting the internal auditory canal. The two arrows indicate the hourglass narrowing of the meatal foramen.
Source: Image used by permission from Eric W Sargent, MD

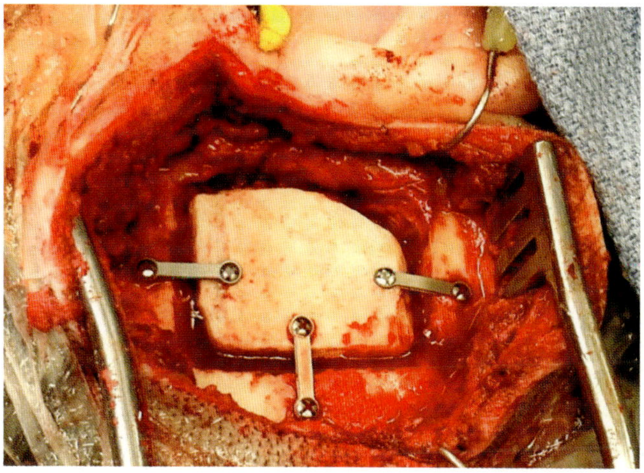

Fig. 13.13: Replacement of the bone flap, secured with titanium microplates, after completion of medial facial nerve decompression.
Source: Image used by permission from Michael J LaRouere, MD

a hydroxyapatite disk or hydroxyapatite cement. The bone flap is replaced and anchored to the skull with titanium micro plates (Fig. 13.13). The temporalis muscle is sutured to the cuff of tissue along the superior temporal line with absorbable suture. The skin is reapproximated with suture or staples. Drains are not used.

TEMPORAL BONE TRAUMA

Blunt or penetrating trauma to the temporal bone is a common cause of facial paralysis. Treatment decisions are made along the same path as Bell's palsy, with a few important departures. The indications for and timing of nerve exploration after temporal bone trauma is complex. Many patients who have suffered a temporal bone fracture are unstable and surgery, even if indicated by obvious disruption and distraction of the fallopian canal on CT, may not be safe for some time due to associated temporal lobe contusions. Furthermore, surgical exploration after temporal bone injury is often frustrated by bleeding from fractures and adherent fibrin clot that can make positive identification of the facial nerve more difficult. The decision to operate in this setting should be balanced with concern about causing more injury amidst the swelling and bleeding of fresh trauma. In temporal bone fractures that breach the labyrinth, resulting in deafness, translabyrinthine decompression with nerve repair simplifies treatment.

In contrast to temporal bone fractures, penetrating extratemporal injuries (e.g. knife wounds) to the parotid and/or face with immediate segmental or total paralysis of the face require surgical exploration and repair within 72 hours to allow identification of injured nerves before Wallerian degeneration makes identification with a nerve stimulator impossible. Beyond 72 hours, identification of the distal nerve end becomes a challenge and typically requires following the nerve from known landmarks near the facial musculature toward the site of laceration.

The evaluation of cases of temporal bone fracture with complete facial paralysis begins with history: is the onset of paralysis immediate or delayed? Unfortunately, otolaryngologists are not consulted immediately in many such cases and the record may not accurately reflect the status of the nerve at presentation.

If facial paralysis is immediate and complete and the patient is medically stable, high-resolution CT is done to establish the site of injury. If there is obvious transection of the nerve on CT, surgery may proceed without electrophysiological testing. Without clear evidence on CT of nerve disruption, absence of voluntary action potentials on facial EMG may suggest benefit from early surgical exploration. If voluntary potentials are present, the patient may be followed with ENoG beginning 72 hours after complete paralysis. If within 2 weeks ENoG deteriorates beyond 90% and facial EMG shows loss of voluntary action potentials, the option of surgical decompression should be discussed with the patient.

Cases of delayed post-traumatic facial paralysis are treated similar to Bell's palsy: monitored with ENoG beginning 72 hours after complete paralysis. Surgery is considered when ENoG deteriorates beyond 90% and voluntary action potentials are lost on facial EMG. Unlike Bell's palsy cases in which it may only occasionally be performed, high-resolution CT is always performed before exploration of a traumatized facial nerve.

The most common site of facial nerve injury in temporal bone fractures is the perigeniculate area (Figs. 13.14 and 13.15). Injuries with complete facial paralysis in this area that meet the electrical testing criteria used for Bell's palsy may benefit from middle cranial fossa decompression or repair. Since temporal bone fractures may injure the facial nerve at more than one site, both middle fossa and transmastoid approaches are usually performed in combination.

SURGICAL STEPS FOR PERIGENICULATE TRAUMA

Step 1: Surgery for perigeniculate trauma is facilitated by first performing a mastoidectomy.

Step 2: Decompression of the tympanic and mastoid segments of the facial nerve is performed if needed.

Step 3: The position of the geniculate ganglion is marked by removing bone of the tegmen tympani over the cochleariform process and heads of the malleus and incus (Figs. 13.16A and B). This fenestrated area of the tegmen is then readily identified when the middle fossa is subsequently exposed from above. In most other respects the incision, management of the temporalis muscle, decompression of the nerve, and repair of the defect is identical to surgery for Bell's palsy. Some tear or crush injuries at the perigeniculate region may be treated with either a nerve graft or a very limited reroutement to achieve a single anastomosis.

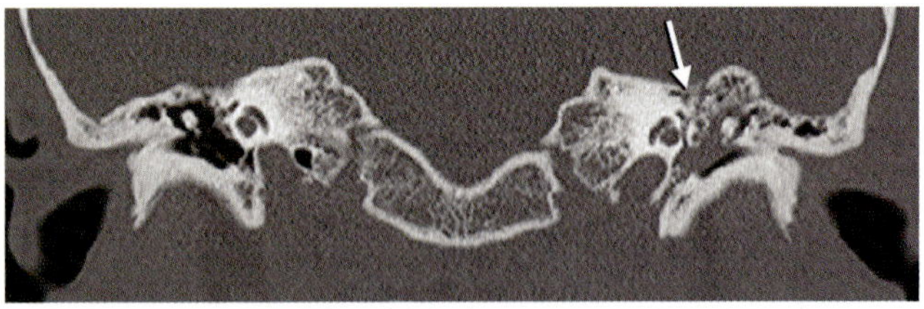

Fig. 13.14: Coronal CT image shows the fractures in the left perigeniculate area (arrow).

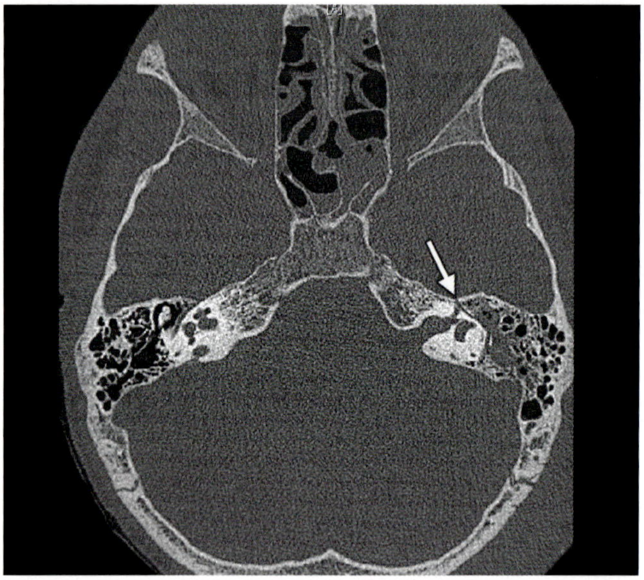

Fig. 13.15: Axial CT image shows the fractures in the left perigeniculate area (arrow).

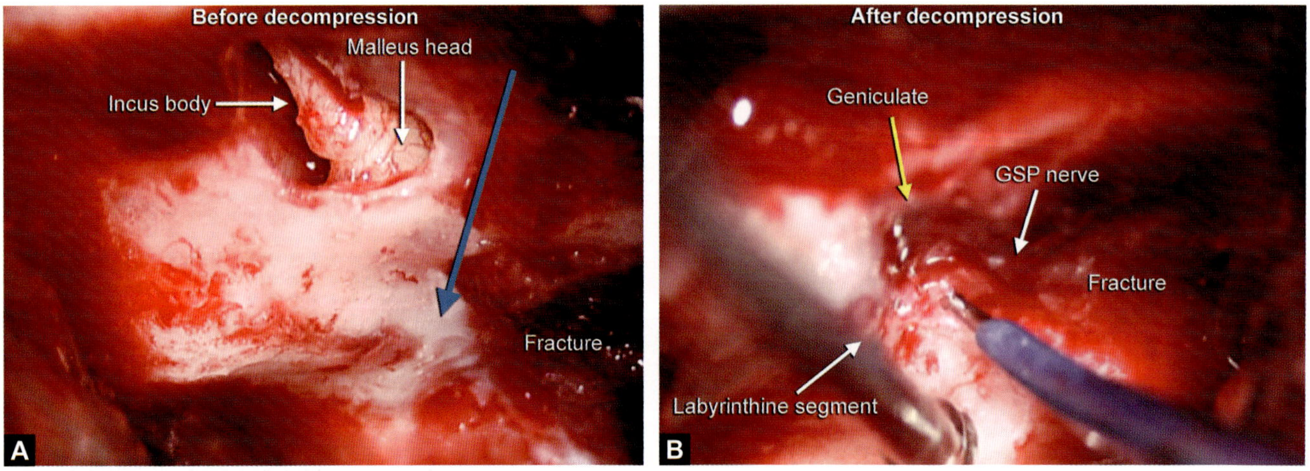

Figs. 13.16A and B: Intraoperative view of the middle fossa decompression showing the floor of the middle fossa with the heads of the ossicles exposed. The inset image is a higher magnification view of the decompressed geniculate ganglion and labyrinthine facial nerve. An upper lid gold weight is placed simultaneously.

Source: Images used by permission from Ilka C Naumann, MD

FACIAL NERVE INJURY IN THE MASTOID

The second most common site of injury is at the second genu that is typically associated with incus displacement (Fig. 13.17). In cases where injury is clearly due to middle ear or mastoid trauma, the middle fossa approach may be omitted.

Figures 13.17 to 13.19 show the sequelae of temporal bone trauma wherein the incus was rotated 90° and driven into the tympanic segment of the facial nerve by a lateral blow. The injury was treated by mastoidectomy with removal of the incus (which was banked in the mastoid for later replacement) and decompression of the tympanic and vertical segments of the nerve. A gold weight was placed simultaneously. Facial nerve function recovered to HBII within 6 months.

SURGICAL STEPS FOR MASTOID FACIAL NERVE DECOMPRESSION

Step 1: Mastoidectomy is performed in the routine fashion. Facial nerve monitoring is employed if there is any possibility of some residual nerve viability.

Step 2: The facial recess is opened widely and the ossicles are identified (Fig. 13.18). Typically, the incus is removed to allow a clear view of the horizontal segment of the facial nerve and the second genu.

Step 3: The facial nerve is decompressed for 5–10 mm on either side of the injury (Fig. 13.19).

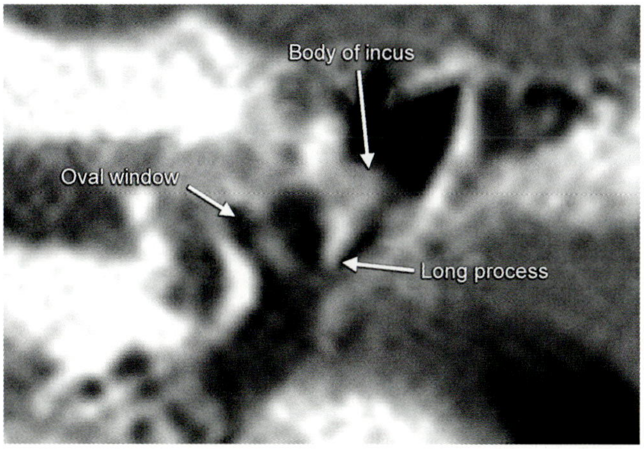

Fig. 13.17: Coronal CT showing rotation of the incus in temporal bone trauma with injury to the left ear horizontal facial nerve segment.

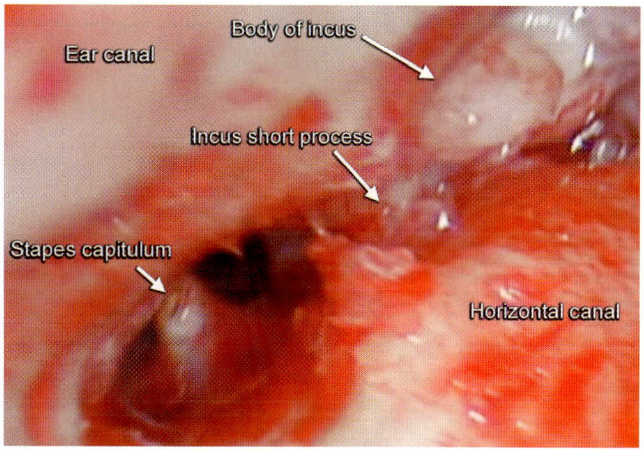

Fig. 13.18: Image before removal of the incus shows that the short process of the incus has been driven into the tympanic segment of the facial nerve.
Source: Image used by permission from Eric W Sargent, MD

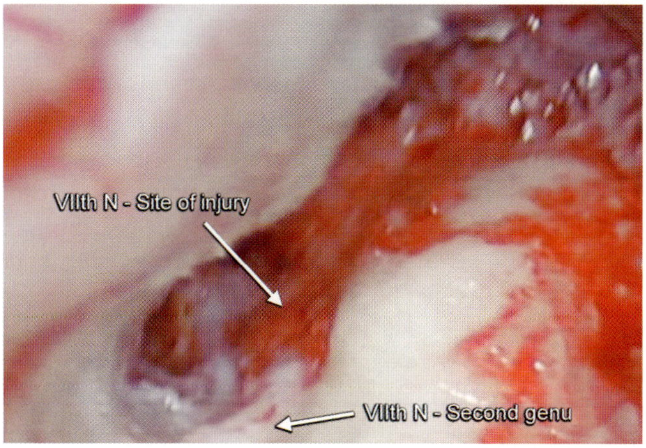

Fig. 13.19: The injured, but intact, tympanic facial nerve and decompression of the nerve proximal and distal to the injury. An upper lid gold weight is placed simultaneously.
Source: Image used by permission from Eric W Sargent, MD

Step 4: The incus can be banked in the mastoid for replacement at a later surgery or replaced in proper orientation to the remaining ossicles and secured with Gelfoam. When possible, we prefer to use a Kartush Incus Strut (Gyrus Olympus, Center Valley, PA) to reconstruct the chain at the time of the facial nerve repair. Ossiculoplasty during the initial operation will hopefully obviate the need for late revision surgery adjacent to an exposed nerve graft.

IATROGENIC NERVE INJURY—MASTOIDECTOMY

Causes of intraoperative facial nerve injury include instrument or drill contact, cautery, and thermal injury with a laser. Stretch injuries are also common when operating at foci where the nerve is tethered, e.g. pons,

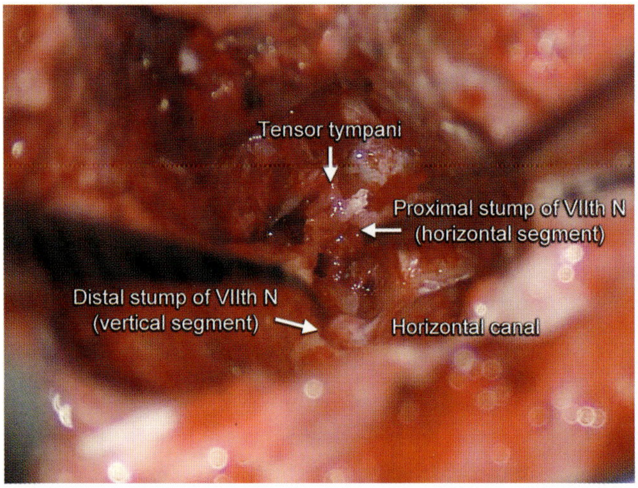

Fig. 13.20: Iatrogenic facial nerve (drill) injury at the second genu, the most common site of injury in mastoidectomy.
Source: Image used by permission from Eric W Sargent, MD

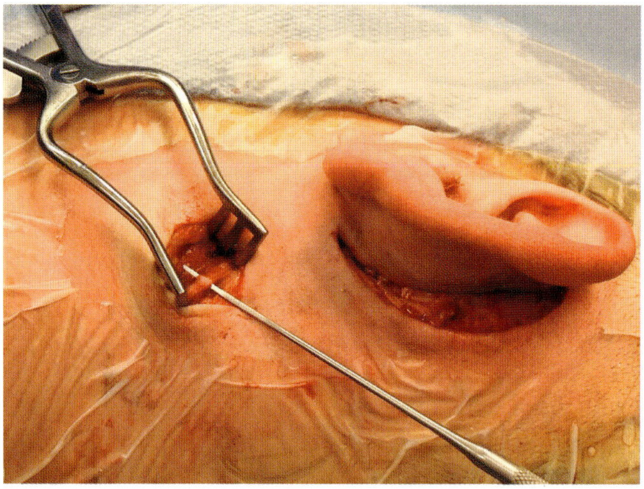

Fig. 13.21: Harvest of great auricular nerve graft in the neck.
Source: Image used by permission from Eric W Sargent, MD

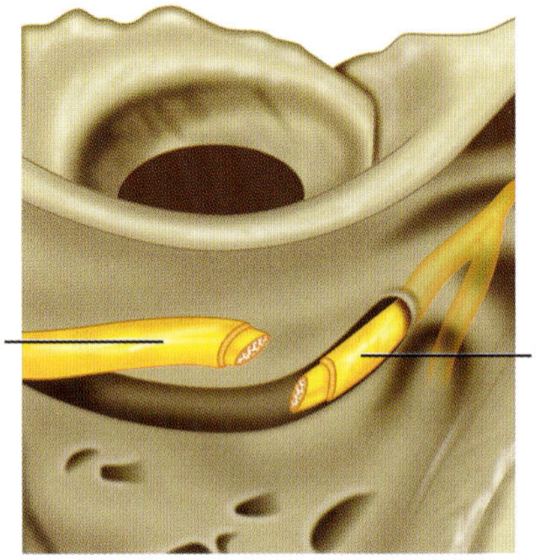

Fig. 13.22: Beveling the ends of the nerve graft and the injured facial nerve at a 45° angle exposes more neural tubules and improves nerve regrowth. Left ear.

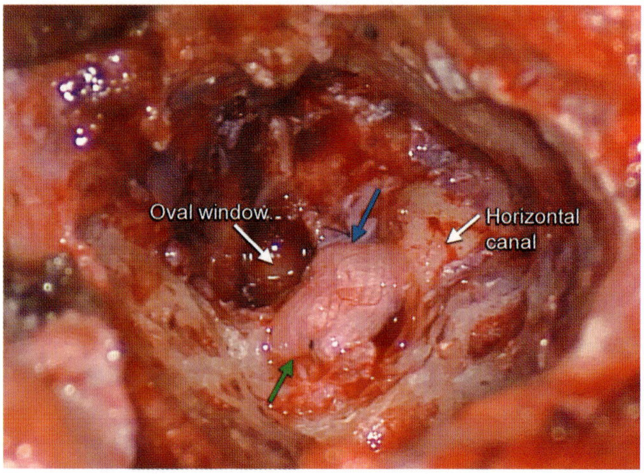

Fig. 13.23: The ends of the graft and facial nerve are sutured with two to three fine nonabsorbable sutures.
Source: Image used by permission from Eric W Sargent, MD

meatal foramen, and stylomastoid foramen. The risk of injury increases when landmarks are obscured by disease, when there is natural or pathological dehiscence of the nerve, or when dissection techniques are unsafe. The risk of injury is decreased by dissection that proceeds in a stepwise fashion using anatomic landmarks. Although no controlled studies confirm that intraoperative monitoring decreases facial nerve injury during routine otologic surgery, following the National Institutes of Health recommendation of intraoperative monitoring for acoustic tumor surgery, surgeons are increasingly using monitoring during mastoid surgery.[20]

The principles of safe mastoid surgery will be covered elsewhere in this volume. Violation of these principles can lead to disaster. Figures 13.20 to 13.23 show a drill injury to the second genu of the facial nerve, the most common site of iatrogenic injury during mastoid surgery.

Accurately assessing facial nerve function in the immediate postoperative period is a sine qua non of patient care following any surgery in which the facial nerve is at risk. Taking inventory of function in all branches of the nerve can be critical information later if delayed facial paralysis develops since many cases of delayed facial paralysis can be managed nonsurgically with steroids. However, if facial weakness or asymmetry in the recovery room is noted, diagnostic pitfalls must be avoided. Complete paralysis may be misinterpreted as incomplete paresis because (a) in children, youthful tone of skin and muscles prevents early drooping, and (b) slow, complete eye closure may be due not to orbicularis contraction (VIIn innervation) but instead due to reflex relaxation of the levator palpebri (IIIn innervation). In these cases, observing active eye closure, rather than passive eyelid lowering, is critical to making an accurate diagnosis.

In cases of suspected facial paralysis after surgery, before deciding management the surgeon should (1) wait until the patient is fully awake to accurately assess function; (2) remove the mastoid dressing that may depress the brow and give the appearance of a "partially functioning" lid; (3) wait for a few hours to allow metabolic clearance of any local anesthetic that may have chemically paralyzed the nerve; and (4) personally assess the patient rather than rely on second-hand assessments.

If paralysis is noted, the surgeon needs to consider where the nerve may have been injured and how severe the injury may be. If exploration seems indicated, the primary surgeon should consider when to repair, how to repair, and who should carry out repair. Even experienced ear surgeons, when faced with the trauma of unexpected facial paralysis after surgery, benefit from consultation with an experienced colleague or subspecialist who can observe and advise on the case or assume management of the complication. If immediate re-exploration is not elected, the surgeon should consider tests that may help to guide future steps, such as electrical testing and CT scan. Steroids should be started.

In deciding when to explore, keep in mind that animal studies suggest that facial nerve grafting can be successful up to 90 days after transection.[21] Thus, there is no physiologic need to operate immediately in the cases of intratemporal transection. The timing of surgical intervention can be based on deliberate evaluation of the site of injury, the experience of the surgeon, the likelihood of reversible neuropraxia versus irreversible neurotmesis, the risks of exploration, and the effects of delayed surgery on the surgical field and distal nerve excitability.

Surgical injuries to the facial nerve in the middle ear and mastoid can be managed using guidelines as follows: (1) simple exposure of the nerve requires no further treatment; (2) contusion or <1/3 transection of the nerve diameter requires decompression of the nerve 5–10 mm on both sides of the injury; (3) if >1/3 of the nerve is transected, neurorrhaphy or nerve grafting is indicated.[22]

The goal of nerve repair is to maximize growth of axons through the anastomosis or graft and minimize synkinesis. Maximum axonal growth to the target motor end plates is accomplished by (a) minimizing fibroblastic growth in the anastomosis, (b) minimizing escape of axons from the anastomosis, and (c) a tension-free anastomosis. No matter how carefully neurorrhaphy or grafting is performed, it is exceedingly rare that facial nerve function will be better than HB III/VI.[22,23]

Direct nerve repair with primary anastomosis is preferable when possible. This minimizes the number of anastomoses that could allow ingrowth of fibroblasts or escape of axons. However, it is frequently not practical in the temporal bone. In some cases, a missing or damaged segment can be managed with reroutement within constraints. However, nerve grafting may be preferable to reroutement since reroutement devascularizes the surviving nerve. In cases of severe nerve injury in the mastoid with segmental loss of nerve, the surgical steps are as follows:

Step 1: Perform a mastoidectomy, if not already done.

Step 2: If surgery is performed within 72 hours of injury, the distal facial nerve can be identified by facial nerve stimulation (Fig. 13.20).

Step 3: The nerve is decompressed on both sides of the injury with a diamond bur and continuous irrigation.

Step 4: A great auricular nerve graft is harvested (Fig. 13.21).

Step 5: The ends of the nerve graft and the injured facial nerve are freshened at a 45° angle (Fig. 13.22), which exposes more neural tubules and improves nerve regrowth.[24] Minimizing fibroblast ingrowth can be aided by trimming excess epineurium and making a tension-free anastomosis.

Step 6: The ends of the graft and facial nerve are sutured with two or three 9-0 nonabsorbable sutures (Fig. 13.23). By carefully coapting the nerve ends with fine nonabsorbable suture both ingrowth of fibroblasts and escape of axons can be minimized.

FACIAL NERVE INJURY IN THE CEREBELLOPONTINE ANGLE

Repair of the facial nerve in the cerebellopontine angle is challenging. Without an epineurium, suture repair of the nerve in this location is rarely optimal. While the use of collagen tube and fibrin glue may help slightly, the outcomes are often unpredictable and unsatisfying, with "fair" return of function in 40–60% and a 20% failure rate.[25-27] The success of nerve repair in injuries distal to the geniculate ganglion is higher.

In tumor cases when hearing has been sacrificed or lost intraoperatively, reconstruction of the facial nerve when a segment of nerve is missing in the cerebellopontine

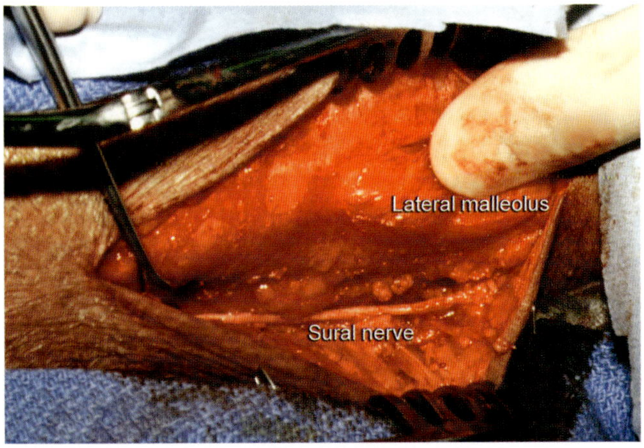

Fig. 13.24: Harvest of a right sural nerve for a long facial nerve graft. The nerve can also be harvested with the aid of an endoscope through a smaller incision.
Source: Image used by permission from Eric W Sargent, MD

angle can be performed with rerouting the nerve from the stylomastoid foramen. This reduces the need for the second anastomosis required for a nerve graft and should yield better preservation of functional nerve fibers. In mastoidectomy cases where nerve injury or sacrifice occurs, primary anastomosis of the nerve may require rerouting over the promontory and the available length is usually <10 mm.

NERVE GRAFTS

An interposition graft is required if tension-free primary repair of the facial nerve is not possible. The great auricular nerve, which has about the same diameter as the facial nerve, is easily harvested through the same incision of many otologic or neurologic procedures. It can also be harvested through an inconspicuous separate incision over the sternocleidomastoid muscle. Harvest of the great auricular nerve results in only an anesthesia of the skin over the parotid gland and mastoid process and both surfaces of the pinna.

In cases where the great auricular nerve is not available as a graft, the anterior branch of the medial antebrachial cutaneous nerve can be used. This nerve, which provides sensation to the medial cutaneous aspect of the arm, can be sacrificed with little donor site morbidity.

When a graft longer than 8–10 cm is needed to provide tension-free anastomosis, a segment of the sural nerve should be used. The sural nerve is found paralleling the saphenous vein, immediately posterior to the lateral malleolus (Fig. 13.24). Sacrifice of the sural nerve causes anesthesia of a small area of the lateral lower leg and lateral dorsum of the foot.

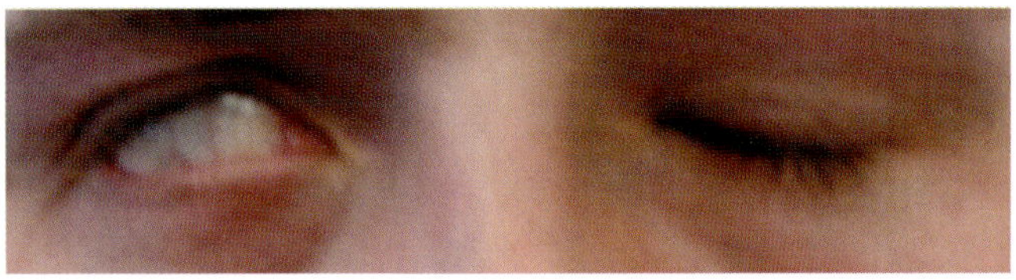

Fig. 13.25: Severe right paralytic lagophthalmos. Note excellent Bell's phenomenon.
Source: Image used by permission from Eric W Sargent, MD

FACIAL REHABILITATION

Patients with facial nerve injury or pathology may not respond to medical or surgical treatment resulting in persistent paralysis or severe paresis, requiring further rehabilitative procedures. Many modalities now in current use, such as free-muscle transfer in long-standing paralysis and injected botulinum toxin for facial spasm that can occur after reinnervation, are beyond the scope of this chapter. Three major rehabilitative procedures will be reviewed.

GOLD WEIGHT IMPLANTATION

As mentioned earlier, protection of the eye is paramount in preventing morbidity due to paralytic lagophthalmos (Fig. 13.25). Short-term, ocular lubricants, taping of the lid, or a temporary tarsorrhaphy are effective temporizing measures. The latter had been a mainstay in the past but tarsorrhaphy is both cosmetically unappealing and suboptimal because it focuses its eyelid narrowing either medially or laterally, whereas the greatest concern is the center of the cornea. Thus, for paralytic lagophthalmos that is not expected to recover within a few weeks, loading the upper lid with an implanted gold or platinum weight is quick, effective, low-risk, and can be performed under local anesthesia with sedation. Unlike tarsorrhaphy, upper lid weighting appropriately has its main benefit over the center of the cornea. Consultation with an ophthalmologist in paralytic lagophthalmos is recommended to minimize the risk of exposure keratitis in patients who do not respond to the aforementioned conservative measures. The risks of gold or platinum weight implantation include infection, bleeding, foreign body reaction, extrusion of the implant, and visual impairment due to corneal astigmatism. Alternative treatments include palpebral springs, titanium chain link implants, and in the most troublesome cases, complete temporary closure of the eyelid with sutures.

Step 1: Before going to the operating room, nonsterile gold or platinum weights are tested on the patient's paralyzed

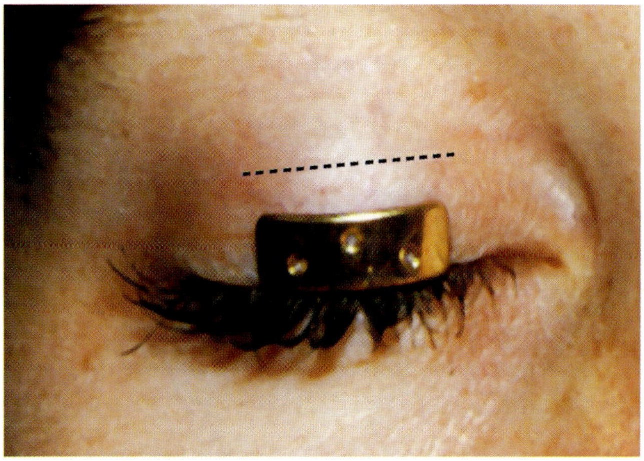

Fig. 13.26: Testing a gold weight in the office or preoperative holding area determines the proper size required. The dotted line indicates the incision in the upper lid.

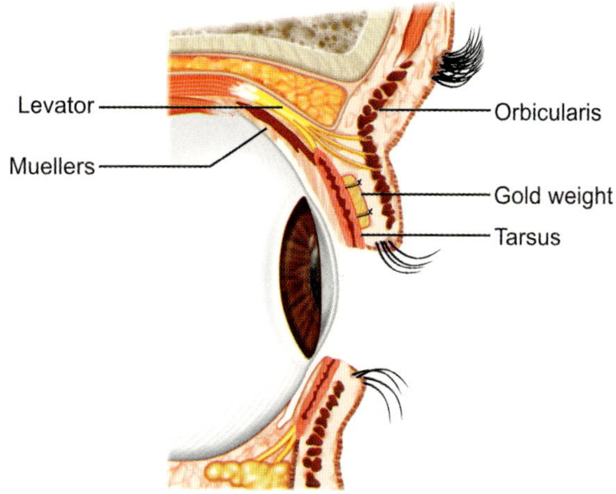

Fig. 13.27: The gold weight is placed parallel to and just above the eyelash line and anchored to the tarsal cartilage with absorbable monofilament suture.

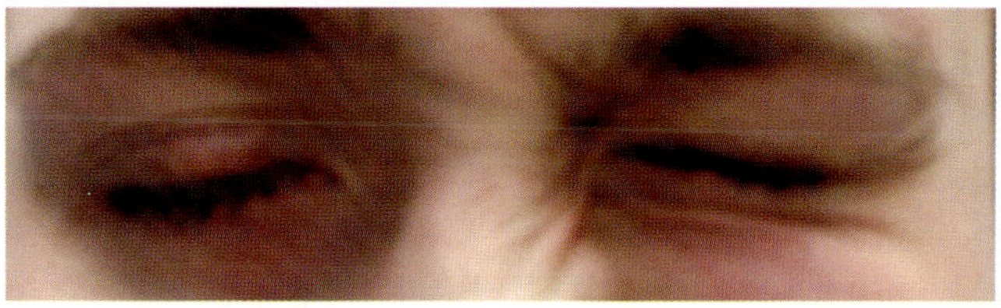

Fig. 13.28: Result of gold weight (0.8g) implantation on patient depicted in Figure 13.25.
Source: Image used by permission from Eric W Sargent, MD

eyelid with the patient seated to find the proper weight. A dab of Mastisol on the weight allows it to temporarily adhere to the skin. For men, the usual weight is 1–1.2 g; for women, the weight is usually 0.8–1.2 g (Fig. 13.26).
Step 2: An approximately 15 mm horizontal incision is made in the supratarsal crease of the upper lid centered in the midpupillary line (Fig. 13.26, dashed line).
Step 3: The skin is elevated to the superior border of the tarsus. Care should be taken to avoid transection of the levator muscle attachments in order to avoid ptosis.
Step 4: A pocket is formed directly on the tarsal plate sufficient to accommodate the weight, leaving a cuff of tissue on the lid margin. Thin tissue over the weight can lead to extrusion of the implant.
Step 5: The weight is placed parallel to and just above the eyelash line (Fig. 13.27).
Step 6: The implant is sutured to the tarsus with 5-0 absorbable monofilament and the pocket is flushed with balanced saline solution (BSS).
Step 7: The orbicularis-levator complex is reapproximated with 5-0 absorbable monofilament and the skin is closed with 5-0 fast-absorbing gut suture.

Postoperative care: The patient should intermittently apply a cold-pack to the lid for 6–12 hours and rest somewhat upright to reduce swelling. Use of ocular lubricants and taping the eye shut at night should continue until the weight is clearly effective since the weight relies on gravity and, when the patient is supine, the weight may actually pull the lid open (Fig. 13.28).

HYPOGLOSSAL-FACIAL NERVE ANASTOMOSIS

When direct nerve repair is not possible, but facial muscles remain viable, neurotization (i.e. use of a donor nerve to reinnervate the facial nerve) is indicated. Typical situations in which this may occur include loss or sacrifice of the proximal trunk of CN VII (as in facial nerve schwannoma or other cerebellopontine angle pathology), destruction of the facial nucleus (e.g. due to pontine hemorrhage), or in cases of internal axonotomesis (e.g. when a nerve appear anatomically intact, but does not functionally recover within 12 months). Although a variety of donor nerves, such as the phrenic and spinal accessory nerves, have been used historically for neurotization, the nerve with the greatest reliability and least donor morbidity is the hypoglossal nerve.[28]

The timing of hypoglossal neurotization is little debated at the present time: in the case of known sacrifice of the facial nerve in the cerebellopontine angle without

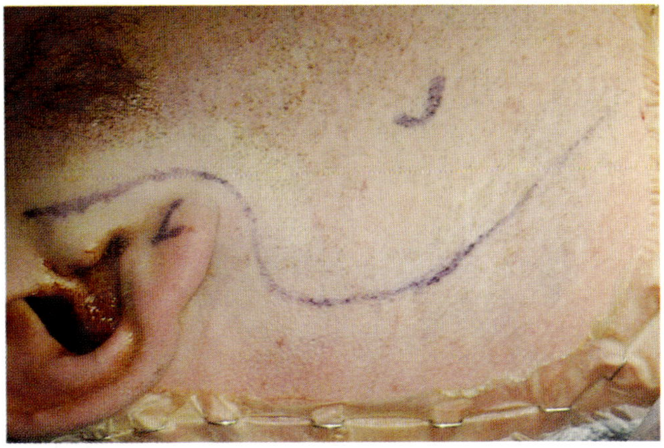

Fig. 13.29: Preauricular and cervical incision for hypoglossal-facial nerve anastomosis.
Source: Image used by permission from Michael J LaRouere, MD

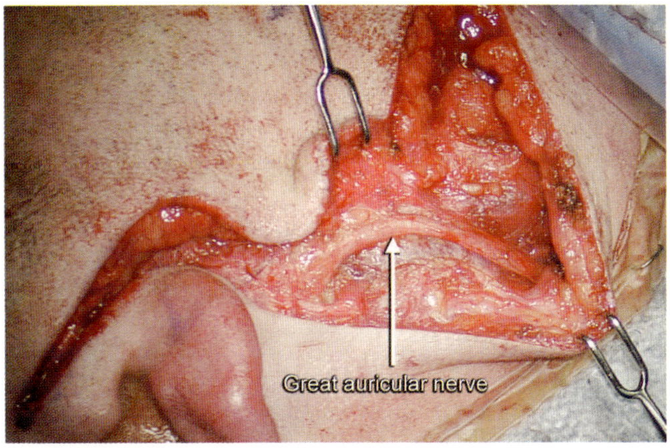

Fig. 13.30: Identification of the great auricular nerve.
Source: Image used by permission from Michael J LaRouere, MD

immediate nerve reanastomosis or grafting, hypoglossal-facial grafting can be performed as soon as the patient's condition permits. In the case of a facial nerve that appears anatomically intact at the end of surgery or has been re-anastomosed or grafted in the cerebellopontine angle and yet does not recover function, hypoglossal-facial grafting should be done no later than 12–18 months after onset of paralysis. Although there are reports of facial nerve recovery as late as 2 years after tumor resection, this is exceedingly rare. Most patients who recover facial nerve function spontaneously from complete facial paralysis will begin to do so between 3 and 4 months after cerebellopontine angle surgery, and usually never after 12 months.[29,30]

Technique—Hypoglossal-Facial Jump Graft with Nerve Interposition

Step 1: An abbreviated parotid incision is made and extended in a submandibular crease two to three finger breadths below the margin of the mandible (Fig. 13.29).
Step 2: The great auricular nerve is identified and harvested (Fig. 13.30).
Step 3: The hypoglossal nerve is found running inferior and posterior to the posterior belly of the digastric muscle (Fig. 13.31).
Step 4: The facial nerve is identified in the triangle created by the tragal pointer (superior), posterior belly of digastric muscle (inferior), anterior face of mastoid prominence (posterior), and mandible (anterior) (Fig. 13.32).
Step 5: The pes anserinus is dissected and the division of the nerve into its two main superior and inferior branches is identified.

There are arguments in favor of anastomosing the entire VIIth nerve trunk to the hypoglossal nerve and, alternatively, to the inferior division of the facial nerve (Fig. 13.33). Our institutional preference is to selectively reinnervate the lower face through an anastomosis that connects the inferior division to the hypoglossal nerve and treating the paralysis of the upper division with gold or platinum weight implantation and brow lift (if needed). In our view, this gives more power in mimetic function to the lower face and avoids the synkinesis inherent to an anastomosis of the entire facial nerve to the hypoglossal nerve. Furthermore, the current technique of using an incision in one-third of the hypoglossal nerve to avoid hemitongue atrophy and associated morbidity may not supply enough nerve to power the entire facial nerve.
Step 6: The anastomosis with the hypoglossal nerve is made by cutting one-third of the way through the superior aspect of the nerve (Fig. 13.34). In doing so, there is adequate motor nerve available for the graft with little or no resulting tongue weakness or atrophy.
Step 7: The great auricular nerve graft is coapted to the posterior (i.e. proximal) end of the cut made in the hypoglossal nerve with two to three perineural sutures (Fig. 13.35). If selective reinnervation of the lower face is selected, the lower division is divided at the pes and sutured with two to three fine sutures to a nerve graft of an appropriate length harvested from the great auricular nerve. It is our experience that the most tension-free

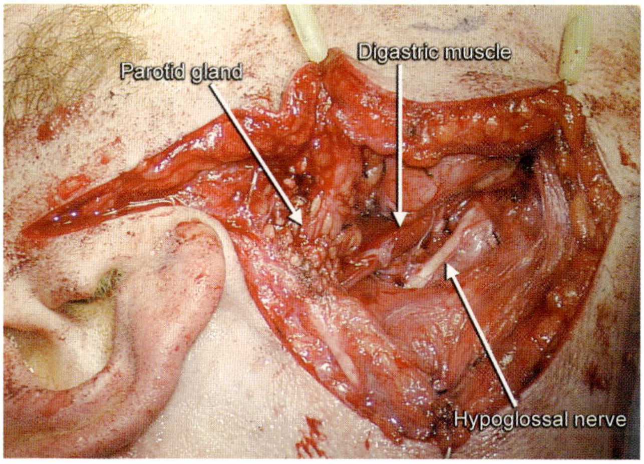

Fig. 13.31: Identification of the hypoglossal nerve.
Source: Image used by permission from Michael J LaRouere, MD

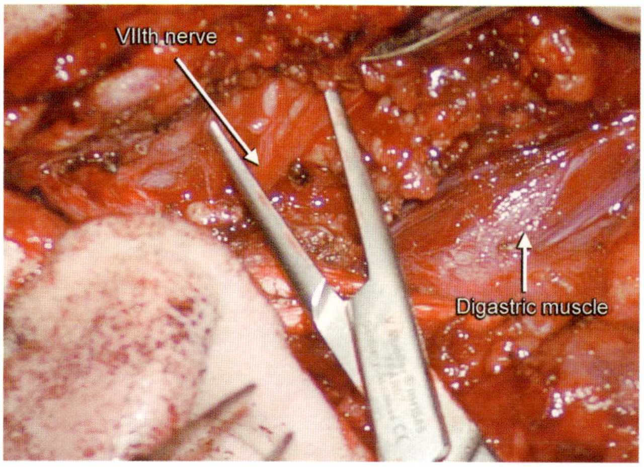

Fig. 13.32: Identification of the facial nerve.
Source: Image used by permission from Michael J LaRouere, MD

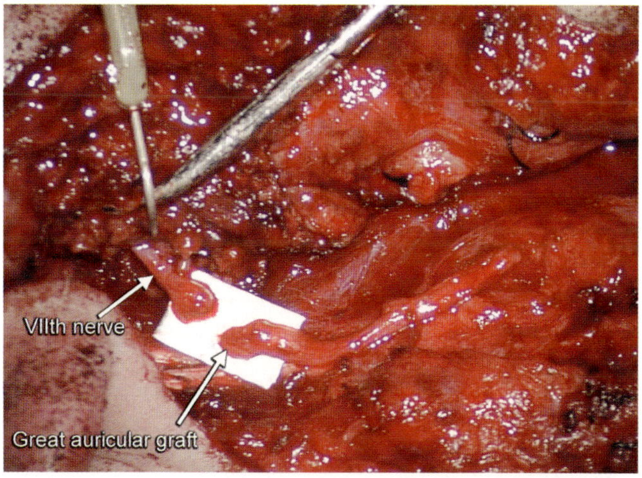

Fig. 13.33: Rotation of the facial nerve toward the nerve graft and hypoglossal nerve is facilitated by dividing the upper division of the nerve.
Source: Image used by permission from Michael J LaRouere, MD

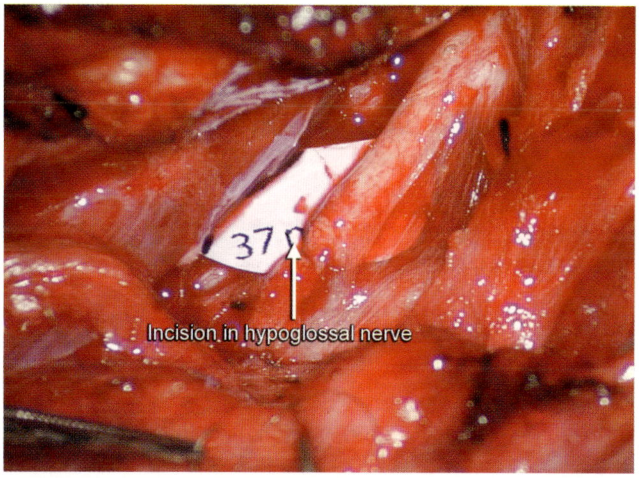

Fig. 13.34: Incision through the upper one third of the hypoglossal nerve.
Source: Image used by permission from Michael J LaRouere, MD

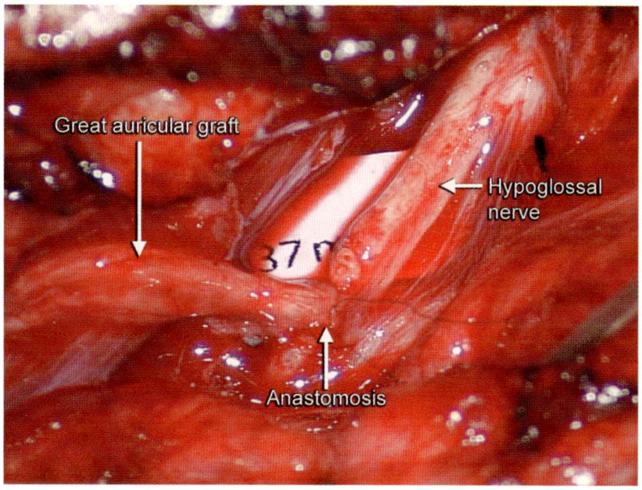

Fig. 13.35: The great auricular nerve graft is sutured to the proximal end of the cut made in the hypoglossal nerve.
Source: Image used by permission from Michael J LaRouere, MD

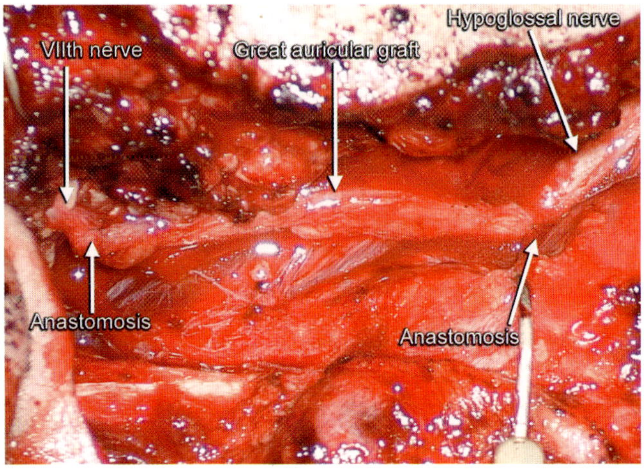

Fig. 13.36: Completed hypoglossal-facial jump graft with great auricular nerve.
Source: Image used by permission from Michael J LaRouere, MD

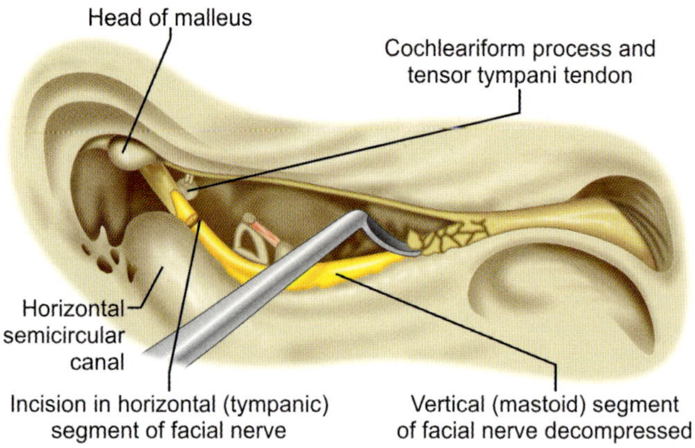

Fig. 13.37: After decompression, the facial nerve in the mastoid is transected in the horizontal segment and rotated into the neck where it is anastomosed to the hypoglossal nerve in a manner identical to Figures 13.35 and 13.36.

anastomosis can be made by running the nerve graft over the posterior belly of the digastric muscle rather than under the muscle (Fig. 13.36).

Technique—Hypoglossal-Facial Jump Graft without Nerve Interposition

An alternative to a jump graft is to insert the entire facial nerve into the hypoglossal nerve.

Step 1: A standard mastoidectomy incision is made behind the postauricular crease and extended toward the neck.

Step 2: Mastoidectomy is performed and the bone of the fallopian canal is removed. Removal of the incus may be required.

Step 3: The facial nerve is dissected from the fallopian canal with a diamond burr and blunt excavator after transecting the tympanic segment, close to the geniculate ganglion (Fig. 13.37).

Step 4: The extratemporal facial nerve trunk is mobilized from the stylomastoid foramen to the pes anserinus.

Step 5: The hypoglossal nerve is identified anatomically and with a nerve stimulator along the posterior belly of the digastric muscle and dissected from its exit at the skull base to the insertion at the tongue musculature.

Step 6: The mobilized facial nerve is rotated toward the hypoglossal nerve and sutured end-to-side in the hypoglossal nerve in a tension-free fashion with 8-0 or 10-0 suture.

Using this technique, Beutner et al. observed improved facial tone in all five patients of their series within 6 months and HB III/VI function 7–16 months after surgery.[31] The technique results in less functional morbidity since the great auricular nerve is not sacrificed and should have more neurotization of facial muscles because a second anastomosis required for the hypoglossal-facial jump graft using a nerve interposition—is not required.

Using either technique, initial restoration of tone begins after 3 months and good movement is observed 6–12 months after surgery.

FACIAL NERVE REHABILITATION—MUSCLE TRANSPOSITION

Temporalis muscle transposition is a reliable way to reanimate the paralyzed face and can provide immediate improvement in appearance while the result of simultaneous nerve grafting is awaited. Muscle transposition can also be the sole means of reanimation of the face if facial paralysis has persisted >18 months and hypoglossal-facial anastomosis will not likely be successful. The muscle is innervated by V3 that joins the muscle on its medial side. The blood supply is from the deep temporal vessels of the external carotid artery. The procedure can be performed at the same time as a hypoglossal-facial jump graft is performed as long as dissection for the muscle transposition is superficial to the facial musculature.

Step 1: A curvilinear preauricular incision is made that extends above the ear and then arcs forward.

Step 2: The zygoma is exposed and thinned with a drill. This will allow the arch to be used as a fulcrum for the

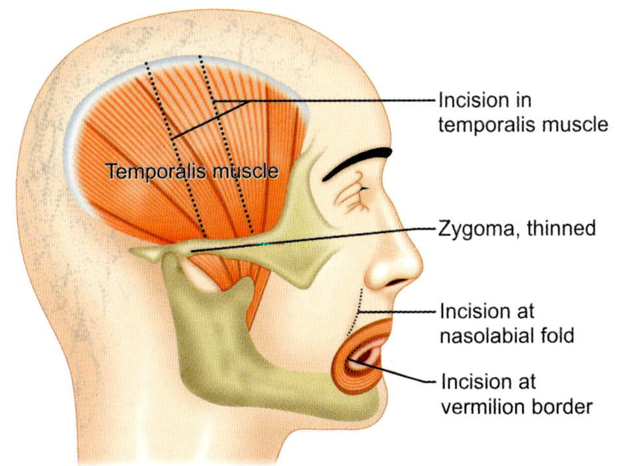

Fig. 13.38: Exposure of the temporalis muscle. Incisions are made to create a 3–4 cm wide strip of muscle and fascia. The zygomatic arch is thinned or drilled down.

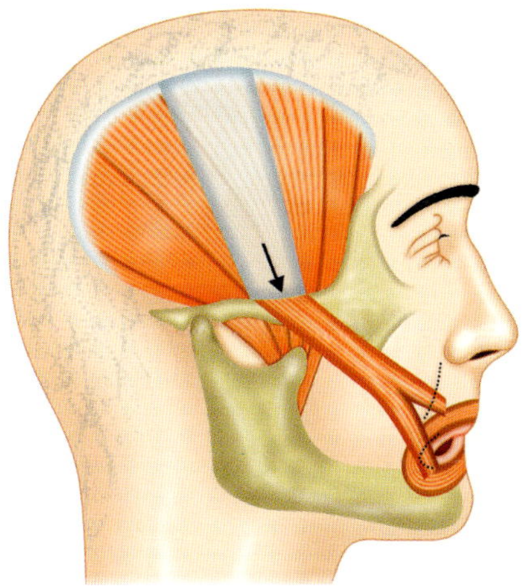

Fig. 13.39: The strip of temporalis is muscle and fascia is tunneled subcutaneously toward the oral commissure.

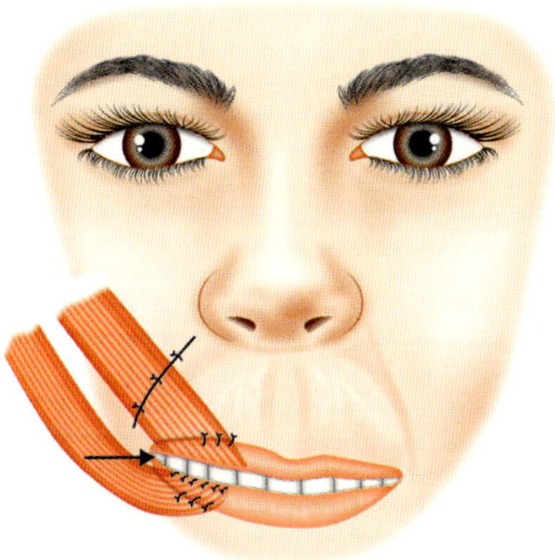

Fig. 13.40: Through incisions in the nasolabial fold and at the vermilion border of the oral commissure, the strips of temporalis muscle and fascia are sutured with permanent suture material to the dermis.

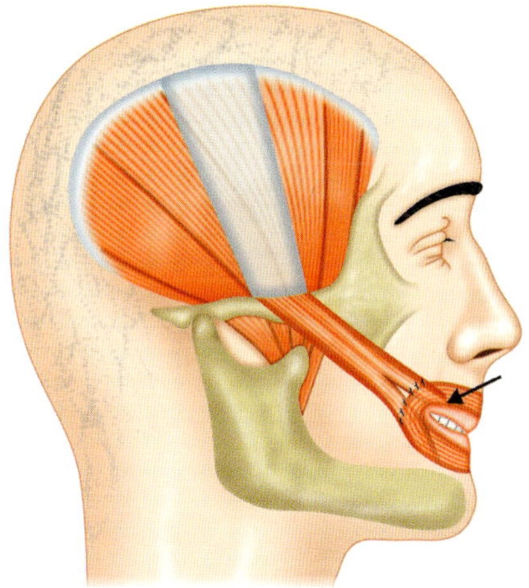

Fig. 13.41: The temporalis muscle/fascia is sutured to dramatically overcorrect the sag of the face to allow for postoperative tissue relaxation.

muscle, but reduce the bulge of the muscle over the arch. Alternatively, the arch can be removed, further reducing the bulge of the muscle (Fig. 13.38).

Step 3: Our preference is to harvest a central 3–4 cm wide strip of muscle with its fascial insertion at the superior temporal line. The fat that overlays the muscle near the zygomatic arch is removed. The defect left by the harvest of the central strip of muscle can be obliterated with fat or by suturing the 2 remaining halves of the temporalis muscle (Fig. 13.39).

Step 4: The muscle is then tunneled subcutaneously toward the oral commissure and nasolabial fold (Fig. 13.40).

Step 5: An incision in the nasolabial fold is made and a semilunar piece of skin may be removed from the fold to create a slightly exaggerated fold. A second incision is made at the vermillion border of the oral commissure.

Step 6: The fascia of the temporal muscle strip is then sutured to the dermis of the nasolabial fold and oral commissure with nonabsorbable suture, such as Ethibond (Ethicon, Inc., Somerville, NJ). If not enough native temporalis fascia is available, a piece of Alloderm (LifeCell Corp., Township of Branchburg, NJ) can be used as an extension (Fig. 13.41).

The critical step in this procedure is to dramatically overcorrect the pull on the face by the transferred muscle so that the entire ipsilateral canine tooth can be seen when the patient is in an upright position in the OR. This is done because tissue relaxation in the postoperative period will gradually lower the lip into a more natural position (Fig. 13.42).

Although there are modifications of the transposition to include the eyelids, as noted, our preference is to

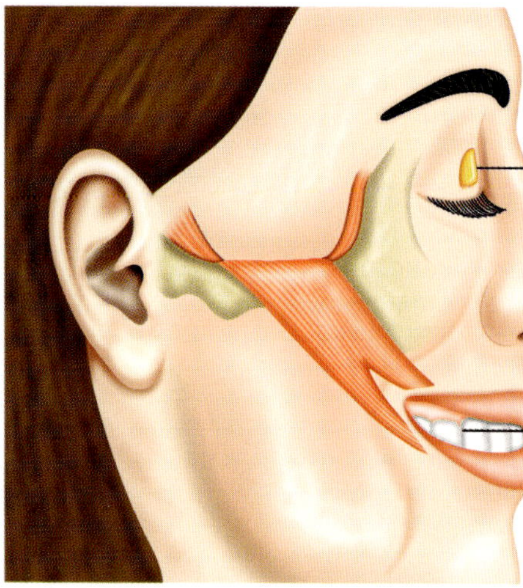

Fig. 13.42: The completed temporalis transposition with gold weight implantation.

reanimate the lower face with temporalis transposition and the upper face separately with a gold or platinum weight and brow lift (when indicated).

After temporalis muscle transposition with or without hypoglossal-facial anastomosis, many patients improve mimetic movement of the face using video or mirror feedback. We also note that when these procedures are combined in the early postfacial nerve injury time frame, trigeminal neurotization may allow innervation into some of the upper facial muscles, thereby improving facial muscle tone wholly separate from the elevation obtained by the temporalis muscle.

REFERENCES

1. Burgess RC, Michaels L, Bale JF, et al. Polymerase chain reaction amplification of herpes simplex viral DNA from the geniculate ganglion of a patient with Bell's palsy. Ann Otol Rhinol Laryngol. 1994;103:775-9.
2. Furuta Y, Furuta S, Chida E, et al. Reactivation of herpes simplex virus type 1 in patients with Bell's palsy. J Med Virol. 1998;54:162-6.
3. Adour KK, Ruboyianes JM, Von Doersten PG, et al. Bell's palsy treatment with acyclovir and prednisone compared with prednisone alone: A double blind, randomized, controlled trial. Ann Oto Rhinol Laryngol. 1996;105:371-8.
4. Sullivan FM, Swan IR, Donnan PT, et al. Early treatment with prednisolone or acyclovir in Bell's palsy. NEJM. 2007;357:1598-607.
5. Sargent EW, Kartush JM, Graham MD. Meatal facial nerve decompression in acoustic neuroma resection. Am J Otol. 1996;16:457-64.
6. Ge XX, Spector GJ. Labyrinthine segment and geniculate ganglion of facial nerve in fetal and adult human temporal bones. Ann Otol Rhinol Laryngol Suppl. 1981;90 (4 Pt 2)1-12.
7. Fisch U. Surgery for Bell's palsy. Arch Otolaryngol. 1981;107:1-11.
8. Gantz BJ. Idiopathic facial paralysis. In: Gates GA (Ed). Current Therapy in Otolaryngology Head and Neck Surgery. Toronto: BC Decker; 1987. pp. 62-6.
9. Gantz BJ, Rubinstein JT, Gidley P, et al. Surgical management of Bell's palsy. Laryngoscope. 1999;109:1177-88.
10. Peitersen E. The natural history of Bell's palsy. Am J Otol. 1982;4:107-11.
11. Aviel A, Marshak G. Ramsay Hunt syndrome: a cranial polyneuropathy. Am J Otolaryngol. 1982;3:61-6.
12. Robillard ZRB, HilsingerJr RL, Adour KK. Ramsay Hunt facial paralysis: clinical analysis of 185 patients. Otolaryngol Head Neck Surg. 1986;95:292-7.
13. Murakami S, Honda N, Mizobuchi M, et al. Rapid diagnosis of varicella zoster virus infection in acute facial palsy. Neurology. 1998;51:1202-5.
14. Morgan M, Nathwani D. Facial palsy and infection: the unfolding story. Clin Inf Dis. 1992;14:263-71.
15. Murakami S, Hato N, Horiuchi J. Treatment of Ramsay Hunt syndrome with acyclovir-prednisone: significance of early diagnosis and treatment. Ann Neurol. 1997;41:353-7.
16. Kartush JM, Linstrom CJ, McCann PM, et al. Early gold weight eyelid implantation for facial paralysis. Otolaryngol Head Neck Surg. 1990;103:1016-23.
17. Maina R, Ducati A, Lanzino G. The middle cranial fossa: morphometric study and surgical considerations. Skull Base. 2007;17:395-404.
18. Kartush JM, Kemink JL, Graham MD. The arcuate eminence: topographic orientation in middle cranial fossa surgery. Ann Otol Rhinol Laryngol. 1985;94:25-8.
19. Sargent EW, Bucholz RD. Middle cranial fossa surgery with image-guided instrumentation. Otolaryngol Head Neck Surg. 1997;117:131-4.
20. NIH Consensus Development Conference Statement on Acoustic Neuroma, Intraoperative Monitoring, Bethesda, MD, December, 1991.
21. Barrs DM. Facial nerve trauma: optimal timing for repair. Laryngoscope. 1991;101:835-48.
22. Weber PC. Iatrogenic complications from chronic ear surgery. Otolaryngol Clin N Am. 2005;38:711-22.
23. Adkins WY, Osguthorpe JD. Management of trauma of the facial nerve. Otolaryngol Clin N Am. 1991;24:587-611.
24. Yamamoto E, Fisch U. Experiments on facial nerve suturing. Otorhinolaryngol Relat Spec. 1974;36:193.
25. Sterkers O, Becherel P, Sterkers JM. Reparation du nerf facial par de la colle de fibrine exclusive. Ann Otolaryngol Chir Cervicofac. 1989;106:176.
26. King TT, Sparrow OC, Arias JM, et al. Repair of facial nerve after removal of cerebellopontine angle tumors: a comparative study. J Neurosurg. 1993;78:720.
27. Barrs DM, Brackmann DE, Hitselberger WE. Facial nerve anastomosis in the cerebellopontine angle. Am J Otol. 1984;5:269.

28. Samii M, Matthies C. Indication, technique and results of facial nerve reconstruction. Acta Neurochir. 1994;130: 125-39.
29. Kunihiro T, Kanzaki J, Shiobara R, et al. Long-term prognosis of profound facial nerve paralysis secondary to acoustic neuroma resection. ORL J Otorhinolaryngol Relat Spec. 1999;61:98-102.
30. Kunihiro T, Kanzaki J, Yoshihara S, et al. Analysis of the prognosis and the recovery process of profound facial nerve paralysis secondary to acoustic neuroma resection. ORL J Otorhinolaryngol Relat Spec. 1994;56:331-3.
31. Beutner D, Luers J, Grosheva M. Hypoglossal-facial-jump anastomosis without an interposition nerve graft. Laryngoscope. 2013;123:2392-6.

CHAPTER 14

Encephaloceles and Related CSF Leaks

Dan Sdrulla, Michael LaRouere

INTRODUCTION

Meningoencephaloceles of the temporal bone and related spontaneous cerebrospinal fluid (CSF) leaks are defined as abnormal connections between the temporal bone, meninges, subarachnoid space and possibly brain, and the underlying mastoid bone. This abnormal communication requires a bony defect in the tegmen, through which the meninges and brain may herniate. Because spontaneous CSF leaks are rare, the exact incidence is not known. Less than 500 cases have been described in literature.

Patient Characteristics

Spontaneous CSF leaks can be either congenital or acquired. Seventy-two percent of spontaneous CSF leaks occur in children and are congenital, while the reminder occur in adults.[1] Meningitis is the presenting symptom in 93% of the pediatric patients, while only 36% of adults with spontaneous CSF leaks present with meningitis.[2,3] In children, sensorineural hearing loss is also often present (82%). In adults, the most common presenting symptoms are conductive hearing loss, ear fullness, nonremitting serous otitis media, or unilateral otorrhea after tube placement.[4-7] In addition to meningitis, chronic otitis media, vertigo, and epilepsy have also been described in spontaneous CSF leak patients.[7-10]

Children with congenital CSF leaks often have otic capsule abnormalities such as a Mondini malformation.[11] Mondini malformations are associated with an abnormally patent lateral IAC which allows the flow of CSF into the inner ear. A second defect in the annular ring of the oval window or in the round window then allows CSF drainage into the middle ear. Other described pathways of CSF egress in the middle ear and mastoid air cells of the pediatric patients are a patent Hyrtl's (tympanomeningeal) fissure, a patent petromastoid canal (housing the subarcuate artery), a patent fallopian canal or patent cochlear or vestibular aqueducts.[12-15] As encephaloceles are not present in these patients, their management is outside the scope of this chapter.

The adult with a spontaneous CSF leak is often obese and has symptoms consistent with idiopathic intracranial hypertension (IIH).[16] From a demographic standpoint, most of these patients are women, with a female to male ratio of 2:1. The average age at diagnosis is 60. These patients have an average BMI higher than that of age matched controls. Further, most patients with spontaneous CSF leaks have symptoms of IIH: headache, pulsatile tinnitus, hypertension, balance problems, or vision complaints.[17] The diagnostic criteria for IIH apply to the majority of spontaneous CSF leak patients, suggesting that this clinical entity may be a subvariant of IIH. Herniation of the subarachnoid space within the sella turcica (empty sella) occurs in up to 80% of spontaneous CSF leak patients, with 20–30% of them exhibiting some level of hypopituitarism.[18] Neuro-ophthalmologic and endocrine evaluations may be indicated in the preoperative workup of the spontaneous CSF leak patient population depending on associated findings.

Pathophysiology

From a pathophysiologic standpoint, two theories have been postulated regarding spontaneous CSF leaks and encephalocele development. In 1990, Gacek demonstrated abnormal arachnoid granulations (AG) in the tegmen of the middle fossa or the posterior fossa.[19] Gacek hypothesized that the abnormal locations of these AG results in decreased outflow to the venous system leading to small CSF accumulations which subsequently induce thinning and erosion of the bone. An alternative theory endorses that congenital bony defects may initially exist.[20] These congenital defects get enlarged by constant CSF pulsations and pressure with resultant bony and dural thinning and herniation.

DIAGNOSTIC TESTING

In the patient with a suspected CSF leak, testing of the draining fluid is confirmatory. B2-transferrin is a protein almost unique to CSF and the standard test for

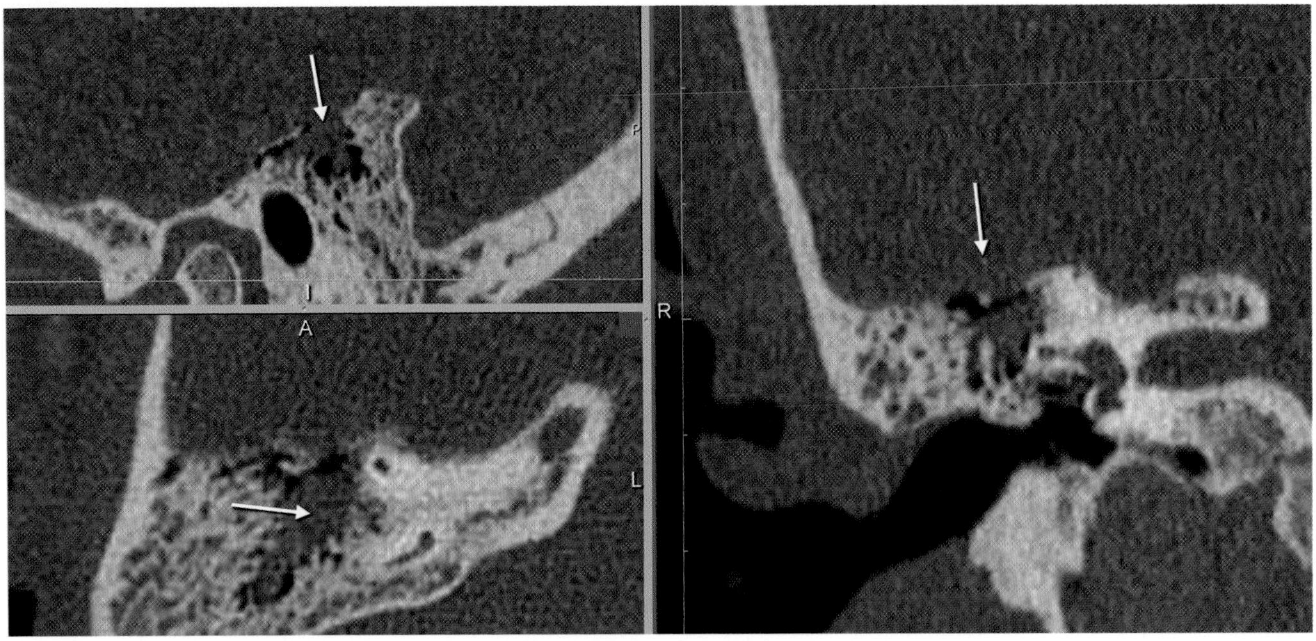

Fig. 14.1: High-resolution computed tomography temporal bone multiplanar reconstruction, right ear, bone windows, demonstrating tegmen dehiscence and opacification of the mastoid air cells. Right panel, coronal cut. Left superior panel, parasagittal cut. Left inferior panel, axial cut. Arrows point at the tegmen destruction suggestive of an encephalocele.

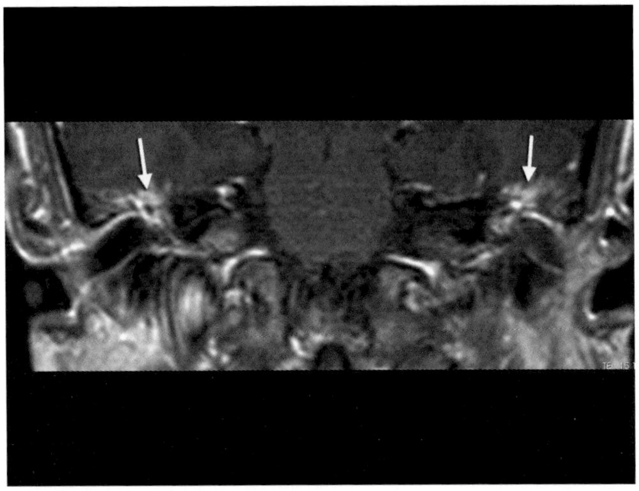

Fig. 14.2: T1 postcontrast MRI of brain, coronal, demonstrating bilateral tegmen dehiscence herniation in the mastoid space (arrows).

positively identifying a CSF leak. A small amount (0.5 mL) of fluid is sufficient for diagnosis. The sensitivity and specificity of B2-transferrin for CSF detection is 94% and 98%, respectively.[21] Once the presence of a CSF leak is suspected, imaging is essential both in evaluating the etiology as well as in facilitating surgical planning. High-resolution computed tomography (HRCT) is often the test of choice, as it best demonstrates bony anatomy and the location of the tegmen defects[22] (Fig. 14.1). Magnetic resonance imaging (MRI) is commonly obtained in conjunction with the HRCT, and reveals the herniation of the meninges and/or brain tissue through the defect (Fig. 14.2).

Superior semicircular canal dehiscences (SSCD) are also much more frequent in this patient population (Fig. 14.3). A study by Allen in 2012 identified a SSCD rate of 15.2% in the spontaneous CSF leak patients, compared to the reported 0.5% SSCD rate in the general population.[22] The presence of SSCD must be assessed on HRCT during preoperative planning, and the presence of vertigo in these patients should be carefully scrutinized. Once identified, if symptomatic, SSCD may be repaired at the time of the encephalocele repair.

SURGICAL MANAGEMENT

Due to the risk of neurological complications such as meningitis, encephalitis, cerebral abscess, or epilepsy, surgical management has been recommended and is the standard of care for spontaneous CSF leaks. Transmastoid, middle cranial fossa, or combined approaches are most common. The unifying concept underlying these approaches is a multilayered repair, combining the use of both soft-tissue layers (autologous fascia, myofascial flaps, or lypophilized homologous dura mater), placed on top of autologous and homologous cartilage, bone, preformed hydroxyapatite (HA), or HA cement.

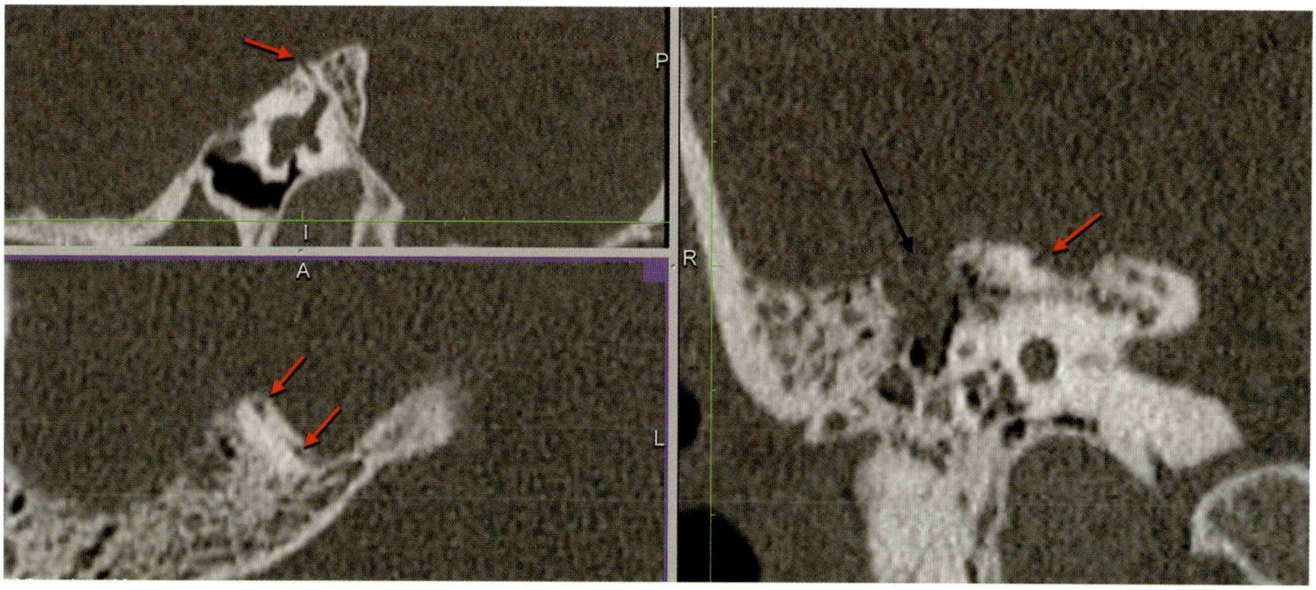

Fig. 14.3: High-resolution computed tomography multiplanar reconstruction, demonstrating the simultaneous presence of a tegmen dehiscence (black arrow), as well as superior semicircular canal dehiscences (red arrows).

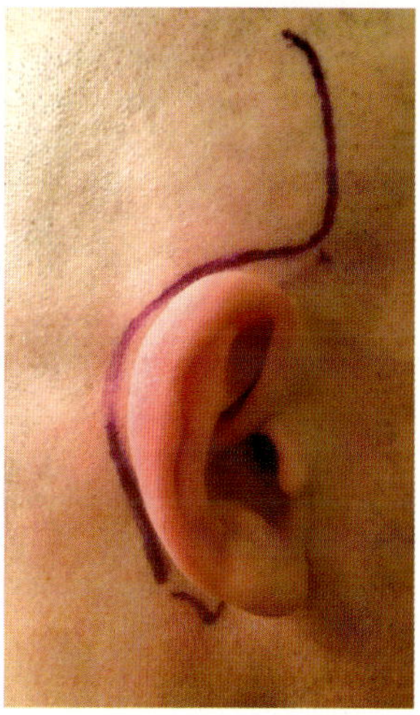

Fig. 14.4: Design of incision for combined transmastoid-middle fossa approach.

The order of the layers is independent of the method of repair: after the encephalocele is either reduced or amputated, the dural defect(s) is identified and covered with one or more soft-tissue layers (dural repair material, temporalis fascia), then the bony defect is directly covered or bridged with HA, bone, or cartilage. In our practice, the repair materials most commonly used are temporalis fascia, Durepair, a dural soft-tissue substitute (Medtronic, Memphis, TN), cartilage for a small bony defect, or HA (either as cement or preformed discs). For single bony defects <2 cm in diameter, the transmastoid approach may suffice. For multiple bony defects, or large defects >2 cm in diameter, a combined transmastoid/middle cranial fossa is our standard approach. The transmastoid approach is performed first, allowing identification of the bony defect(s) location, isolation of the herniated tissue from the ossicular chain, and reduction or amputation of the bulk of herniated tissue (which is nonfunctional) from the mastoid cavity.

Perioperative Considerations

Given that a transmastoid approach may need to be converted to a combined approach based on the mastoid findings, intraoperative monitoring of cranial nerves VII and VIII is performed for all our encephalocele repair procedures.

Surgical Technique

Transmastoid Approach

Step 1: The incision is designed such as to incorporate a postauricular incision (for the transmastoid approach), which may then be extended superiorly to allow middle fossa exposure (Fig. 14.4). The field is prepped and draped in the standard fashion to allow for both options.

Step 2: A standard canal wall up mastoidectomy is performed (*see* Mastoidectomy chapter for technique).

Step 3: A large fascia graft is obtained (*see* Tympanoplasty chapter for technique), and set aside for later use.

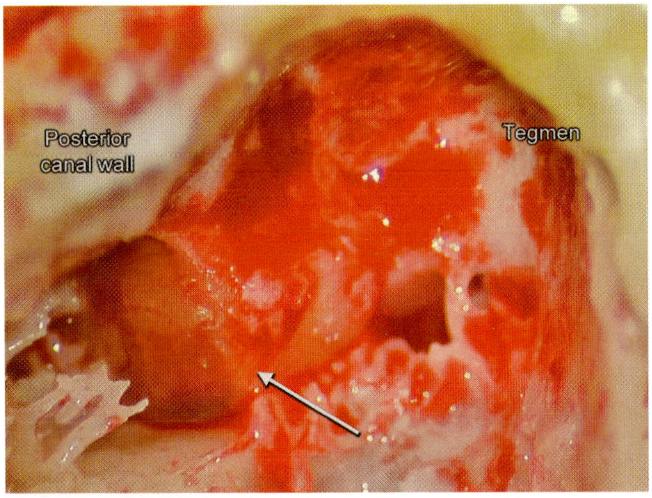

Fig. 14.5: Initial view of encephalocele in the mastoid (arrow).

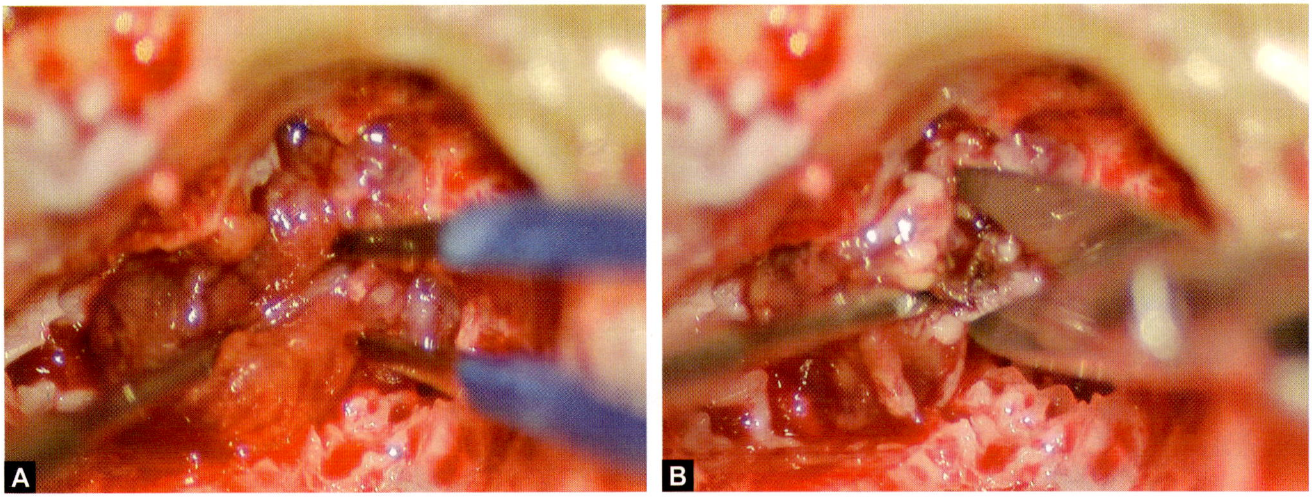

Figs. 14.6A and B: Resection of the encephalocele using (A) bipolar cautery and (B) bayonet scissors.

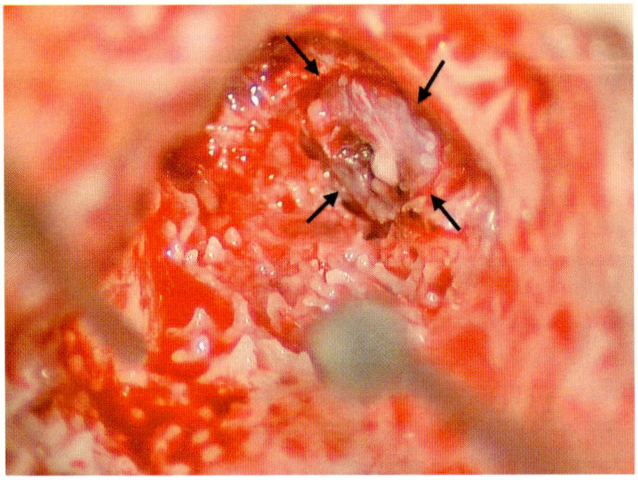

Fig. 14.7: Tegmen bony defect edges (arrows) once all the mastoid air cells surrounding the encephalocele have been exenterated.

Step 4: The encephalocele is identified within the mastoid cavity (Fig. 14.5).

Step 5: The bony spicules enclosing the encephalocele are slowly removed with either a curette or a high-speed diamond drill, advancing superiorly toward the tegmen. Bipolar cautery followed with bayonet scissors are sequentially used to resect the most dependent part of the encephalocele, allowing further superior visualization toward the tegmen (Figs. 14.6A and B).

Step 6: The tegmen defect is identified, and all the herniated tissue resected (Fig. 14.7).

Step 7: The dural defect edges are identified, and an 8-0 nylon suture is placed across both sides of the dural defect (Fig. 14.8). An initial piece of Durepair is appropriately trimmed, fitted medial to the bony defect (Fig. 14.9A), and tied in place (Fig. 14.9B).

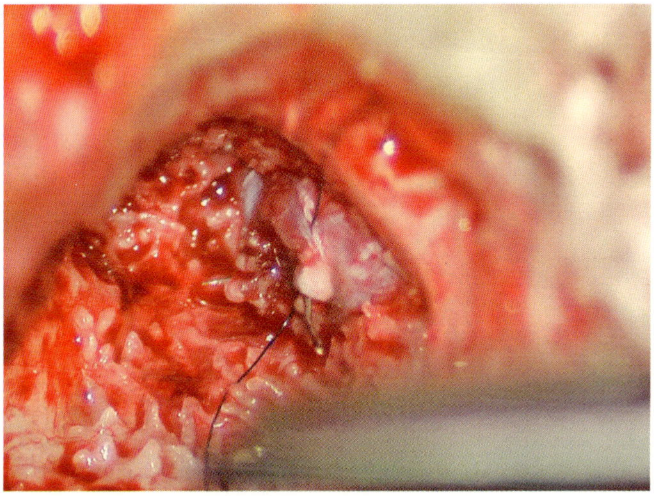

Fig. 14.8: 8-0 nylon suture placed through the edges of the dural defect. This will later secure the layer in place.

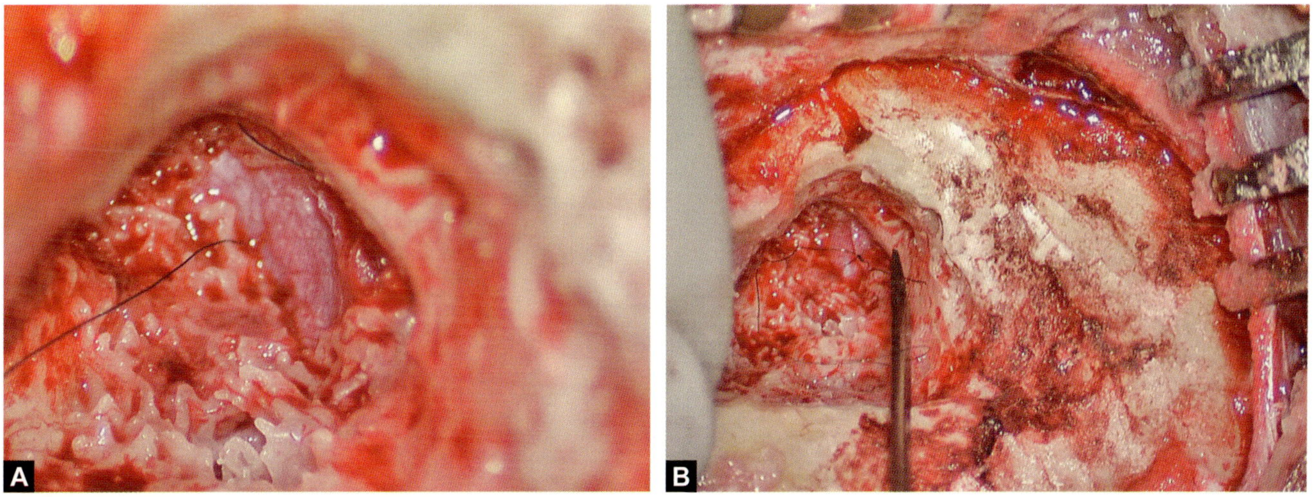

Figs. 14.9A and B: First layer of Durepair (A) before and (B) after being tied in place over the dural defect.

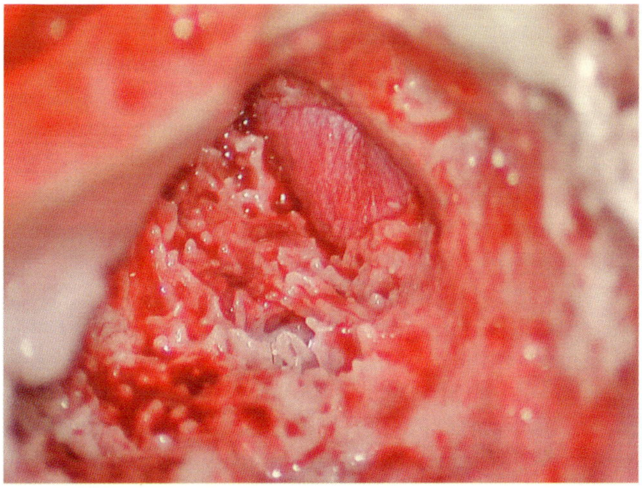

Fig. 14.10: Second layer of Durepair placed medial to the bony defect.

Step 8: A second layer of Durepair is trimmed and medially placed to span the entire bony defect (Fig. 14.10).

Step 9: The harvested temporalis fascia is now fitted to the bony defect and placed medial to it (Fig. 14.11).

Step 10: Two large pieces of saline-soaked Gelfoam are placed over the antrum to occlude it and protect the ossicles from application of HA cement (Fig. 14.12).

Step 11: The HA cement is then applied over the tegmen bony defect, allowed to set (Fig. 14.13), then the Gelfoam pieces removed. An alternative to the HA cement is the medial placement of preformed HA discs to span the bony defect (Fig. 14.14).

Step 12: The wound is then copiously irrigated and closed in standard fashion.

Step 13: If a post-tympanostomy tube perforation is present, this is repaired. A small postauricular incision is

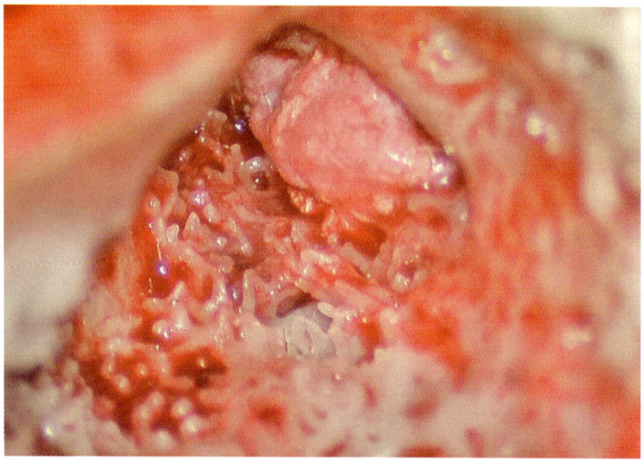

Fig. 14.11: Temporalis fascia layer placed medial to the bony defect.

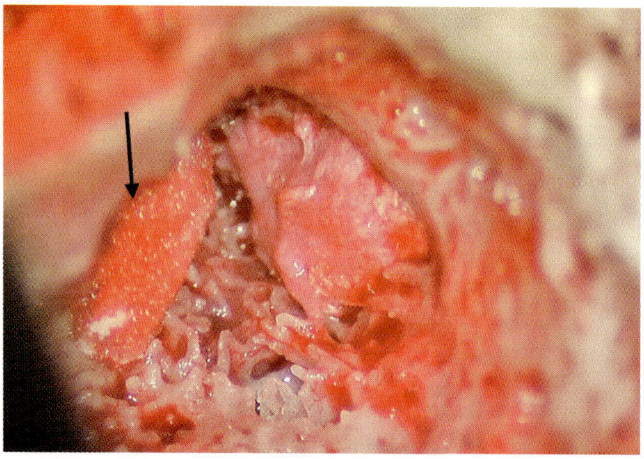

Fig. 14.12: Gelfoam (arrow) placement over the antrum protecting the ossicular chain and the middle ear space from any hydroxyapatite cement leaking prior to setting.

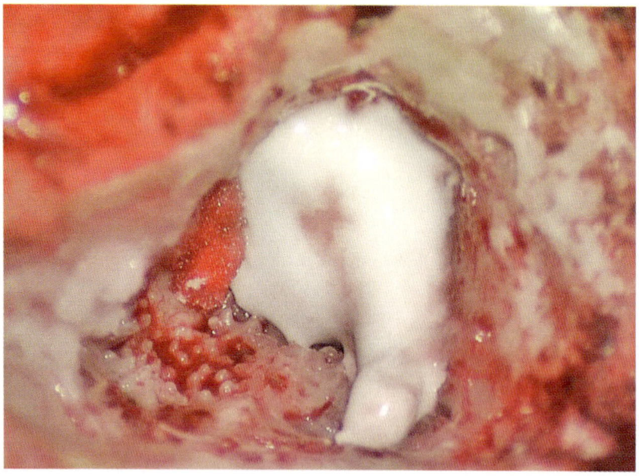

Fig. 14.13: Hydroxyapatite cement application sealing the tegmen bone defect.

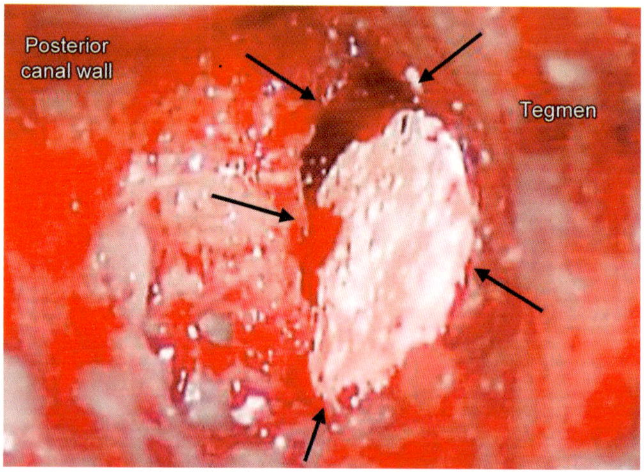

Fig. 14.14: Preformed hydroxyapatite (HA) disc placed medial to the bony defect (arrows) as an alternative option to HA cement.

made, subcutaneous fatty tissue harvested, trimmed to size and placed half medial, half lateral to the tympanic perforation, such that the graft dumbbells across the perforation.

Step 14: A Glasscock dressing is placed.

Middle Fossa Approach

Special considerations: 25–50 g of mannitol may be given 15–30 minutes prior to beginning elevation of the dura from the tegmen. The patient should also be hyperventilated at the same time, bringing the pCO_2 to 28. This allows a reduction in the CSF pressure and relaxes the tension of the dura during its elevation from the tegmen, facilitating the view of the middle fossa floor and potential tegmen defects.

Step 1: If only the middle fossa approach is intended, a 5–7 cm vertical incision is designed approximately 1 cm anterior to the helical crus, with the inferior end just superior to the tragus (Fig. 14.15). For the transmastoid-middle fossa combined approach, the inferior end of the incision curves posteriorly and continues with a standard mastoidectomy incision, 1 cm posterior to the postauricular groove, toward the mastoid tip (Fig. 14.4). This allows the intraoperative flexibility of starting only with the transmastoid approach, and extending the incision superiorly if the combined approach is deemed necessary based on the mastoid findings.

Step 2: Skin flaps are elevated anteriorly and posteriorly, revealing the temporalis muscle and its fascia (Fig. 14.16).

Step 3: A large temporalis fascia graft is harvested and set aside for later use (Fig. 14.17).

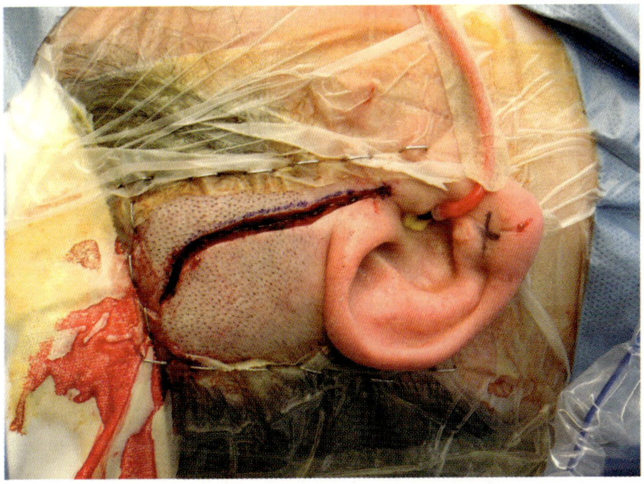

Fig. 14.15: Middle cranial fossa preauricular incision.

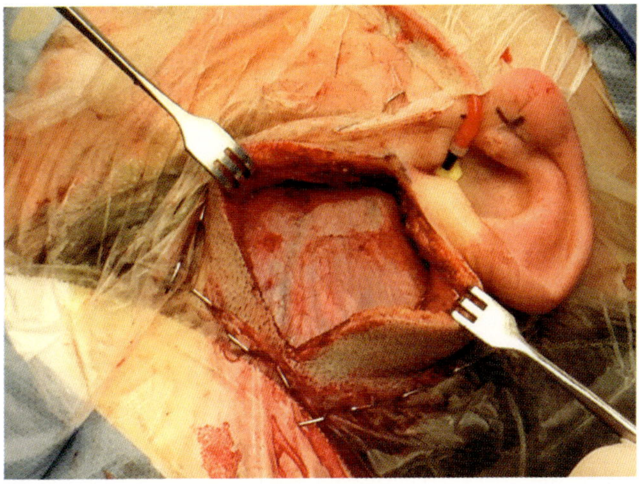

Fig. 14.16: Skin flaps elevated and retracted, revealing the temporalis muscle.

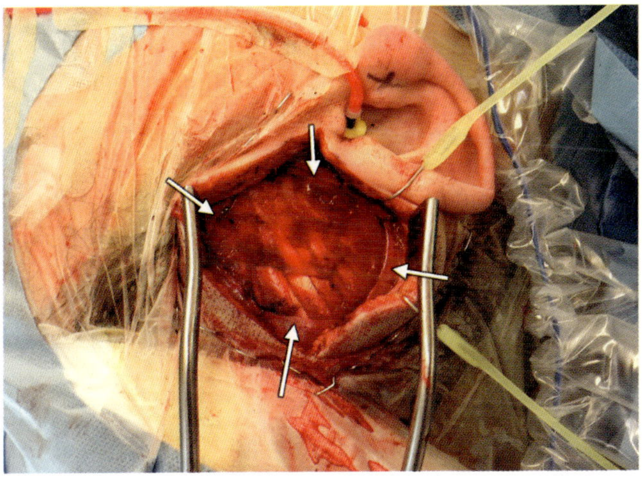

Fig. 14.17: Temporal muscle fascia defect (arrows) after harvest of the fascia graft.

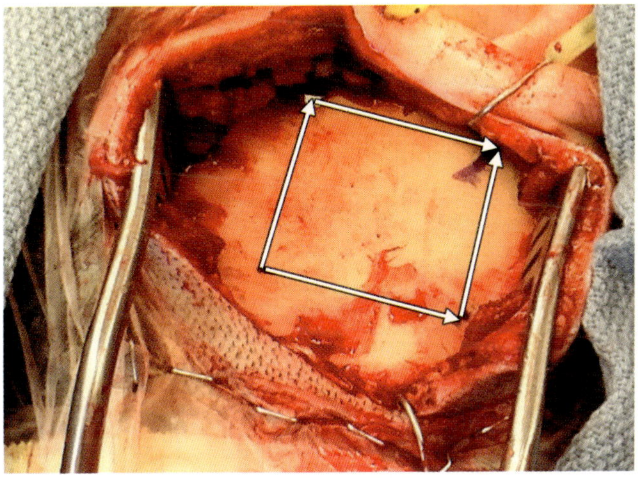

Fig. 14.18: Retraction of the muscle edges reveals the squamosa of the temporal bone. The edges of the craniotomy window are marked.

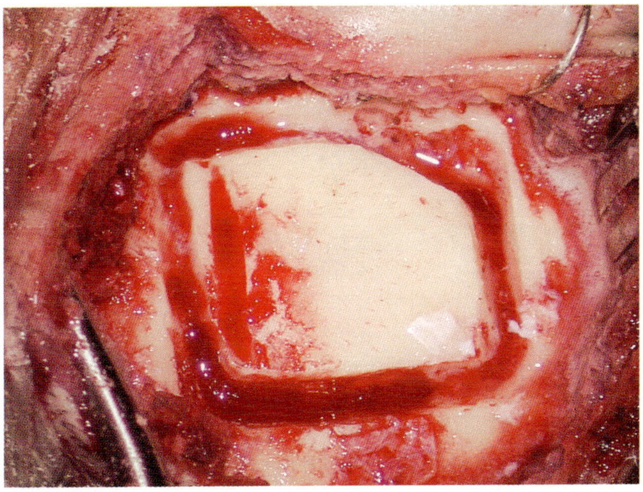

Fig. 14.19: The bone flap during drilling.

Step 4: The temporalis muscle and periosteum are divided and retracted, revealing the squamosa (Fig. 14.18).

Step 5: A square, 5 × 5 cm, craniotomy window is designed, with the inferior edge of the window at the level of the root of the zygoma (defining the approximate level of the tegmen), and the anterior vertical edge of the bone window 1 cm anterior to the helical crus (Fig. 14.18). A 4 mm cutting bur followed by a 3 mm diamond bur is used to drill the bony window (Fig. 14.19). The skull thickness varies along the edges of this bony window, and care is taken to avoid dural defects during drilling.

Step 6: Once the bony window is circumferentially released from the surrounding bone, a freer elevator is used to separate it from the medial dura (Fig. 14.20). The removed bone flap is set aside for replacement at the end of the case.

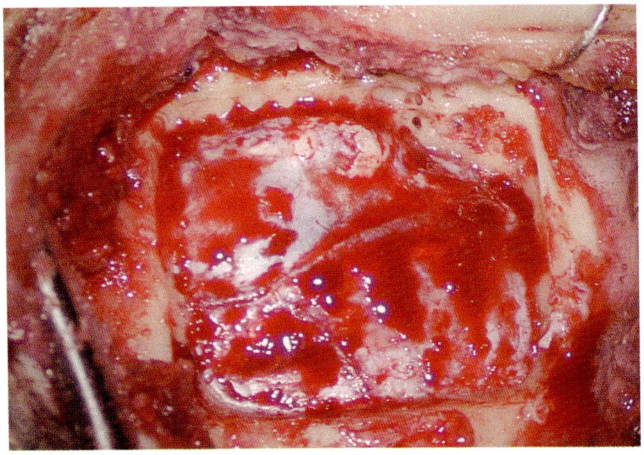

Fig. 14.20: Intact dura after removal of the bone flap with a freer elevator.

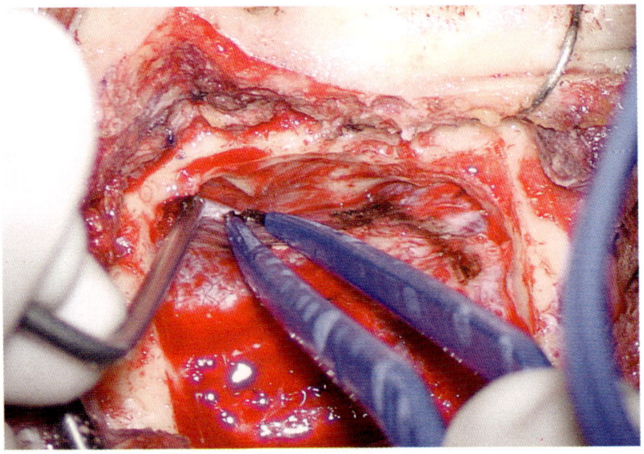

Fig. 14.21: During elevation of the dura from the middle fossa floor, bleeding from bridging veins is controlled with bipolar cautery.

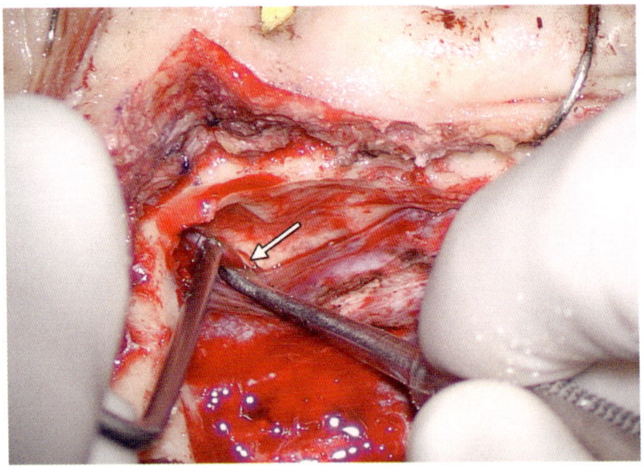

Fig. 14.22: Location of a superior semicircular canal dehiscence is identified during dural elevation.

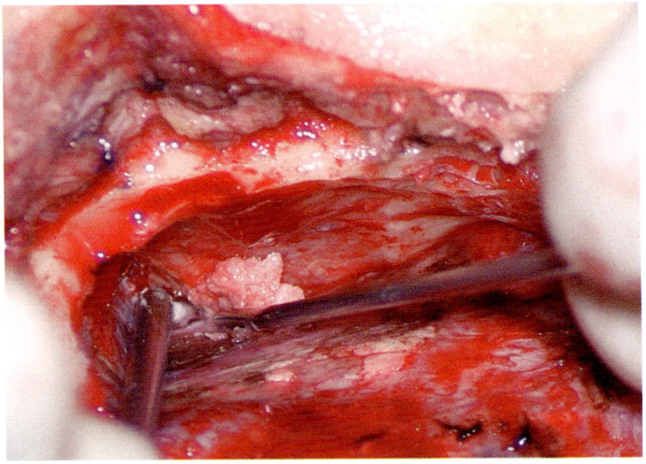

Fig. 14.23: Bone pate is used to pack the dehiscent semicircular canal.

Step 7: The dura is then slowly freed from the tegmen. Bridging veins are bipolared (Fig. 14.21). If a SSCD is encountered (Fig. 14.22), it is immediately packed with bone dust and fascia (Fig. 14.23).
Step 8: The encephalocele is then reduced, and the temporalis fascia previously harvested is placed to span both the encephalocele defect and the SSCD (Fig. 14.24). Durepair may also be used at this point, by itself or in conjunction with temporalis fascia.
Step 9: One or more preformed HA discs are then used, placed medial to the fascia and lateral to the Durepair, spanning the encephalocele defect (Fig. 14.25). The size of the HA disc is chosen such to completely cover the tegmen defect. If multiple defects exist, more than one HA disc may be used.
Step 10: The dura is then released over the multilayered closure (Fig. 14.26).
Step 11: The bone flap is replaced and secured to the surrounding bone with titanium plates and screws (Fig. 14.27).
Step 12: The temporalis muscle and the subcutaneous tissues are then closed with 3-0 Vicryl sutures, while the skin is reapproximated with 3-0 prolene sutures.
Step 13: A mastoid pressure dressing is then applied.

POSTOPERATIVE CARE

Patients who undergo encephalocele repair using the transmastoid approach do not require neurosurgical intensive care unit (NICU) monitoring. The Glasscock dressing is removed on postoperative day 1, and the patient is often discharged that day. Middle cranial fossa encephalocele repair patients are admitted to the NICU for close monitoring. If stable, they are transferred to a step-down unit on postoperative day 1. Daily electrolytes are obtained, and

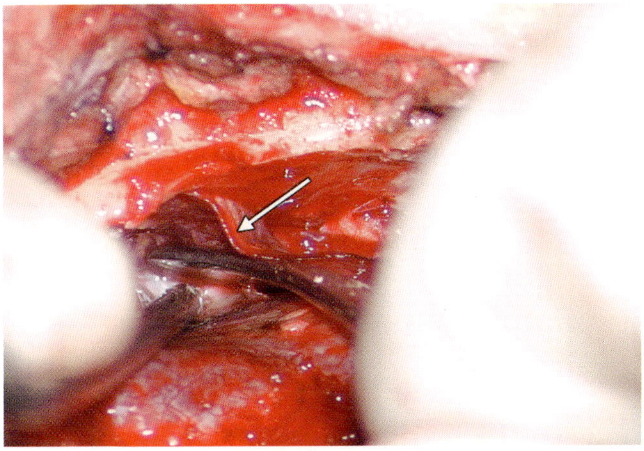

Fig. 14.24: Temporalis fascia graft (arrow) is placed from a medial to lateral aspect, with care being taken to span both the tegmen dehiscence and the superior semicircular canal dehiscence.

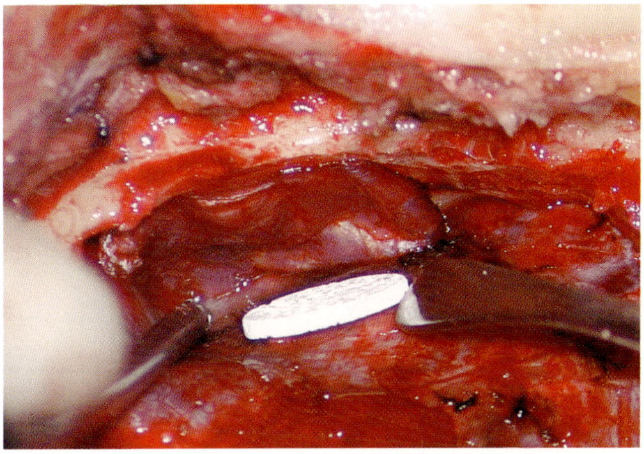

Fig. 14.25: Placement of a 10 mm preformed hydroxyapatite disc over the areas of the superior canal dehiscence and tegmen dehiscence.

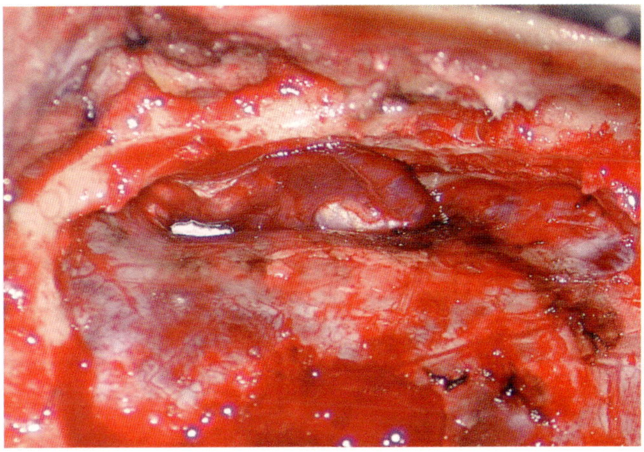

Fig. 14.26: Dura is released over the multilayered closure of the defect.

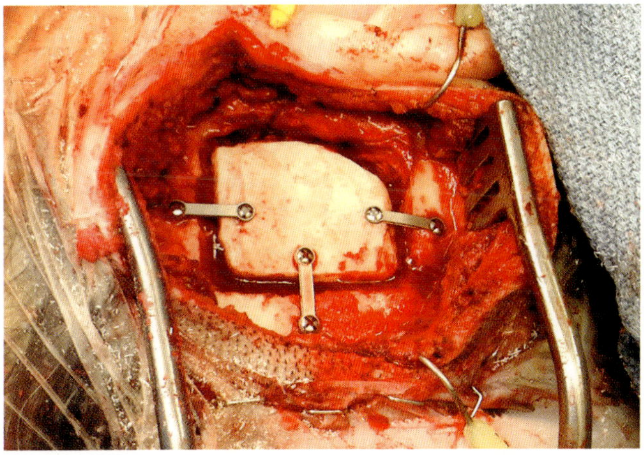

Fig. 14.27: Bone flap replaced and secured in place with titanium plates and screws.

serum sodium is closely monitored for the development of hyponatremia. The mastoid dressing is replaced on postoperative day 1, and removed on postoperative day 3. Usually, the patient is discharged on postoperative day 2 or 3. w

COMPLICATIONS

Recurrence of a CSF leak is the most common complication. Published recurrence rates vary around 5-15%. Transmastoid only series have described higher rates of CSF leak recurrences than middle fossa or combined approaches. This is not difficult to conceive, given that the anatomy of the mastoid cavity varies (sclerotic, anterior sigmoid sinus in relation to the posterior ear canal wall) and that the encephaloceles may be multiple or anteriorly located in the epitympanum over the heads of the ossicles. Careful assessment of the tegmen defect with imaging is paramount. Planning for a combined approach and starting transmastoid allows the greatest flexibility in optimizing the surgical approach to each encephalocele's anatomical location and intraoperative findings.

Postoperative sensorineural hearing loss occurs at a rate of <10% and is seen following middle fossa or combined approaches.[23] It is of particular importance to assess for SSCD preoperatively with imaging and during the repair (Figs. 14.3 and 14.28). Aggressive elevation of the dura from the middle fossa floor or suctioning of fluid from a SSCD may lead to this complication. If such a leak is noted, packing the dehiscent canal with bone pate and fascia without suctioning may prevent hearing loss.

Meningitis following encephalocele repair is rare, occurring around 1%.[24] Often the onset of meningitis is

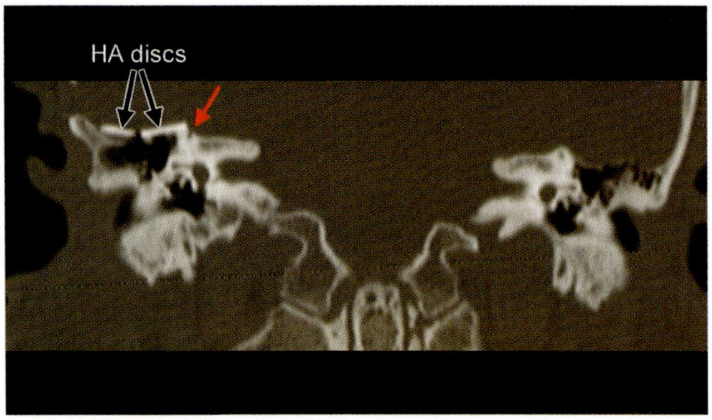

Fig. 14.28: Postoperative high-resolution computed tomography coronal slice at the level of the prior tegmen dehiscence, demonstrating the aerated mastoid, the postoperative location of the hydroxyapatite (HA) discs (black arrows) and the proximity to superior semicircular canal dehiscences (red arrow).

a sign predictive of CSF leak recurrence. One study identified the use of titanium mesh in the repair as increasing the risk of meningitis.[25]

Facial nerve paresis and postoperative seizures have also been described, but are also rare. A dehiscent facial nerve at the geniculate ganglion may be injured during a middle fossa repair. Postoperative epilepsy has been described in one patient after middle fossa encephalocele repair and was well controlled with anticonvulsant medications.

REFERENCES

1. Kutz JW Jr, Husain IA, Isaacson B, et al. Management of spontaneous cerebrospinal fluid otorrhea. Laryngoscope. 2008;118(12):2195-9.
2. Wetmore SJ, Herrmann P, Fisch U. Spontaneous cerebrospinal fluid otorrhea. Am J Otol. 1987;8(2):96-102.
3. Jahrsdoerfer RA, Richtsmeier WJ, Cantrell RW. Spontaneous CSF otorrhea. Arch Otolaryngol. 1981;107(4):257-61.
4. Brown NE, Grundfast KM, Jabre A, et al. Diagnosis and management of spontaneous cerebrospinal fluid-middle ear effusion and otorrhea. Laryngoscope. 2004;114:800-5.
5. Leonetti JP, Marzo S, Anderson D, et al. Spontaneous transtemporal CSF leakage: a study of 51 cases. Ear Nose Throat J. 2005;84:702-4, 6.
6. Pappas DG Jr, Hoffman RA, Cohen NL, et al. Spontaneous temporal bone cerebrospinal fluid leak. Am J Otol. 1992; 13:534-9.
7. Nahas Z, Tatlipinar A, Limb CJ, et al. Spontaneous meningoencephalocele of the temporal bone: clinical spectrum and presentation. Arch Otolaryngol Head Neck Surg. 2008;134:509-18.
8. Gubbels SP, Selden NR, Delashaw JB Jr, et al. Spontaneous middle fossa encephalocele and cerebrospinal fluid leakage: diagnosis and management. Otol Neurotol. 2007;28:1131-9.
9. Lundy LB, Graham MD, Kartush JM, et al. Temporal bone encephalocele and cerebrospinal fluid leaks. Am J Otol. 1996;17:461-9.
10. Mayeno JK, Korol HW, Nutik SL. Spontaneous meningoencephalic herniation of the temporal bone: case series with recommended treatment. Otolaryngol Head Neck Surg. 2004;130:486-9.
11. Park TS, Hoffman HJ, Humphreys RP, et al. Spontaneous cerebrospinal fluid otorrhea in association with a congenital defect of the cochlear aqueduct and Mondini dysplasia. Neurosurgery. 1982;11(3):356-62.
12. Jegoux F, Malard O, Gayet-Delacroix M, et al. Hyrtl's fissure: a case of spontaneous cerebrospinal fluid otorrhoea. AJNR Am J Neuroradiol. 2005;26:9636.
13. Phelps PD, Proops D, Sellars S, et al. Congenital cerebrospinal fluid fistula through the inner ear and meningitis. J Laryngol Otol. 1993;107:492-5.
14. Phelps PD. Congenital cerebrospinal fluid fistulae of the petrous temporal bone. Clin Otolaryngol. 1986;11:79-92.
15. Weber PC, Perez BA, Bluestone CD. Congenital perilymphatic fistula and associated middle ear abnormalities. Laryngoscope. 1993;103(2):160-4.
16. Schlosser RJ, Woodworth BA, Wilensky EM, et al. Spontaneous cerebrospinal fluid leaks: a variant of benign intracranial hypertension. Ann Otol Rhinol Laryngol. 2006;115(7):495-500.
17. LeVay A, Kveton J. Relationship between obesity, obstructive sleep apnea, and spontaneous cerebrospinal fluid otorrhea. Laryngoscope. 2008;118:275-8.
18. Prichard C, Isaacson B, Oghalai J, et al. Adult spontaneous CSF otorrhea: correlation with radiographic empty sella. Otol Head Neck Surg. 2006;134:767-71.
19. Gacek RR, Gacek MR, Tart R. Adult spontaneous cerebrospinal fluid otorrhea: diagnosis and management. Am J Otol. 1999;20:770-6.
20. Rao A, Merenda D, Wetmore S. Diagnosis and management of spontaneous cerebrospinal fluid otorrhea. Otol Neurotol. 2005;26:1171-5.
21. Lund VJ1, Savy L, Lloyd G, et al. Optimum imaging and diagnosis of cerebrospinal fluid rhinorrhoea. Laryngol Otol. 2000;114(12):988-92.
22. Allen KP, Perez CL, Isaacson B, et al. Superior semicircular canal dehiscence in patients with spontaneous cerebrospinal fluid otorrhea. Otolaryngol Head Neck Surg. 2012; 147(6):1120-4.
23. Son HJ, Karkas A, Buchanan P, et al. Spontaneous cerebrospinal fluid effusion of the temporal bone: repair, audiological outcomes, and obesity. Laryngoscope. 2014; 125(5):1204-8.
24. Sanna M, Fois P, Russo A, et al. Management of meningoencephalic herniation of the temporal bone: personal experience and literature review. Laryngoscope. 2009; 119(8):1579-85.
25. Carlson ML1, Copeland WR 3rd, Driscoll CL, et al. Temporal bone encephalocele and cerebrospinal fluid fistula repair utilizing the middle cranial fossa or combined mastoid-middle cranial fossa approach. J Neurosurg. 2013; 119(5):1314-22.

CHAPTER 15

Endoscopic Neurotologic Surgery

Pradeep Setty, Daniel R Pieper

INTRODUCTION

The surgical endoscope was first designed in 1879 by Max Nitze[1] and first utilized for cerebellopontine angle (CPA) pathology in 1917 when Doyen used it to perform a trigeminal neurectomy.[2] Built with multiple lenses and a light at the tip, these initial endoscopes never gained significant traction in CPA surgery due to their limited magnification and illumination. The operative microscope, introduced in the 1960s, provided improved visualization and lighting, especially to the deep, dark recesses of the skull base, thereby limiting use of the endoscope to endonasal and intraventricular approaches. Despite these improvements, however, the microscope did have its limitations. It struggled to provide appropriate visualization around corners due to the linear nature of the light source located outside the surgical field. This lack of illumination limited the surgeon's ability to adequately visualize all necessary structures in the CPA and created the need for larger cranial openings and significant cerebellar retraction in order to compensate for these shortcomings.

By the 1990s, technical advancements in illumination and image resolution allowed for the endoscope to be introduced as an adjunct to the operative microscope to enhance visualization of CPA corridors previously unseen with microscopy alone.[3-6] Initially, fully endoscopic procedures were unable to be performed due to the need to operate with precise bimanual dexterity adjacent to the essential neurovascular structures of the CPA, precluding the surgeon from holding the endoscope during dissection. In addition, unlike endonasal endoscopy where the surgical field can accommodate two surgeons and four hands working in coordination, the limited space of the lateral suboccipital space impedes this. As a result, endoscopy was relegated to an adjunct in CPA surgery with its use limited to inspection of the neurovascular structures while microscopy remained the mainstay for surgical dissection. The development of multijoint, polyaxial, pneumatic arms to hold the surgical endoscope in

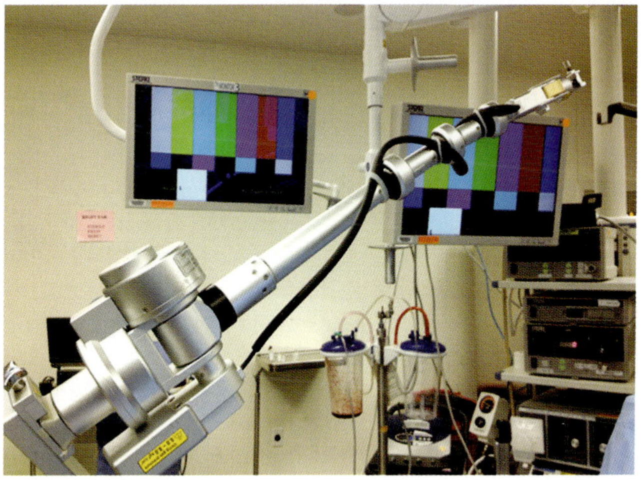

Fig. 15.1: View of the polyaxial, multijointed pneumatic holding arm in its outstretched position. Compressing the yellow button at the end of the holder allows the surgeon to easily move the endoscope, while releasing it stabilizes the endoscope in a fixed, rigid position.

place revolutionized endoscopic surgery in the CPA. These pneumatic holding arms allow the surgeon to constantly change trajectory throughout all planes of motion and relock into a stable configuration with the depression and release of a single button creating the ability to reposition the endoscope with one hand (Fig. 15.1).

Shahanian et al. were the first to describe a fully endoscopic approach to the CPA for microvascular decompression (MVD) in trigeminal neuralgia and hemifacial spasm.[7,8] Since then, several others have reported successful results performing MVDs in a fully endoscopic manner.[9-12] In addition, the fully endoscopic approach has been reported for neurectomies,[13-15] resection of epidermoid cysts[16-18] as well as resection of vestibular schwannomas and meningiomas of the CPA without the aid of an operating microscope.[14,19-24] The benefits of performing CPA surgery in a fully endoscopic technique is the wider field of view that allows for improved visualization of the neurovascular structures from cranial nerve (CN) III superiorly at the level of the incisura through the foramen magnum, while minimizing the cranial opening and essentially eliminating all cerebellar retraction. As a result, it is less necessary to sacrifice venous structures and the patient is provided with decreased operative time, postoperative pain, cerebellar symptoms, cranial neuropathies, hospital length of stay, and recovery time.

Despite the significant improvements made with endoscopy, several limitations and disadvantages still exist. Absence of the interpeduncular and/or prepontine cisterns due to mass effect or elevated intracranial pressure is considered a contraindication to endoscopic CPA surgery. While this should not affect the ability to perform a fully endoscopic MVD, it is essential to consider when evaluating preoperative radiographs prior to any cyst or neoplasm resection. Another factor to consider is the overheating of vital structures in the CPA due to the close proximity of the light source. A thin sleeve over the endoscope to allow frequent, intermittent irrigation to cooling the tip can minimize heat transfer and allow for the procedure to be performed safely. Unlike microsurgery where surgical instruments work in series along the optical trajectory of the microscope lens, the surgeon must work in parallel to the endoscope. In addition, the working corridor is small and limited by the cerebellum and petrous bone, which unfortunately precludes the use of bayonetted instruments. Instead a set based on the principle of rotational pistol-grip instruments, as well as straight-shafted dissectors must be used. However, the biggest challenge to overcome is the loss of depth perception when visualizing the procedure on a 2D monitor. This point is especially valid in the CPA, as damage from inadvertent contact to vital structures in this area can have led to catastrophic events, resulting in a steep learning curve for surgeons who are new to this technique. As a result, it is essential that surgeons are comfortable with the anatomy of the CPA and have significant experience in handling the endoscope in the laboratory or in other surgical approaches prior to attempting use of the endoscope in the CPA.

MICROVASCULAR DECOMPRESSION

Several authors have described successful results of MVD performed in a fully endoscopic manner for both trigeminal neuralgia and hemifacial spasm;[7-12] however, there is no contraindication for this technique to be used in MVDs or cranial neurectomies of any CN in the CPA. Prior to the decompression, a thorough 360° inspection of the root entry zone should be performed in order to account for all potential vascular entities. The offending vessels should then be dissected from the surrounding arachnoid bands to allow adequate mobility, which minimizes inadvertent vascular injury during placement of the pledget (Figs. 15.2A to D). It is imperative that the endoscope not be withdrawn if significant bleeding is encountered, as recannulation of the CPA will be difficult. Instead, in this event, the endoscope should be left in place and copious amounts of irrigation along with either bipolar cautery or gentle pressure should be used to provide adequate hemostasis. In the case of MVD for hemifacial spasm, pre- and poststimulation threshold is recommended in order to evaluate the integrity of the nerve prior to closure. An electrical recording of CN VII at a direct stimulation of 0.05 mA is generally consistent with a favorable facial nerve response.

VESTIBULAR NEURECTOMY

Modern endoscopes, combined with high-definition monitors and HD capable cameras surpass the detail visualized by the operating microscope. This provides a major advantage in performing vestibular neurectomy as delineation of the vestibular and cochlear portions of CN VIII are essential for success in this procedure (Figs. 15.3A to D). In addition, CN VII and nervus intermedius should also be identified prior to the neurectomy in order to avoid injury. The superior visualization of the endoscope allows better identification of these structures, and thereby, improves the likelihood of a successful result while minimizing the chance of injury to the adjacent neurovascular structures. During the neurectomy, continuous brainstem auditory evoked potentials (BAER) monitoring is performed to assess the cochlear nerve.

TUMOR RESECTION

The fully endoscopic technique can also be utilized for resection of extra-axial CPA angle tumors such as vestibular schwannomas (Figs. 15.4A and B), meningiomas (Figs. 15.5A to F), and epidermoid cysts (Figs. 15.6A to D). The advantage that the endoscope provides in these cases is the improved visualization of the neural structures splayed along the tumor capsule, allowing for early identification of the cochlear nerve in hearing preservation cases. In addition, the endoscope allows the surgeon to visualize structures ventral to the tumor, such as CN VII, prior to resection, minimizing risk of facial nerve injury. In addition, the 30° endoscope enhances visualization out along the IAC during the retrosigmoid approach,

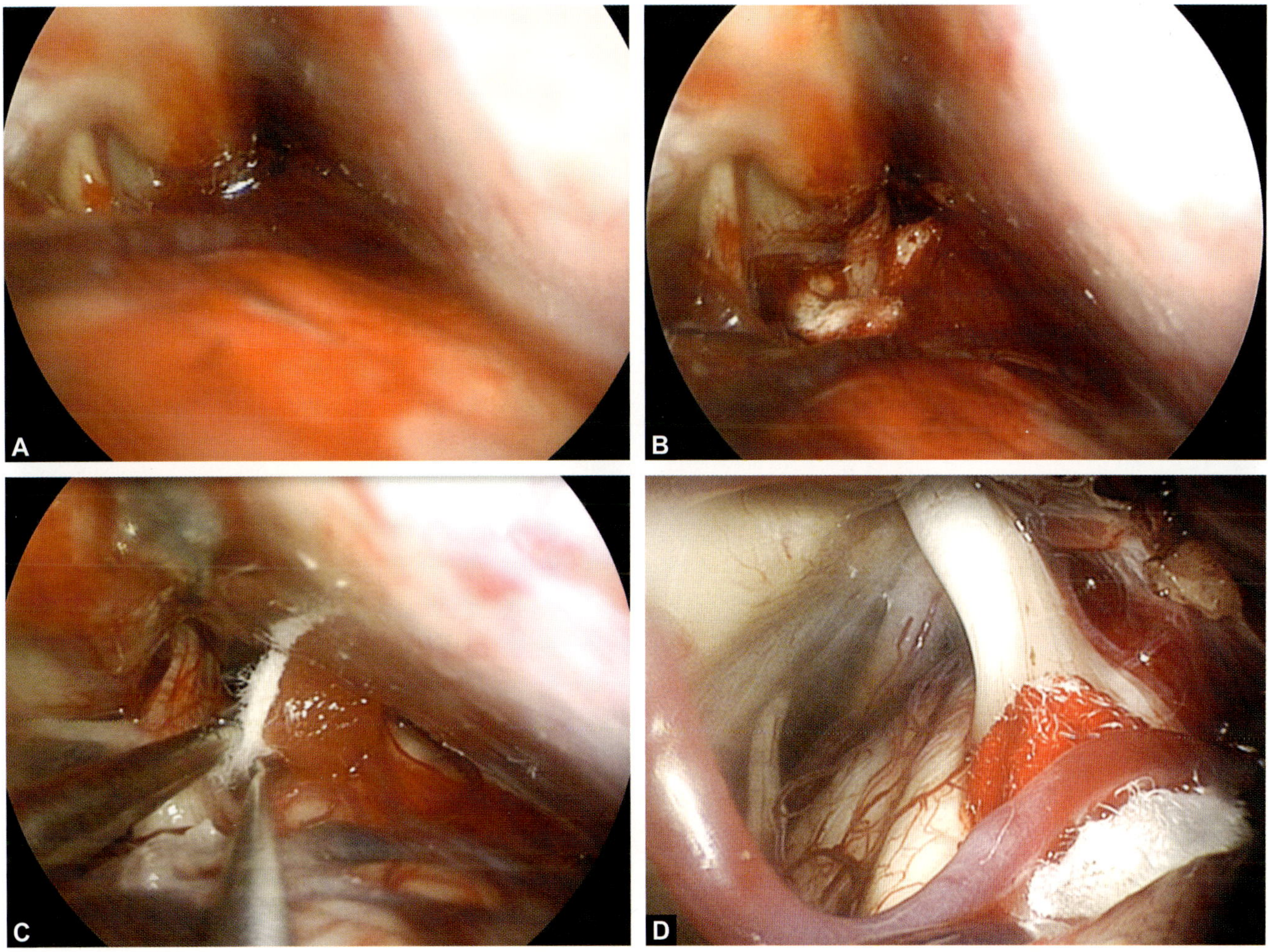

Figs. 15.2A to D: (A) Endoscopic view of the cerebellopontine angle prior to cerebrospinal fluid (CSF) egress. (B) Endoscopic view of the cerebellopontine angle post-CSF egress. (C) Endoscopic view of the microvascular decompression being performed in a bimanual fashion. (D) Intraoperative image after the microvascular decompression has been performed on cranial nerve (CN) V. A pledget is seen separating CN V from two separate vessels at the root entry zone.

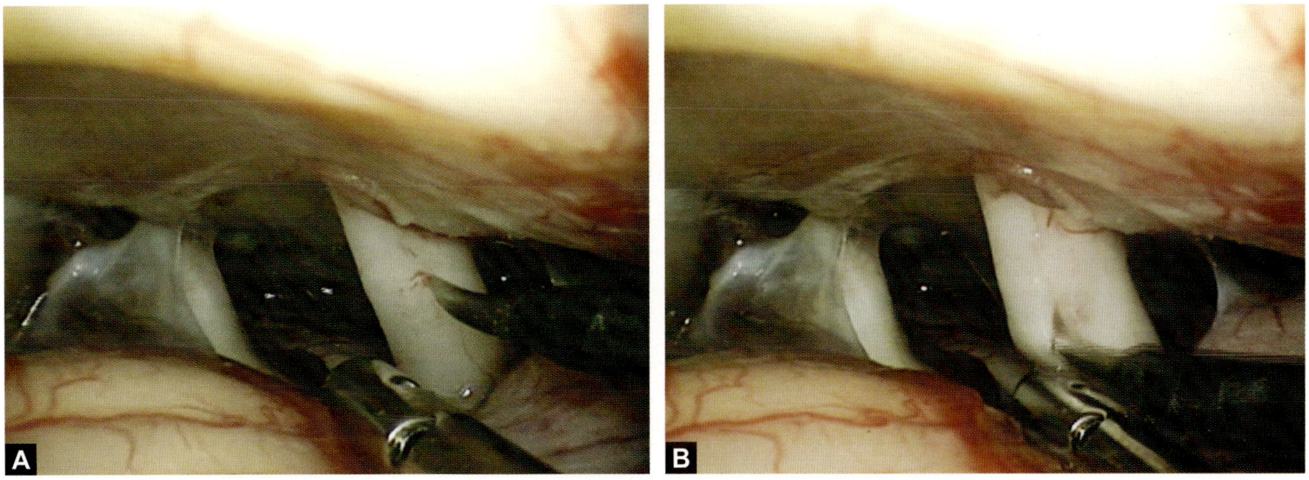

Figs. 15.3A and B: (A) Intraoperative, endoscopic view of cranial nerve (CN) VIII with a microdissector demarcating the division of the superior and inferior vestibular nerves. (B) Separation of the superior and inferior vestibular nerves.

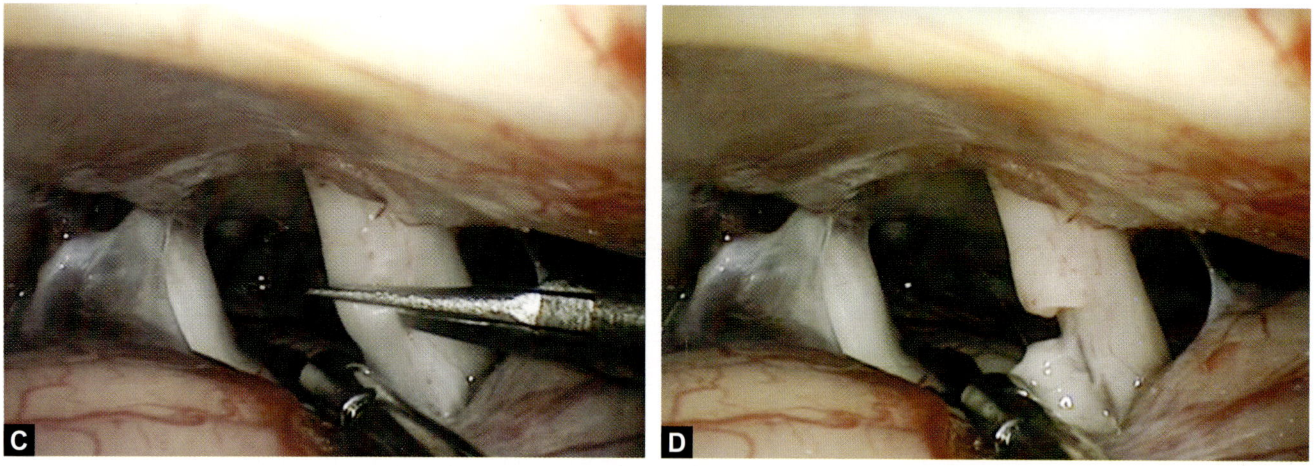

Figs. 15.3C and D: (C) View of the superior vestibular nerve being sectioned. (D) Final view of CN VIII after the superior vestibular nerve has been fully sectioned.

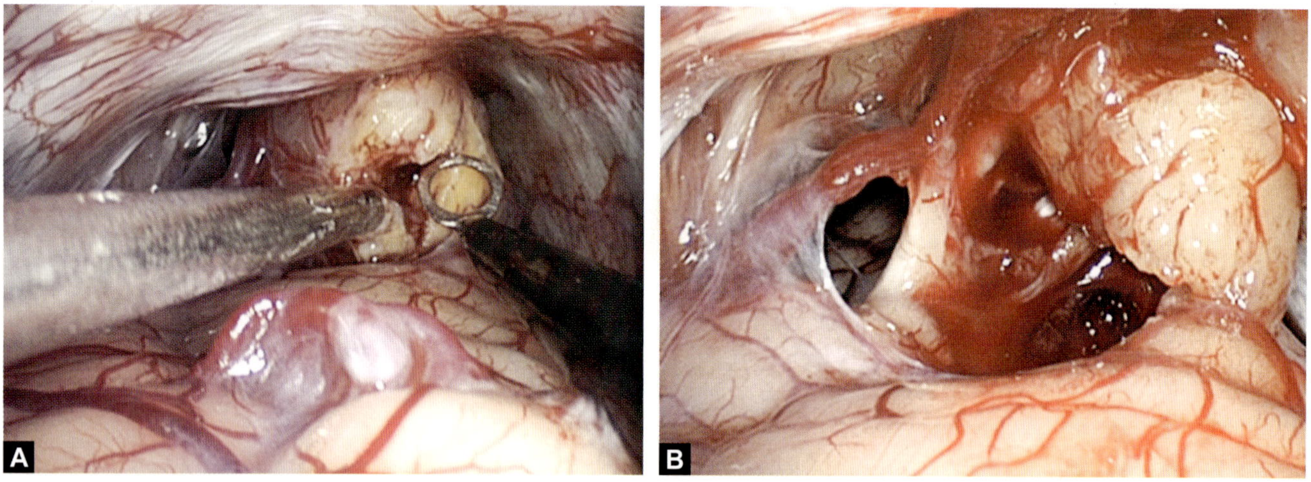

Figs. 15.4A and B: Intraoperative, endoscopic view of vestibular schwannoma resection.

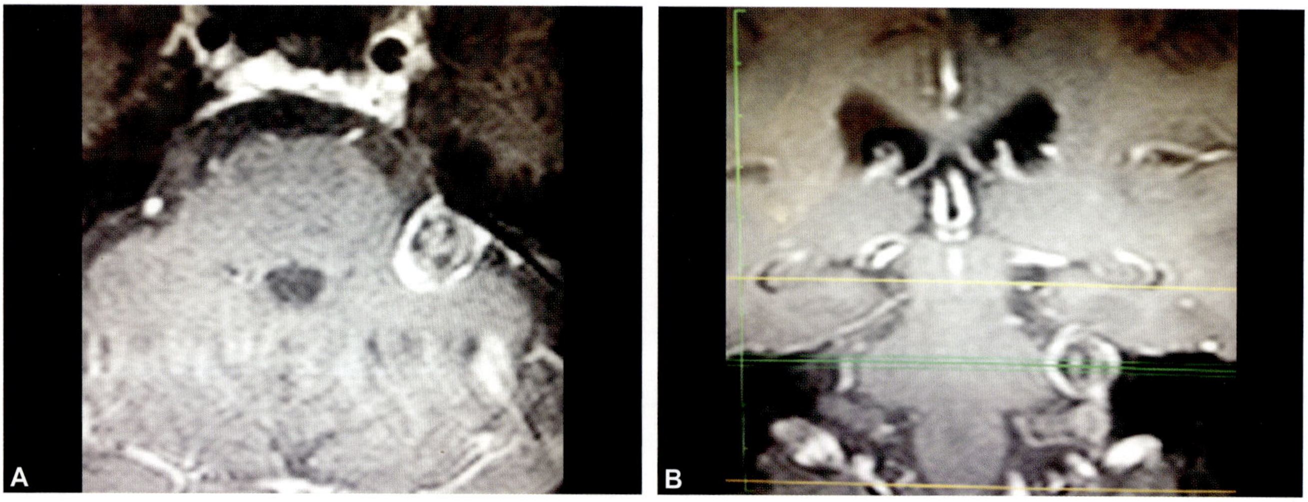

Figs. 15.5A and B: (A) Preoperative T1 axial with gadolinium identifying a 2.0 × 1.5 cm meningioma in the left cerebellopontine angle (CPA). (B) Preoperative T1 coronal with gadolinium.

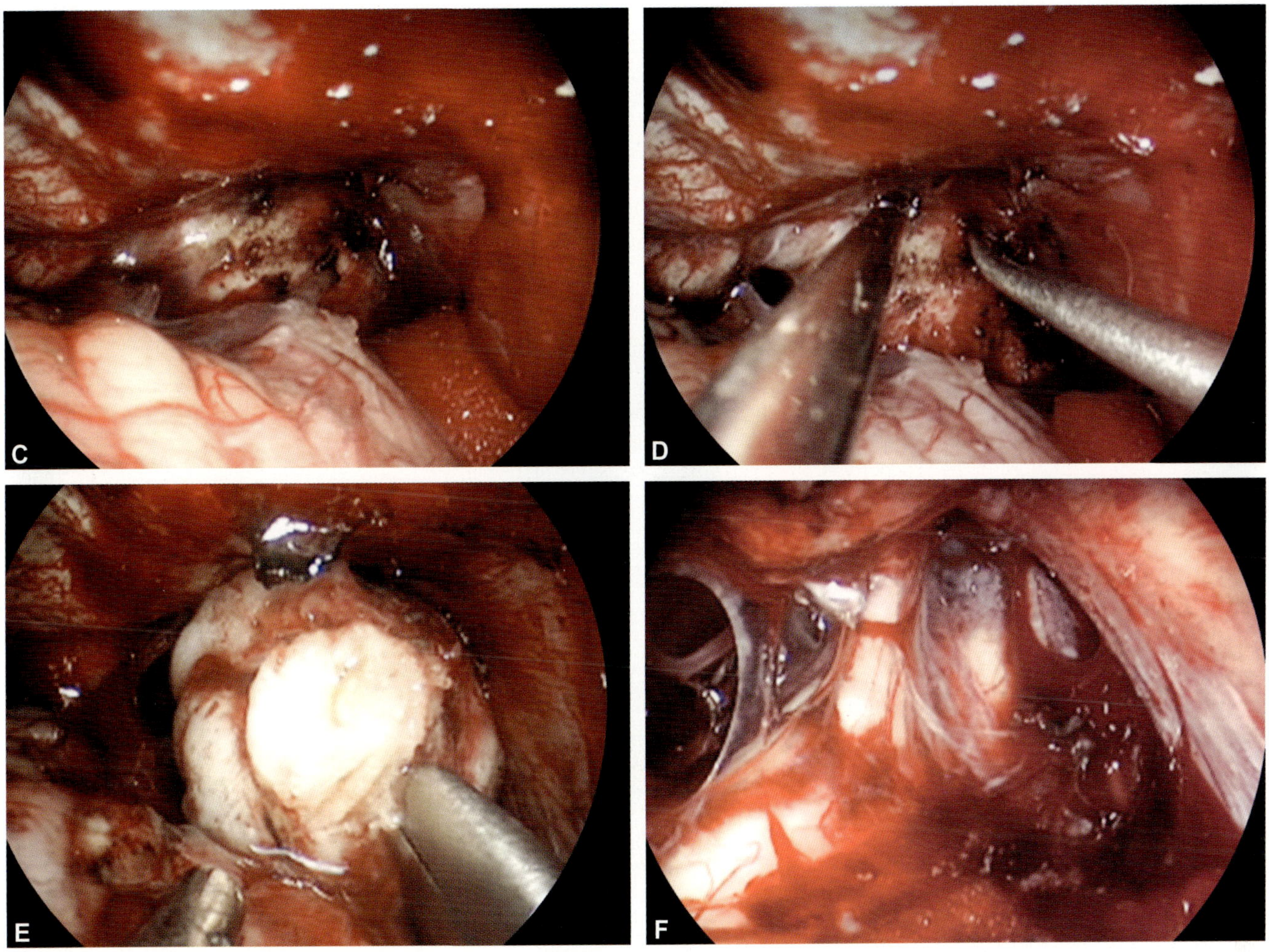

Figs. 15.5C to F: (C) Intraoperative endoscopic view of a 2.0 × 1.5 cm meningioma located in the left CPA prior to resection. The cerebellum is located inferiorly, the petrous temporal bone superiorly and the tentorium is located to the right. (D) Endoscopic view of bimanual dissection of tumor from the surrounding structures. Note that no retractors are present and no retraction of the cerebellum is necessary. (E) The tumor has been dissected free of all structures and is being removed from the CPA. (F) Intraoperative, endoscopic view of the CPA after gross total resection has been achieved.

minimizing the amount of bone removal at the porous acousticus. Tension to the neural structures is also minimized as virtually no retraction is applied to the cerebellum. With the advent of endoscopic ultrasonic aspirator and laser technology, limitations encountered early on in endoscopy are diminishing.

SURGICAL TECHNIQUE

Step 1: The monitor for the endoscope is placed in a direct line of site for the surgeon. The pneumatic holding arm is positioned to allow the surgeon a wide range of freedom for the placement of the endoscope. The patient's head is immobilized. This is especially important as no paralytics can be used to allow for intraoperative facial nerve monitoring and any movement by the patient during the procedure can cause the endoscope or instruments to impale the brainstem. The head is elevated to 30° above the horizontal (Fig. 15.7) and the patient is given 1–2 gm/kg of mannitol and 20 mg furosemide followed by lowering of the $Paco_2$ to 28 mmHg. Monitoring electrodes are utilized depending on the cranial nerves likely to be encountered; this usually includes the facial nerve and BAER, but can include endotracheal tube monitoring electrodes, SSEP, CN XI and XII.

Step 2: Next, the transverse-sigmoid (TS) junction must be approximated for the location of the incision. The transverse sinus is located by marking a line between the root of the zygoma and the external occipital protuberance. The sigmoid sinus can be estimated as parallel and just

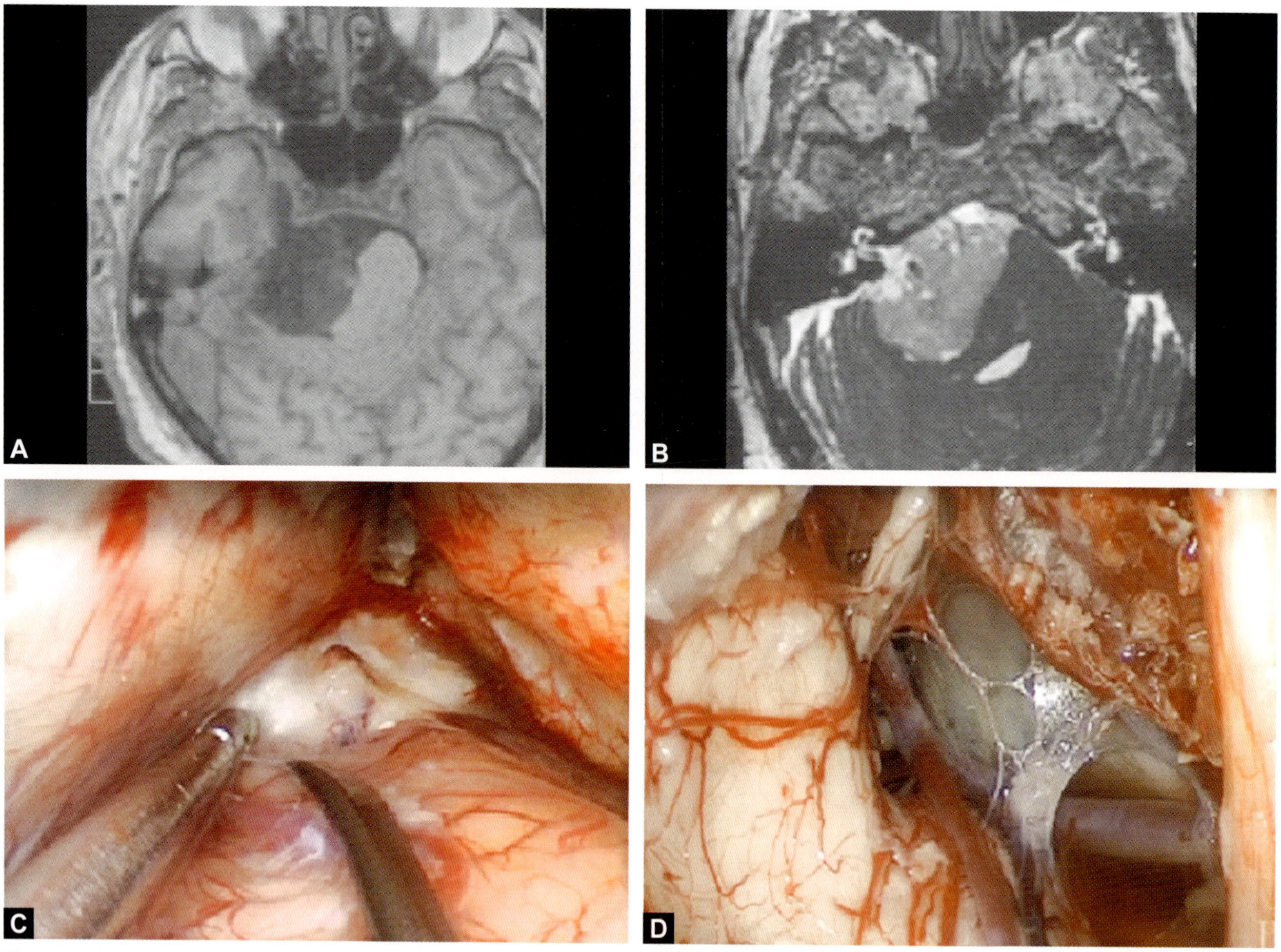

Figs. 15.6A to D: (A) Preoperative T1 axial MRI demonstrating a cerebellopontine angle (CPA) epidermoid cyst. (B) Preoperative T2 axial MRI. (C) Intraoperative, endoscopic view of a CPA epidermoid cyst. (D) Intraoperative, endoscopic view of the CPA after gross total resection.

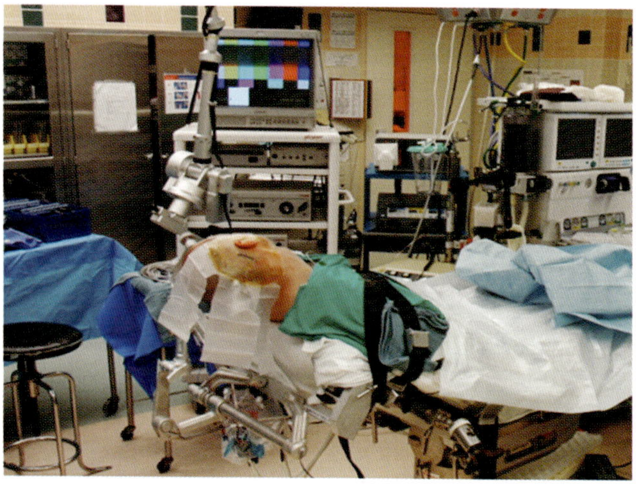

Fig. 15.7: Preoperative setup of the operating room. The pneumatic holding arm and HD monitor are positioned directly in line with each other so that the surgeon has a direct view of the video screen while operating.

lateral to the posterior mastoid groove. The intersection of these two lines demarcates the approximation of the TS junction (Fig. 15.8). A 3–4 mm oblique incision is then made over this location, parallel to the hairline for cosmetic purposes. Monopolar cautery is then utilized to dissect down to the skull exposing the asterion and occipitomastoid suture. Fishhooks are used instead of self-retaining retractors due to their low profile (Fig. 15.9).

Step 3: After asterion and the occipitomastoid suture are identified, a high-speed drill is used to create a 14 mm craniectomy just inferior to asterion and two-thirds posterior, one-third anterior to the occipitomastoid suture. The posteroinferior edge of the TS junction is skeletonized and located in the superolateral portion of the cranial defect (Fig. 15.9). The dura is then opened in a curvilinear fashion paralleling the TS junction, reflecting the dural flap inferior and medially. Care must be taken to allow for an adequate cuff of dura for later closure.

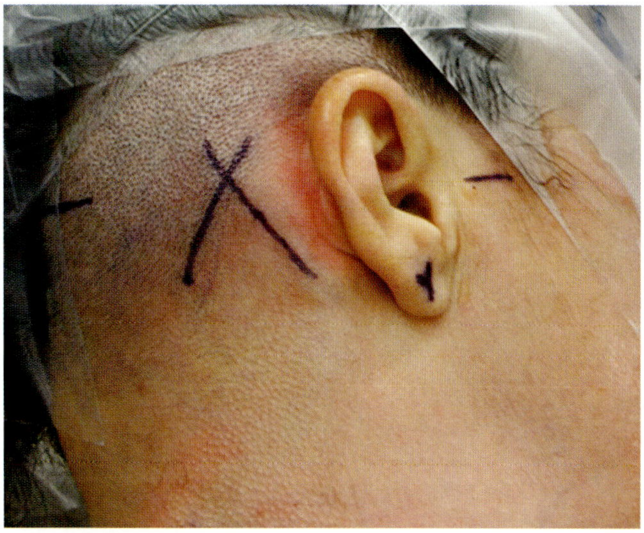

Fig. 15.8: The external occipital protuberance is marked on the left and the root of the zygoma is marked on the right. In the center, a line is drawn parallel and just lateral to the posterior mastoid groove while another line demarcates the hairline.

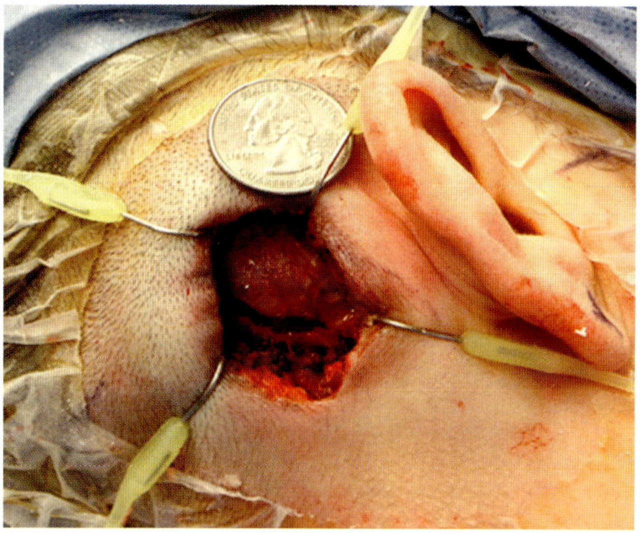

Fig. 15.9: A 14 mm retrosigmoid craniectomy has been performed with a 24 mm coin placed nearby for size reference. Using the asterion and occipitomastoid suture as landmarks, the posteroinferior aspect of the junction between the transverse and sigmoid sinuses is exposed. Note the fishhooks retracting the skin edges to maximize the incision, while maintaining a low profile.

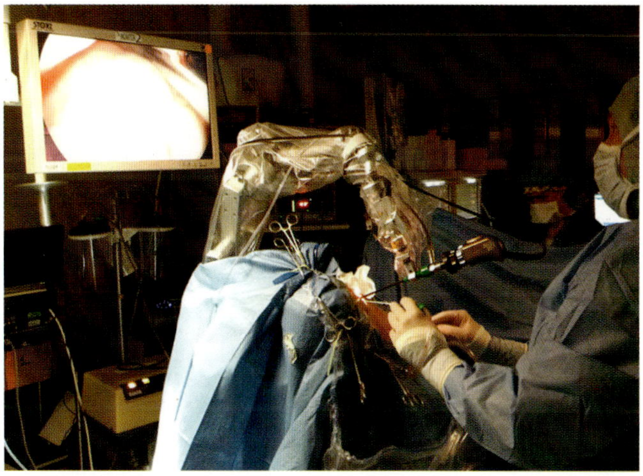

Fig. 15.10: Operative setup with the holding arm arched over the patient's head and holding the endoscope in a rigid position, allowing the surgeon to operate with bimanual dexterity. The HD monitor is in direct sight for the surgeon.

Step 4: Initially, a 4 mm, 0°, rigid endoscope is cannulated along the tentorium and petrous temporal bone (Fig. 15.10). A 2.7 mm endoscope will provide a smaller footprint, but also decreases the field of view. The petrosal veins are usually encountered and must be either cauterized and cut or mobilized to access the cerebrospinal fluid (CSF) cisterns. The endoscope is then advanced past the CN VII/VIII complex until the arachnoid of the prepontine cistern or cisterna magna is encountered and opened, allowing CSF release and further brain relaxation. Once an adequate amount of CSF egress has occurred, an appropriate working corridor between the cerebellum and petrous bone should be present, allowing visualization of the ventrolateral brainstem. Depending on the procedure being performed, different structures can be inspected, including the CN root entry zone for MVDs as well as the facial and cochlear nerves for tumor resection. In addition, the 30° endoscope can be utilized for inspection ventral to tumors and into the internal auditory canal. At this point, the procedure should essentially be unchanged from a microscope-assisted procedure except that endoscopic aspirators, bipolars (Fig. 15.11), and dissectors are utilized. We prefer using insulated microdissectors (Fig. 15.12) during the procedure, as this allows continuous feedback during the procedure minimizing the risk of neural injury.

Step 5: Once the procedure is completed, CPA is inspected and all bleeding is stopped with gentle pressure or coagulation. The endoscope is then removed and a watertight dural closure is performed. If a watertight closure is not possible, a dural substitute or fascial graft can also be used (Fig. 15.13). Once, the dural closure is completed, the bone defect is filled with hydroxyapatite bone cement (Fig. 15.14). The wound is then closed in a layered fashion.

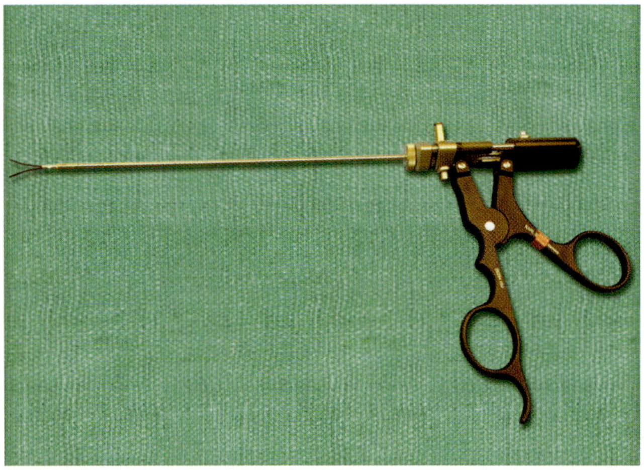

Fig. 15.11: View of the endoscopic bipolar with the pistol-gripped design.

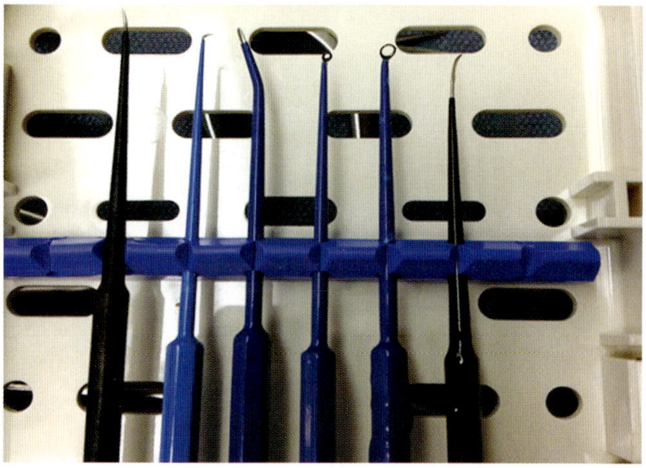

Fig. 15.12: View of the endoscopic insulated microdissectors with neuromonitoring capabilities.

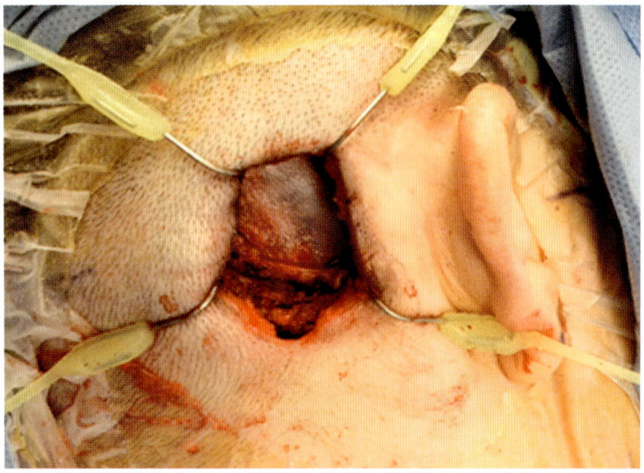

Fig. 15.13: Dural closure using dural on-lay substitute.

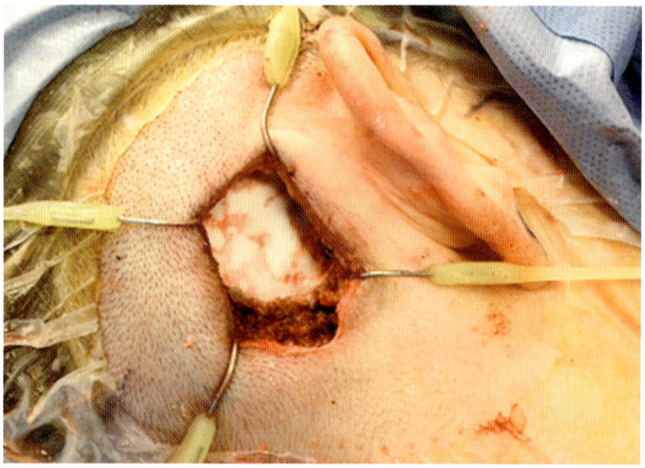

Fig. 15.14: The craniectomy defect has been filled in with hydroxyapatite.

REFERENCES

1. Mouton WG, Bessell JR, Maddern GJ. Looking back to the advent of modern endoscopy. 150th birthday of Maximilan Nitze. World J Surg. 1998;22:1256-8.
2. Doyen E. Surgical Therapeutics and Operative Techniques, Vol I. London: Balliere, Tindall, and Cox; 1917. pp. 599-602.
3. O'Donoghue GM, O'Flynn P. Endoscopic anatomy of the cerebellopontine angle. Am J of Otology. 1993;14(2):122-5.
4. Magnan J, Chays A, Lepetre C, et al. Surgical perspectives of endoscopy of the cerebellopontine angle. Am J Otology. 1994;15:366-70.
5. Wachym PA, King WA, Meyer GA, et al. Endoscopy in neuro-otologic surgery. Otolaryngol Clin North Am. 2002;35(2): 297-323.
6. Takemura Y, Inoue T, Morishita T, et al. Comparison of Microscopic and Endoscopic Approaches to the Cerebellopontine Angle. World Neurosurg. 2013;pii:S1878-8750(13) 00827-9.
7. Eby JB, Cha ST, Shahinian HK. Fully endoscopic vascular decompression of the facial nerve for hemifacial spasm. Skull Base. 2001;11:189-97.
8. Jarrahy R, Eby JB, Cha ST, et al. Fully endoscopic vascular decompression of the trigeminal nerve. Minim Invas Neurosurg. 2002;45:32-5.
9. Artz GJ, Hux FJ, LaRouere MJ, et al. Endoscopic vascular decompression. J Otol Neurotol. 2008;29:995-1000.
10. Yadav YR, Parihar V, Agarwal M, et al. Endoscopic vascular decompression of the trigeminal neuralgia. Minim Invasive Neurosurg. 2011;54:110-4.
11. Halpern CH, Lang SS, Lee JY. Fully endoscopic microvascular decompression: our early experience. Minim Invasive Surg. 2013;2013:739432.
12. Setty P, Volkov AA, D'Andrea KP, et al. Endoscopic vascular decompression for the treatment of trigeminal neuralgia: clinical outcomes and technical note. World Neurosurg. 2014;81(3-4):603-8.

13. Wackym PA, King WA, Barker FG, et al. Endoscope-assisted vestibular neurectomy. Laryngoscope. 1998;108:1787-93.
14. Miyazaki H, Deveze A, Magnan J. Neuro-otologic surgery through minimally invasive retrosigmoid approach: endoscope assisted microvascular decompression, vestibular neurotomy, and tumor removal. Laryngoscope. 2005;115:1612-7.
15. Cutler AR, Kaloostian SW, Ishiyama A, et al. Two-handed endoscopic-directed vestibular nerve sectioning: case series and review of the literature. J Neurosurg. 2012;117:507-13.
16. Schroeder HWS, Oertel J, Gaab MR. Endoscope-assisted microsurgical resection of epidermoid tumors of the cerebellopontine angle. J Neurosurg. 2004;101:227-32.
17. Divitiis O, Cavallo LM, Dal Fabbro M, et al. Freehand dynamic endoscopic resection of an epidermoid tumor of the cerebellopontine angle: technical case report. Neurosurgery. 2007;61:ONSE239-40.
18. Krass J, Hahn Y, Karami K, et al. Endoscopic assisted resection of prepontine epidermoid cysts. J Neurol Surg A Cent E Neurosurg. 2014;75(2):120-5.
19. Magnan J, Chays A, Cohen JM, et al. Endoscopy of the cerebellopontine angle. Rev Laryngol Otol Rhinol (Bord). 1995;116(2):115-8.
20. Goksu N, Bayazit Y, Kemaloglu Y. Endoscopy of the posterior fossa and endoscopic dissection of acoustic neuroma. Neurosurgical Focus. 1999;6(4):15.
21. Wackym PA, King WA, Poe DS, et al. Adjunctive use of endoscopy during acoustic neuroma surgery. Laryngoscope. 1999;109:1193-201.
22. Shahanian HK, Eby JB, Ocon M. Fully endoscopic excision of vestibular schwannomas. Minim Invasive Neurosurg. 2004; 47(6):329-32.
23. Shahanian HK, Ra Y. 527 Fully endoscopic resections of vestibular schwannomas. Minim Invasive Neurosurg. 2011; 54(2):61-7.
24. Pieper DR. The endoscopic approach to vestibular schwannomas and posterolateral skull base pathology. Otolaryngol Clin North Am. 2012;45(2):439-54.

CHAPTER

16 Implantable Hearing Appliances

Robert S Hong, Seilesh Babu

INTRODUCTION

The provision of hearing via bone conduction is an excellent solution for hearing loss in certain scenarios where conventional hearing amplification cannot be performed. For example, some patients have hearing loss in the context of a chronically draining ear, with the otorrhea blocking the transmission of sound by a conventional hearing aid through the ear canal. Others may have a severe enough hearing loss in a single ear that the amplification of sound by a conventional aid provides little utility. Bone conduction hearing provides a potential solution for conductive or mixed hearing loss, as well as single-sided deafness, by bypassing the normal mechanisms of sound transmission through the ear. The mechanical vibration of the skull bone provided by a bone conduction device is thought to provide hearing via a number of mechanisms, including (1) vibrating the air within the external auditory canal to drive the tympanic membrane, (2) directly vibrating the ossicular chain, and (3) directly compressing the fluids within the inner ear. In so doing, bone conduction devices provide patients with a sensation of hearing essentially indistinguishable from hearing via normal air conduction, with excellent sound quality and minimal distortion.

There are a number of delivery systems available that provide hearing via bone conduction, each with their own advantages and disadvantages. While in all cases, the microphone to pick up the sound is near the impaired ear, the site at which the mechanical vibration of the skull is delivered varies from device to device. These sites include (1) within the ear canal at the bony portion of the external auditory canal [TransEar (Ear Technology Corporation, Johnson City, Tennessee)], (2) within the mouth via the upper teeth [SoundBite Hearing System (Sonitus Medical, San Mateo, California)], (3) across the skin of the skull with the device secured against the head using a headband [BAHA Softband (Cochlear Bone Anchored Solutions AB, Sweden); Ponto Softband (Oticon Medical AB, Sweden)], and (4) at the bone found just behind the auricle [BAHA (bone-anchored hearing appliance)]. The first three devices mentioned are advantageous in that they do not require surgery; however, each has other potential drawbacks, including patient discomfort at the location where the device is placed and in the case of the Softband, significant damping of sound transmission by the soft tissues. In this chapter, we focus on the fourth solution mentioned, the BAHA (Fig. 16.1).

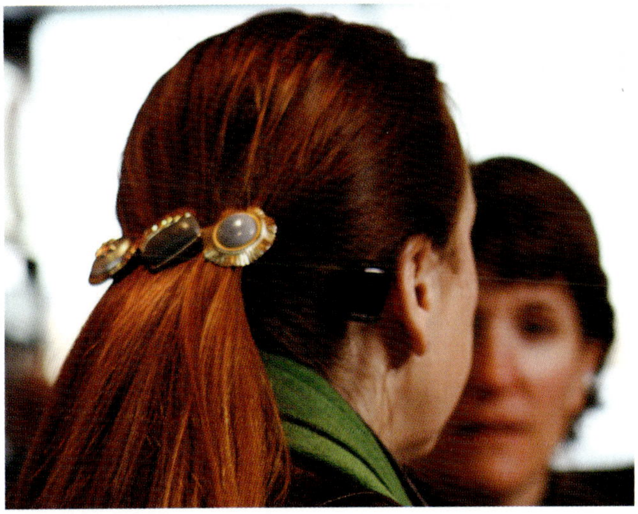

Fig. 16.1: Appearance of a BAHA implant worn behind the ear. *Courtesy*: Cochlear Americas, ©2014 Cochlear Americas

To date, over 100,000 patients have received a BAHA device worldwide. The BAHA provides bone conduction hearing via the vibration of a sound processor that clips onto an osseointegrated titanium abutment located posterior to the auricle. Osseointegration of the implant to the surrounding bone, facilitated by osteocytes, occurs over the course of weeks to months and is the key to the success of the procedure. Failure of osseointegration may result in the inability of the abutment to tolerate the load produced by the vibrations of the BAHA leading to implant extrusion. Advantages of the BAHA over other devices include the ability to provide a relatively more powerful bone conduction stimulus to the skull, the need to wear only a single device in a single location, and near universal health insurance coverage for the device in the United States.

There are two primary BAHA devices currently in the market: (1) Cochlear Baha (Cochlear Bone Anchored Solutions AB, Sweden) and (2) Ponto (Oticon Medical AB, Sweden). Both devices are similar in how they function, relying on a vibrating sound processor placed on an osseointegrated abutment located behind the ear to provide bone conduction hearing. The devices differ in the exact shape and configuration of both the abutment and sound processor. However, in our experience, patients express similar satisfaction with both devices. Thus, we offer both devices to our qualified patients with equal enthusiasm.

PATIENT SELECTION

All patients considering BAHA implantation should have a formal audiogram with both pure tone and speech discrimination testing to establish the degree and type of hearing loss. Tuning forks should also be used (Weber and Rinne exams) to corroborate audiometric findings. In general, patients who are candidates for the BAHA can be divided into two groups: (1) conductive or mixed hearing loss and (2) single-sided (sensorineural) deafness.

Conductive or Mixed Hearing Loss

Patients who have a conductive or mixed hearing loss where the conductive component of the hearing loss is at least 30 dB may benefit from a BAHA. The hearing loss may be either unilateral or bilateral, though patients with bilateral hearing loss should have relatively symmetric bone conduction thresholds (within 10–15 dB of one another) for benefit to be obtained in both ears. In cases of mixed hearing loss, the sensorineural component of the hearing loss should be no worse than a moderate hearing loss. However, patients with bone conduction thresholds on the poorer end of the candidacy spectrum need to be aware that they may need a larger and more powerful speech processor, including potentially a body-worn device, for the BAHA to be effective.

There are a number of scenarios where the BAHA may be considered for conductive or mixed hearing loss. One of the most common is the patient who is unable to tolerate a conventional hearing aid. This may be because the patient has chronic drainage from the ear that blocks the transmission of sound by a conventional aid, experiences chronic irritation from having the hearing aid within the ear canal, or experiences significant acoustic feedback with the device. Some of these patients may have had prior attempts at surgical correction of hearing loss that have been unsuccessful (such as patients with end-stage chronic ear disease) or deferred attempts at surgery because of the risk involved (such as with otosclerosis in an only hearing ear). BAHA has also been advocated as a treatment for hearing loss in Down syndrome in children, when patients have failed conventional hearing aids and pressure equalization tubes.[1,2]

Another scenario is that of congenital aural atresia, where the ear canal is not patent, preventing usage of a conventional hearing aid. Because a bone conduction device bypasses the normal pathway of sound transmission to the ear, it can provide hearing to these patients. All patients with *bilateral* congenital aural atresia should initially in infancy have hearing provided via a bone conduction device, typically a Softband device (as the BAHA is not approved by the US Food and Drug Administration for children younger than 5 years of age). As the children grow older, they may consider outer and middle ear reconstruction surgery to address their conductive hearing loss, or alternatively, may elect to have placement of a surgically implanted BAHA. Additionally, patients with *unilateral* congenital aural atresia will also experience benefit from a BAHA. Traditionally, children with unilateral aural atresia were not provided with a bone-conduction device as it was believed that a single hearing ear was good enough. However, more recent evidence has suggested that lack of a second hearing ear may lead to poorer academic performance and greater speech and learning difficulties.[3,4]

Single-sided Deafness

Patients who have single-sided deafness and essentially normal hearing in the contralateral ear are also candidates for the BAHA. These patients find minimal to no benefit from conventional hearing amplification in the deaf ear. In the contralateral ear, the pure tone average of bone conduction thresholds (taken at 500 Hz, 1 kHz, 2 kHz, and 3 kHz) should be 20 dB HL or better. In contrast to patients who receive the BAHA for unilateral conductive hearing loss, where the information is presented to the same ear as the hearing loss, those with single-sided deafness rely on the BAHA to route sound from the deaf side to the contralateral normal cochlea. Possible etiologies of single-sided deafness include idiopathic sudden sensorineural hearing loss, vestibular schwannoma, Meniere's disease, temporal bone trauma, viral infections, and congenital etiologies.

Contraindications

There are no absolute contraindications for the BAHA. Patients who receive the BAHA need to have adequate bone volume and bone quality for placement and osseointegration of the titanium abutment. As such, children younger than 5 years of age have not been approved by the US Food and Drug Administration for the BAHA, though there have been reports from outside the United States of children being implanted younger without complications.[5] Conditions that may lead to a higher risk of implant failure due to lack of osseointegration include those who have previously received radiation to the surgical field, and those with bone diseases such as fibrous dysplasia or Paget's disease.

Concern for a higher risk of postoperative wound healing issues may be present in those who exhibit poor general hygiene, poorly controlled diabetics, those with skin problems, smokers, and those with a tendency toward hypertrophic scarring or keloids. Relative contraindications include inability to followup for programming and maintenance of the device, disinclination to use the device, and inability to follow instructions. The need for magnetic resonance imaging (MRI) is not a contraindication, as the titanium implant is considered MRI safe and the BAHA sound processor can be removed from the abutment before undergoing imaging.

PREOPERATIVE COUNSELING AND INFORMED CONSENT

A thorough discussion of the risks, benefits, and alternatives to the BAHA is presented to all patients prior to surgery. Patients with a conductive or mixed hearing loss should explore the alternatives of observation, a conventional hearing aid, and surgical correction of hearing loss (such as via ossicular chain reconstruction when appropriate) with their otolaryngologist. Patients with single-sided deafness are asked to consider all potential options, including observation, the CROS (contralateral routing of signals) hearing aid, the SoundBite hearing system, and the BAHA.

Patients are counseled that they need to have realistic expectations and that the BAHA does not restore normal hearing, though many patients find that the BAHA helps particularly in challenging listening situations when sound is presented to the side with hearing impairment. All patients are asked to undergo a BAHA simulation using a bone conduction oscillator placed against the skin of the skull. We have found that the simulator helps patients understand the benefit they may receive from the BAHA and provides them with realistic expectations.

Preoperative imaging is typically not important to the success of BAHA implantation. However, a CT scan may be considered prior to surgery in children to assess the thickness of the bone and determine the safest location for implantation. Children with craniofacial abnormalities may be more likely to have thin bone or a low-laying middle fossa tegmen.

Risks of surgery are discussed with the patient and include local numbness, hair loss, skin irritation, skin overgrowth, infection, pain, bleeding, and implant extrusion. Intracranial complications such as cerebrospinal fluid (CSF) leak or subdural hematoma are rare but can occur, particularly if the bone where the abutment is to be placed is thin (such as in children). Patients are also informed that should they decide in the future that they do not want the device and want it removed, that the abutment can be removed and the procedure reversed.

SURGICAL TECHNIQUES

General Considerations

Multiple techniques have been described for performing BAHA surgery. The traditional method of BAHA implantation is the "skin flap" technique, which involves the use of a dermatome to take a pedicled split thickness skin graft centered around the abutment site. The underlying soft tissue is then debulked, the BAHA implant placed, and the skin graft sutured back in place around the abutment at the end of the case. However, this technique has fallen out favor as newer techniques have evolved in recent years, which have led to reduced operating times, faster healing, and fewer wound complications.[6] At our institution, we no longer employ the "skin flap" technique. Instead, we use one of two newer techniques—(1) the "linear incision" technique and (2) the minimally invasive "punch" technique—both of which will be described in this chapter. The decision on which technique to use is made intraoperatively, based on scalp thickness and surgeon preference, with the "punch" technique often favored in patients with thinner scalps due to shorter operating times and similar outcomes.

A second important surgical decision is whether to perform the BAHA implantation in one stage or two stages. The vast majority of BAHA surgeries are performed in one stage. However, in patients where osseointegration of the implant is a concern, the surgery may be performed in two stages. The first stage involves placement of the implant fixture into the bone, without the percutaneous abutment. The second stage occurs 6 months later, and involves attachment of the abutment to the implant. Staging the surgery provides maximum opportunity for osseointegration of the implant by preventing interruption in stability during this critical initial time period, such as by accidental trauma to the percutaneous abutment. Patients in whom a two-stage procedure may be considered include those with thin cortical bone (<3 mm), young children (<9 years of age), those who have been previously irradiated, and those with poor bone quality.

One final consideration is whether or not to place a sleeper implant at the time of surgery. A sleeper implant is a second implant that is placed (without its percutaneous abutment) at the same time as the primary implant, often during the first stage of a two-stage procedure. Young children who are undergoing BAHA implantation should have a sleeper placed, as they have a slightly higher risk of implant extrusion than the general population due to the thinness of their cortical bone. This allows for minimization of the time without a BAHA device should the primary implant extrude, as the secondary implant will already be osseointegrated and available for use pending a second-stage procedure.

Anesthesia

BAHA implantation is most commonly performed under local anesthesia with or without intravenous sedation. However, general anesthesia may be considered for those who may not tolerate local anesthesia with sedation, including pediatric patients, claustrophobic patients, and those who may have had previous bad experiences with surgery under intravenous sedation.

Surgical Preparation

Step 1: The patient is placed in a supine position with the head turned away from the operative side while supported by a headrest. The operating table is turned 180° away from the anesthesia team. The surgery can be performed with the surgeon either in a standing or sitting position.
Step 2: Preoperative antibiotics are administered.
Step 3: Identify and mark the planned location of BAHA implantation. The ideal location of the implant is posterosuperior to the ear canal, just above the level of the temporal line and in line with the top of the pinna. A 5.5 cm line drawn from the external auditory canal extending posterosuperiorly at an angle of 45° helps to identify the implant site (Fig. 16.2). The dummy sound processor template should be used to check the marked site to

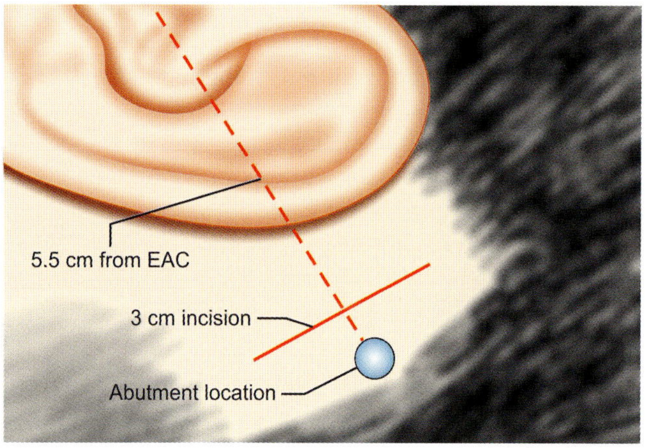

Fig. 16.2: Location of BAHA implantation. The BAHA implant should be placed ~5.5 cm posterosuperior to the external auditory canal. Shown here is the planned incision for the "linear incision" technique. The incision is ~3 cm in length and located anterior to the implant site.

ensure that the sound processor will not touch the auricle. For patients who often wear eyeglasses/sunglasses or hats, the dummy template should also be used to ensure the BAHA will not interfere with these and the location of implantation should be adjusted accordingly.
Step 4: Assessment of scalp thickness at implantation site. This should be done prior to injection of local anesthesia, as the injection will inflate the measured values. The scalp thickness can be estimated by palpation of the skin. Alternatively, it may be measured by placing a small-gauge hypodermic needle perpendicularly through the skin at the implant site until bone is reached, and determining the depth of needle insertion. The assessment of scalp thickness helps to determine (1) if the "linear incision" versus "punch" technique is more appropriate and (2) the length of the BAHA abutment that will need to be placed. A technique with minimal to no soft-tissue debulking, such as the "punch" technique, may be selected in patients with thinner scalps.

Surgical Technique—"Linear Incision" Technique

Step 1: Shave the hair in area around the planned implantation site.
Step 2: Mark the linear incision—A vertical line approximately 3 cm in length and located 1 cm anterior to and centered by the planned BAHA site should be drawn (Fig. 16.2).
Step 3: Inject local anesthesia—One percent lidocaine in 1:100,000 epinephrine is used at our institution. Additional local should be available on the field for use as needed.

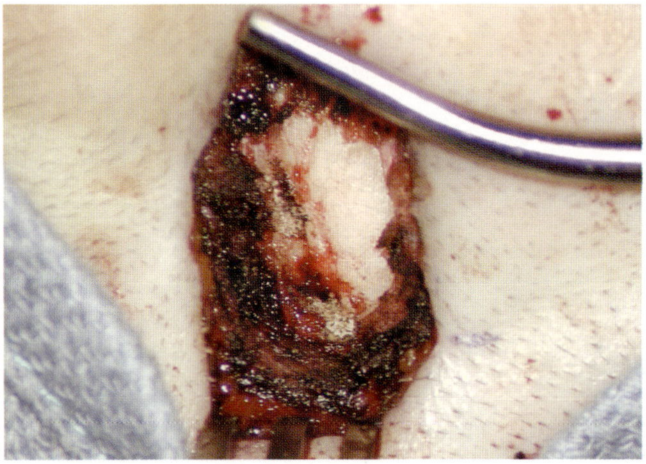

Fig. 16.3: Soft-tissue debulking. The soft tissue has been debulked circumferentially around the incision, with significant undermining of the skin in all directions.

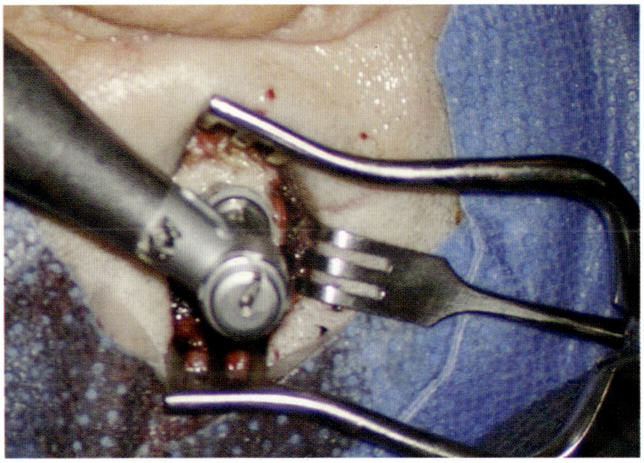

Fig. 16.5: Drilling. The BAHA drill is placed perpendicular to the bone and bone is removed under irrigation.

Step 4: Perform sterile prep and draping of the surgical site.

Step 5: Make incision—A #15 blade is used to make the incision through the skin and subcutaneous tissue.

Step 6: Debulk soft tissue (Fig. 16.3)—A #15 blade is used to separate the skin from the underlying soft tissue in a 360° fashion, extending several centimeters in each direction from the incision. A self-retaining retractor and skin hooks are used to provide countertraction and improve visibility. A pickup and a pair of scissors are then used to remove the soft tissue in a piecemeal fashion down to the level of the periosteum, with electrocautery used sparingly as needed for hemostasis. Special attention is paid to performing adequate debulking posterior and superior to the incision, as these are the most important areas.

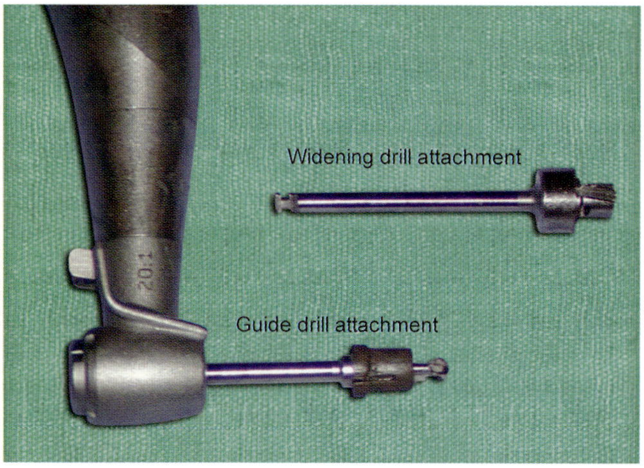

Fig. 16.4: BAHA drill. The drill for performing BAHA surgery has multiple attachments, including one for the guide drill, widening drill, and implant placement (not shown).

Step 7: Drill with guide drill—A 1 × 1 cm cruciate incision is made in the periosteum at the planned site of implantation. The periosteum is elevated off the underlying bone to allow the drill to rotate freely without catching the adjacent soft tissue. The guide drill with the 3 mm spacer is used at 2,000 rpm to drill a 3 mm deep hole at the implantation site (Fig. 16.4). The drilling should be performed perpendicular to the bone and under irrigation (Fig. 16.5). A blunt dissector should be used to palpate the depth of the hole for exposed dura or sigmoid sinus. If no exposure is palpated, the spacer is removed and drilling is continued to increase the depth to 4 mm. Occasionally, a CSF leak can occur if the dura is violated; if this occurs, placement of the implant into the drilled hole is typically sufficient to seal the leak. Alternatively, the hole can be sealed with bone wax or soft tissue and an alternative implant site can be chosen. Bleeding due to violation of the sigmoid sinus can be addressed in a similar manner as a CSF leak.

Step 8: Drill with the widening drill—The widening drill (3 or 4 mm, depending on the depth reached in Step 7) is used to widen the hole and create a countersink (Fig. 16.4). Drilling is performed at 2,000 rpm in line with the original hole and under irrigation. The depth of the countersink should be no more than 0.5 mm, just deep enough to be visible to the naked eye and often corresponding to a hard stop felt during drilling (Fig. 16.6). Over-countersinking may lead to implant instability.

Step 9: Placement of implant (Fig. 16.7)—For purposes of terminology, the titanium BAHA implant will be considered as having two components: (1) the fixture and (2) the abutment (Fig. 16.8). The fixture is the component that is threaded flush against the bone and will

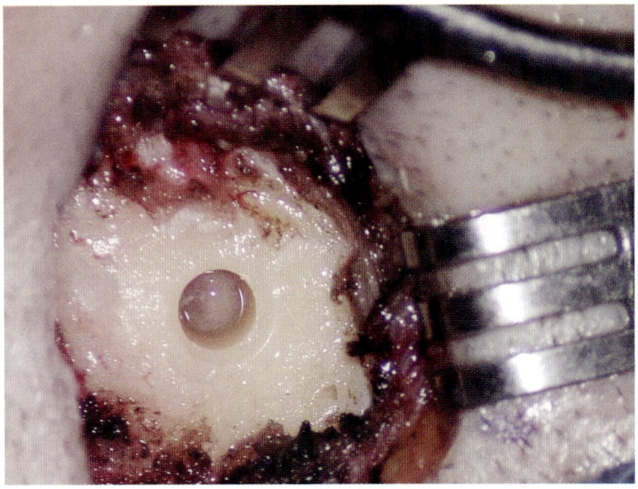

Fig. 16.6: Countersink. The widening drill has been used to create a countersink, which should be visible with the naked eye as a faint bony ring around the deeper primary hole when completed.

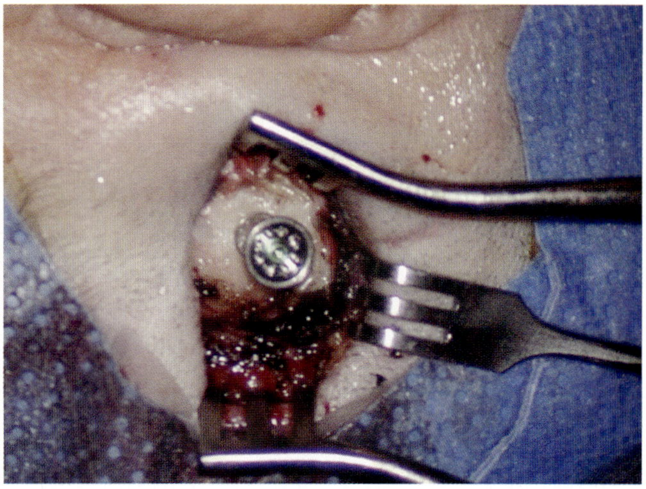

Fig. 16.7: Implantation. The BAHA implant after the fixture has been threaded into the bone, with the abutment protruding outward.

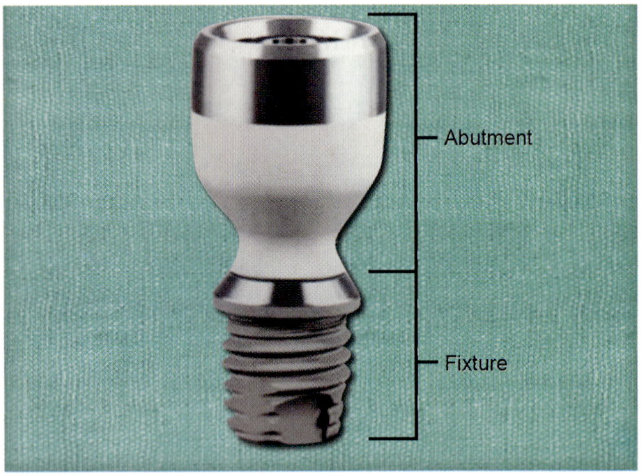

Fig. 16.8: The BAHA implant that is placed intraoperatively consists of two components: (1) the fixture and (2) the abutment. The fixture has two standard lengths (3 and 4 mm lengths) and is threaded into the bone. The abutment has multiple lengths and is chosen based on scalp thickness. Shown here is the titanium Cochlear Baha DermaLock implant, which is partially coated with white hydroxyapatite for potentially better integration with the dermis.
Courtesy: Cochlear Americas, © 2014 Cochlear Americas

osseointegrate. Either a 3 or 4 mm length fixture is available, with selection based on the depth of the drilled hole. The abutment is the component that extends outward from the bone. Multiple abutment lengths are available (ranging from 6 mm to 12 mm). Longer abutments are more appropriate for thicker scalps, though at our institution we almost exclusively use longer abutments in adult patients as this results in fewer postoperative complications (such as issues with skin overgrowth).

If the implantation is to occur in a single stage, as is most commonly done in adults, an implant with the appropriate BAHA fixture and abutment lengths is selected. The abutment inserter (a special attachment placed on the drill) is used to pick up the implant at the abutment end. Care is taken to avoid touching the titanium fixture, as foreign body contamination may lead to poorer osseointegration. The drill is set to a torque of 20–40 Ncm, with a lower torque used for soft or compromised bone. The implant is placed perpendicular to the bone in alignment with the previously drilled hole using the insertion device. If alignment is incorrect, the drill may be placed in reverse to loosen the implant and allow for realignment. Irrigation is not performed until after the first threads of the implant are inserted into the bone, to prevent the irrigation solution from being compressed into the marrow spaces of the bone. The drill will stop automatically and beep when the preset torque is achieved. If the implant still appears somewhat loose, it can be tightened manually with the multi-wrench rotated in a clockwise manner. If this is insufficient, an alternative implant site can be chosen, and placement of the implant is performed at a lower torque setting.

If the implantation is to occur in two stages, for the first stage, an implant consisting of only the BAHA fixture is placed. The implant inserter is used to place the fixture into the bone, after which a cover screw is placed over the fixture to protect it from tissue overgrowth. For young children, a second sleeper fixture is also placed about 1 cm posterior-superior to the primary implant. In the second stage (which occurs 6 months later), the cover

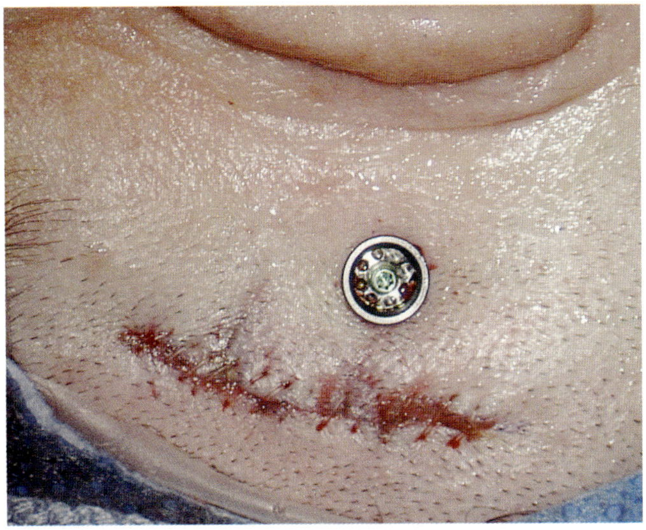

Fig. 16.9: Closure. A skin punch has created a separate hole through the skin for the abutment. Often, the incision is placed anterior to the abutment, though in this case, it is located posteriorly.

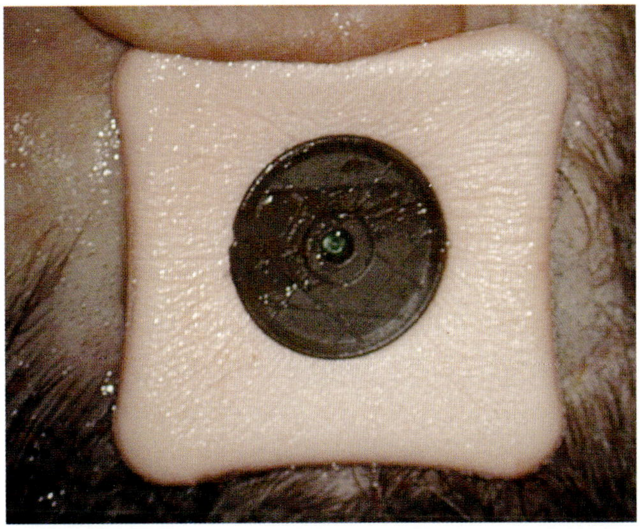

Fig. 16.10: Dressing. The dark healing cap has been snapped in place over the Allevyn dressing and onto the abutment. It is left in place for at least 1 week after surgery.

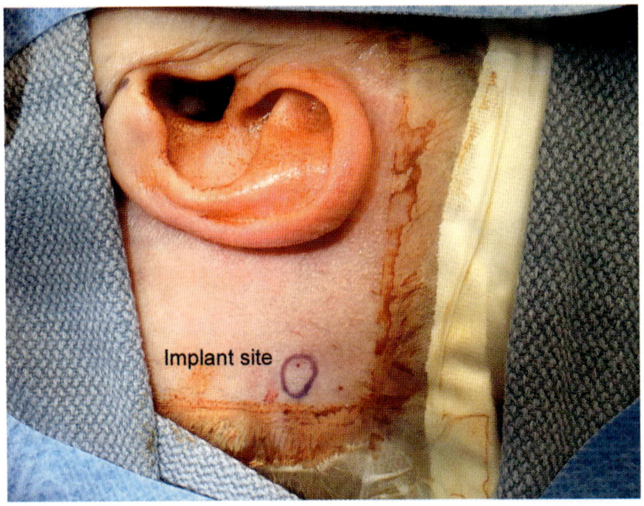

Fig. 16.11: BAHA implant site. The planned location for the BAHA implant is marked posterosuperior to the external auditory canal, at the level of the top of the pinna. No additional incision is needed for the "punch" technique.

screw is then removed and the percutaneous abutment is connected to the fixture. Additionally, when a two-stage procedure is planned, significant soft-tissue debulking (as described in Step 6) is typically deferred in stage 1 and performed during stage 2, after osseointegration of the implant has occurred.

Step 10: Closure—A 4 mm biopsy punch is used to create a hole in the skin for the abutment to fit through. This is typically located about 1 cm anterior or posterior to the incision (Fig. 16.9). A small relaxing incision can be made on each side of the punch defect if needed to allow the abutment to be placed through the skin. The incision is then closed in a multilayer fashion, with vicryl suture for the deeper layer and fast-absorbing gut for the skin.

Step 11: Dressing—A nonadhesive hydrocellular polyurethane dressing (Allevyn) is placed over the skin and around the abutment (Fig. 16.10). The healing cap is then snapped over the dressing onto the abutment to provide local pressure and prevent hematoma formation. A mastoid dressing is then placed over the BAHA site.

Surgical Technique—"Punch" Technique

Step 1: Shave the hair in area around the planned implantation site.

Step 2: Confirm the implantation site (Fig. 16.11).

Step 3: Inject local anesthesia. One percent lidocaine in 1:100,000 epinephrine is used at our institution. Additional local should be available on the field for use as needed.

Step 4: Perform sterile prep and draping of the surgical site.

Step 5: Perform punch. Apply a 5 mm biopsy punch through the skin, soft tissue, and down to the periosteum (Fig. 16.12). Remove the soft tissue from the skin punch. A small incision can be made with a #15 blade in either direction from the punch if additional visualization is needed.

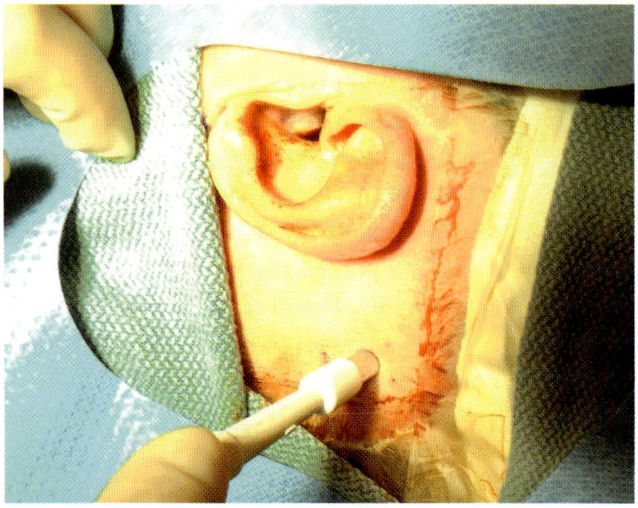

Fig. 16.12: Perform punch. A 5 mm biopsy is used to remove the skin and soft tissue at the BAHA implantation site.

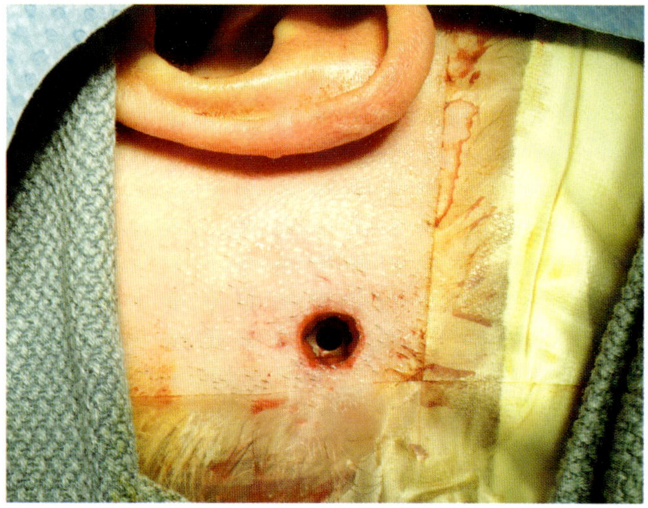

Fig. 16.13: Drilling. The guide drill and widening drill have been used to prepare the bone for implantation.

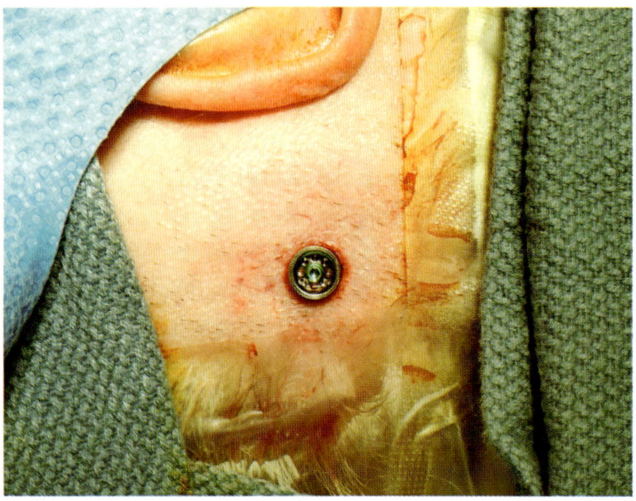

Fig. 16.14: Implantation. The BAHA implant has been placed through the punch site. In contrast to the "linear incision" technique, there is no additional incision to be closed at the end of the case.

Step 6: Note that unlike with the "linear incision" technique, no undermining and debulking of the soft tissue is necessary.

Steps 7–9: Perform drilling of guide hole, creation of countersink, and placement of BAHA implant in same manner as described with "linear incision" technique (Figs. 16.13 and 16.14).

Step 10: Closure—Suturing is typically not necessary, though can be used if incisions of a significant size were created in Step 5 to help with visualization through the biopsy punch hole.

Step 11: Dressing—Place dressing in same manner as described in Step 11 of the "linear incision" technique.

POSTOPERATIVE CARE

BAHA surgery is performed on an outpatient basis. The mastoid dressing is removed on postoperative day 1 and the patient is asked to keep the healing cap on the abutment. At the 1-week postoperative visit, if the soft tissue around the abutment is well seated, the healing cap is removed. If there is any concern that the tissue may overgrow the implant, the dressing is removed but the patient is asked to continue to wear the healing cap. Patients are instructed to use mild soap, water, and a soft brush to keep the implant site clean.

The hookup of the sound processor to the BAHA implant traditionally occurs 3 months after surgery following a single-stage procedure. However, a number of studies have suggested that earlier loading of the BAHA implant can be performed without compromising implant stability, as early as 4–6 weeks after surgery.[7,8] In contrast, in children or patients with compromised bone, at least 6 months is allowed for osseointegration of the implant before performing hookup.

COMPLICATIONS

The most common postoperative complication is local inflammation or infection of the tissue surrounding the abutment. Patients are instructed on meticulous wound care, asked to apply antibiotic ointment to the site, and if infection is suspected, given a course of oral antibiotics. If infection persists, a culture is taken and the abutment may be removed. A new abutment is placed several weeks later after the skin has healed and the infection resolved.

Some patients may also experience skin overgrowth around the abutment, preventing the sound processor from seating firmly on the abutment. This is addressed with steroid ointment and/or injections applied locally. If this continues to be an issue, revision surgery may be performed with excision of the overgrown skin and replacement of the abutment with a longer one.

Rarely, a BAHA implant may extrude due to failure of osseointegration. The risk of implant extrusion can be minimized by avoiding improper handling of the titanium fixture intraoperatively, using copious irrigation during drilling and implantation, using an appropriate torque setting during implantation, avoiding trauma to the abutment once placed, and if indicated, electing to perform the procedure in two stages and waiting longer for BAHA hookup. One sign of a loose implant is pain when touching the implant. Should implant extrusion occur, an alternative site of implantation should be chosen at least 1 cm away from the original site with the appropriate precautions as described above.

RECENT DEVELOPMENTS IN BAHA SURGERY

Over time, the trend in BAHA surgery has been toward less invasive surgery, with the thought that this may lead to fewer postoperative wound care issues.[9-12] Thus, the "punch" technique, which removes a volume of soft tissue similar to that of the implant itself, has been gaining in popularity. However, the punch technique is difficult to perform in patients with thicker scalps, where visualization in the deep hole that is created is poor and mobility of the drill is limited. As a compromise toward less invasive surgery, the "linear incision" technique can be utilized but performed without soft-tissue debulking. BAHA manufacturers have trended toward designing abutments of longer lengths to allow patients with thicker and thicker scalps to have their surgery performed with limited to no debulking.

Manufacturers have also been exploring different materials beyond titanium to see if this may decrease postoperative healing complications. The Cochlear Baha series now has a DermaLock Abutment in which the titanium surface that is expected to contact the soft tissue is coated in hydroxyapatite. It is theorized that this may result in less reactivity and better integration between the dermis and abutment, though outcomes remain to be determined.

Finally, there has been growing interest in BAHA devices that do not involve the placement of a percutaneous abutment, but rather where the implanted portion of the device is completely underneath the skin. These devices utilize magnets to connect the external sound processor to the internal implant. Sophono (Boulder, Colorado) received FDA clearance in June, 2011 for its abutment-free Alpha Bone Conduction Hearing System, and the implant has been FDA cleared as MRI safe (up to 3 Tesla). Recently, Cochlear received FDA clearance in December, 2013 for its abutment-free Baha Attract system. These abutment-free devices are not able to deliver the same level of hearing amplification as those with abutments (due to the damping effect of the skin and soft tissue), but have improved cosmesis and potentially, fewer soft-tissue complications.

REFERENCES

1. McDermott AL, Williams J, Kuo MJ, et al. The role of bone anchored hearing aids in children with Down syndrome. Int J Pediatr Otorhinolaryngol. 2008;72:751-7.
2. Sheehan PZ, Hans PS. UK and Ireland experience of bone anchored hearing aids (BAHA) in individuals with Down syndrome. Int J Pediatr Otorhinolaryngol. 2006;70:981-6.
3. Jensen DR, Grames LM, Lieu JE. Effects of aural atresia on speech development and learning: retrospective analysis from a multidisciplinary craniofacial clinic. JAMA Otolaryngol Head Neck Surg. 2013. [Epub ahead of print].
4. Kesser BW, Krook K, Gray LC. Impact of unilateral conductive hearing loss due to aural atresia on academic performance in children. Laryngoscope. 2013;123:2270-5.
5. Dun CA, de Wolf MJ, Mylanus EA, et al. Bilateral bone-anchored hearing aid application in children: the Nijmegen experience from 1996 to 2008. Otol Neurotol. 2010;31:615-23.
6. Mudry A. Bone-anchored hearing aids (BAHA): skin healing process for skin flap technique versus linear incision technique in the first three months after the implantation. Rev Laryngol Otol Rhinol (Bord). 2009;130:281-4.
7. McLarnon CM, Johnson I, Davison T, et al. Evidence for early loading of osseointegrated implants for bone conduction at 4 weeks. Otol Neurotol. 2012;33:1578-82.
8. Wazen JJ, Gupta R, Ghossaini S, et al. Osseointegration timing for Baha system loading. Laryngoscope. 2007;117:794-6.
9. Goldman RA, Georgolios A, Shaia WT. The punch method for bone-anchored hearing aid placement. Otolaryngol Head Neck Surg. 2013;148:878-80.
10. Hultcrantz M. Outcome of the bone-anchored hearing aid procedure without skin thinning: a prospective clinical trial. Otol Neurotol. 2011;32:1134-9.
11. Husseman J, Szudek J, Monksfield P, et al. Simplified bone-anchored hearing aid insertion using a linear incision without soft tissue reduction. J Laryngol Otol. 2013;127 (Suppl 2): S33-8.
12. Wilkinson EP, Luxford WM, Slattery WH, 3rd et al. Single vertical incision for Baha implant surgery: preliminary results. Otolaryngol Head Neck Surg. 2009;140:573-8.

CHAPTER

17

Stereotactic Radiosurgery for Vestibular Schwannomas

Eric L Slattery, Ann Maitz, Peter Y Chen, Dennis I Bojrab

INTRODUCTION

Stereotactic radiosurgery is an option in the management of many benign cranial base tumors including vestibular schwannomas (acoustic neuromas) and paragangliomas (glomus tumors). The literature, however, consists of many retrospective studies with their inherent biases. The same is true of the surgical and observational protocols. Long-term prospective outcome studies with blinded independent results are needed as a strong supplement on which to base clinical treatment. This chapter discusses and describes stereotactic radiosurgery in general and the procedure of one stereotactic radiosurgery technology, Gamma Knife, specifically. A brief discussion of the principles and outcomes of stereotactic radiosurgery is also presented, although the reader is directed to Hahn and Bojrab as a recent work focusing on principles and outcomes.[1]

HISTORY

Lars Leksell first imagined the concept of stereotactic radiosurgery with multiple radiation sources directed at a target in the 1950s. This technology was later termed Gamma Knife radiosurgery. Gamma Knife's first clinical usage occurred in 1967, treating a patient with a craniopharyngioma. Leksell quickly saw its utility with vestibular schwannomas, given the benign nature of the disease and the high morbidity associated with surgery at the time. The first FDA-approved clinical Gamma Knife unit in the United States was installed at the University of Pittsburgh in 1987. Since then the modality has become widespread and several upgrades to the technology have occurred.

Other forms of stereotactic radiosurgery have evolved. Elekta's Gamma Knife utilizes well-collimated beams of radiation from 201 cobalt-60 sources that are directed through ports in an annular array, allowing the beams to converge and deliver a much higher dose to the target than to the surrounding structures. The precise delivery of the beam is increased by direct fixation of a head frame attached with surgical pins to the cranium of the patient. Linear accelerators (LINAC)-based systems, such as Trilogy and Accuray's CyberKnife, both utilize high-energy X-rays. Instead of multiple sources aimed at a centrally designated target, the LINAC-based systems rotate the treatment beam of the unit around the target in a variable number of rotational arcs. Currently fixed-head frame systems are available for some of these LINAC-based systems (e.g. the Trilogy system), which improve accuracy. Proton radiation has also been used. Protons are heavily charged particles that cause damage directly. They are positively charged and have a much higher mass than electrons. When a proton beam strikes the target, it goes to its maximum depth and delivers almost all of its energy, which results in a rapid drop off of its energy level and limits tissue damage past the target of interest. Protons make use of the Bragg-Gray peak where the entry route into the tumor receives little radiation and the deposition of the energy is at the "peak". Both Gamma Knife and LINAC-based technologies are found in many centers throughout the United States, while proton radiation, at the writing of this chapter, is found at only a few centers. Figure 17.1 shows some of the current available technologies.

PRINCIPLES OF STEREOTACTIC RADIOSURGERY

Radiation damage occurs when radiation exerts its effects on the biologic process of cell division and causes death. Traditionally, radiation has been delivered using high-energy photon beams and is delivered in multiple sessions. This technique is known as external beam radiation. Radiation causes excitation of electrons in the molecules of cells, leading to increased free radical production resulting in damage to DNA. Cells with a higher mitotic index are preferentially damaged by radiation. DNA damage prevents entry into the cell cycle and can lead to

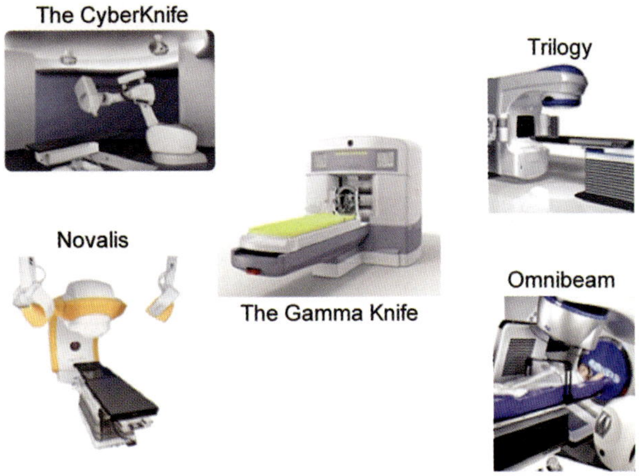

Fig. 17.1: Various forms of stereotactic radiotherapy.

programmed cell death called apoptosis. Radiation damage to the phospholipids of the cell membrane also occurs. In a LINAC system, X-rays arise from an interaction between an electron and the target. In the Gamma Knife system, gamma rays are produced when the contents of the nucleus of an atom returns to its energy state from an excited level and is called gamma decay.

Stereotactic radiosurgery relies on multiple routes of radiation that intersect at a target, creating an additive effect to the target with low radiation to the surrounding tissue. Unlike conventional radiotherapy, which consists of photon beam radiation that is typically delivered over multiple sessions, stereotactic radiosurgery delivers a large dose of radiation in a single setting (Gamma Knife or LINAC-based systems). LINAC-based systems can also deliver a fractionated regimen, given over days or weeks and takes advantage of radiobiologic principles to reduce late toxicity while maintaining tumor control. Fractionation theoretically reduces the postirradiation complications to the surrounding cranial nerves. Fractionation is advantageous in rapidly dividing tumor cells because of multiple hits at various cells in division. Stereotactic radiosurgery usually involves a high dose of radiation delivered in one fraction from a specially equipped linear accelerator or a specialized unit using multiple cobalt-60 sources.

The source of radiation varies in stereotactic modalities. In the Gamma Knife radiosurgery system, the radiation source is from 201 fixed cobalt-60 sources that emit photons. The use of different size collimators (4, 8, 14, or 18 mm tungsten collimators with circle apertures are used to create varied focal volumes) and blocking conforms the radiation to the shape of the tumor. In LINAC-based systems, the source of radiation is high-energy photons, which is similar to external beam techniques. The difference is that conformal dosing is achieved by moving the treatment gantry and collimating leaves. In both systems, there are radiation beams that intersect at the target. These two systems can target within the millimeter to submillimeter range. One of the distinct advantages of stereotactic radiosurgery in skull base tumors over stereotactic radiotherapy is the use of the stereotactic frame. This is applied to the outer table of the skull allowing the localization in three dimensions to be fixed from the imaging segment of the procedure through the treatment. As with all treatments that rely on stereotaxy for localization, the procedure is dependent on imaging, which can introduce error. Another source of imprecision can include the mechanical inaccuracy of the treatment delivery unit, which can compound the total procedural inaccuracy. This mechanical accuracy is assessed at the time of acceptance testing, commissioning and at annual calibration thereafter. Some units are required to be tested more frequently by law, and usually the medical physics team will test the treatment delivery units monthly.

Current radiation doses are lower than what were previously used. Typically doses for Gamma Knife radiosurgery are prescribed at the 50% isodose line, meaning that tumors within this planned area will obtain 50% or greater of the prescribed dose. Usually, the 50% isodose line is the marginal dose that is thought to exert the optimal biologic effect on the tumor. The radiation dose rapidly falls off beyond the 50% isodose line, minimizing radiation effect to the normal or unaffected areas. Thirty years ago, 16–20 Gy was routinely used at the 50% isodose line for stereotactic radiosurgery for vestibular schwannomas. Complications including hearing loss and facial weakness were seen at these doses, and thus marginal doses were lowered to approximately 12.5 Gy at the 50% isodose line at most centers, with very low complication rates.

INDICATIONS

Current indications for stereotactic radiosurgery of the lateral skull base include vestibular schwannomas, skull base paragangliomas, and meningiomas. This chapter focuses on vestibular schwannoma treatment, as it is the most common application of stereotactic radiosurgery for the lateral skull base. Tumors considered for stereotactic radiosurgery are generally less than 3 cm in any dimension. In general, tumors with smaller volumes are better treated with stereotactic radiation. The relationship to adjacent structures to a tumor should be

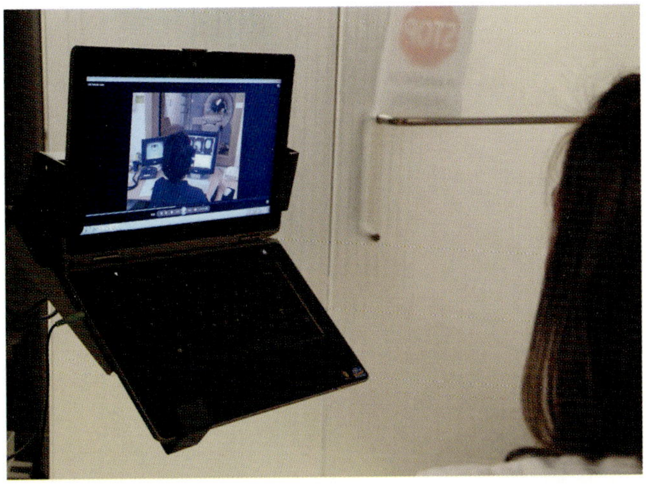

Fig. 17.2: Informational video regarding the procedure watched by the patient prior to treatment.

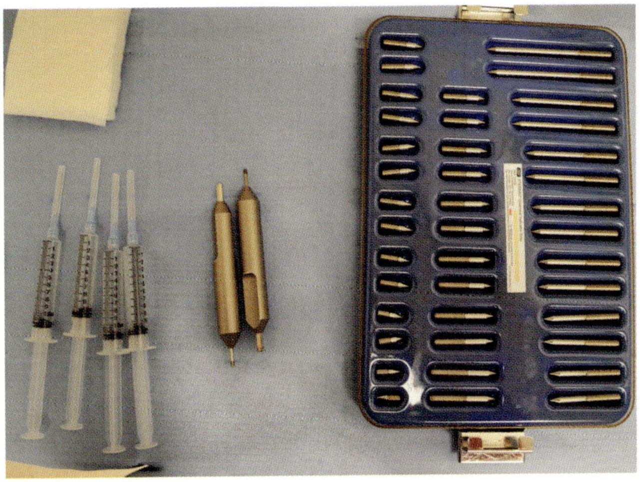

Fig. 17.3: Tray for head frame placement.

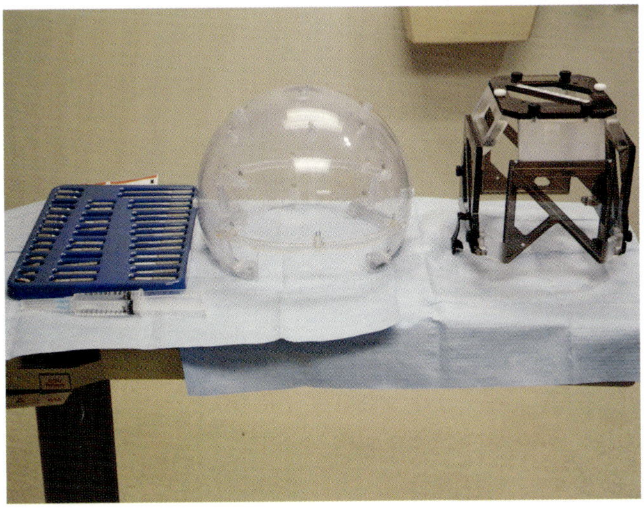

Fig. 17.4: Tray and head frames.

assessed. Stereotactic radiation to tumors that are compressing the brain or brainstem should be avoided due to potential effects of radiation on the brainstem and resultant swelling of the tumor causing potential brainstem compression after treatment. Elderly patients and those with medical comorbidities that preclude surgery are typical candidates for stereotactic radiosurgery. Stereotactic radiosurgery can be used as primary therapy, or following subtotal microsurgical resection. Stereotactic radiation has become a potent therapy in dealing with the multiple intracranial tumors in neurofibromatosis II (NF2). There is some concern for potentially higher malignant transformation following radiation in NF2, but the literature remains controversial at this time.[2] Consideration for tumor edema, which commonly happens after stereotactic radiation, should be accounted for prior to treatment. Furthermore, the literature suggests that although surgery following stereotactic radiotherapy is an option, the surgery has been reported to be more difficult.

PROCEDURE FOR GAMMA KNIFE STEREOTACTIC RADIOSURGERY

Comparable outcomes in tumor control have been reported for the various stereotactic radiosurgery techniques. Treatment procedures for individual technologies vary. Here, we outline the procedure for the Elekta Gamma Knife 4C specifically. This model utilizes a head frame that must be attached to the patient's head.

Placement of the Head Frame

The procedure is performed as an outpatient procedure. Prior to the placement of the head frame and treatment, the patient watches an instructional video detailing the experience (Fig. 17.2) and is given topical anesthetic cream to put on their forehead to lessen the pain of the local anesthetic injections. The patient is given a mild sedative prior to placement of the head frame.

Step 1: The setup tray and frames needed are placed in the room (Figs. 17.3 and 17.4).

Step 2: The areas where local anesthetic is to be injected is cleaned with Betadine (Fig. 17.5).

Step 3: The frame is initially placed on the head prior to pin placement. The authors' preferred technique is to place an earplug, which allows alignment of the frame (Fig. 17.6). An alternative method is to place the frame via a fiducial box.

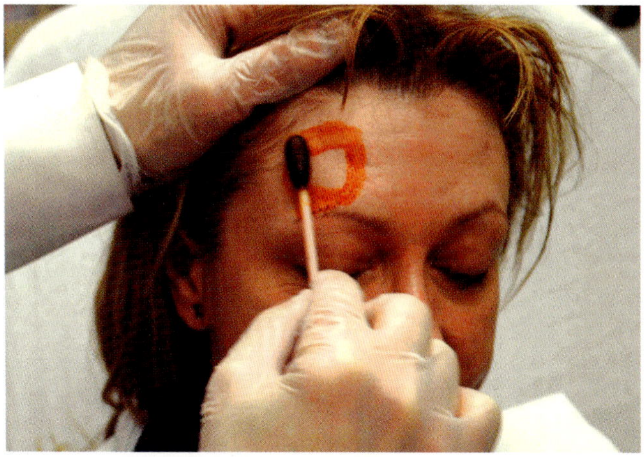

Fig. 17.5: Applying Betadine to planned pin sites.

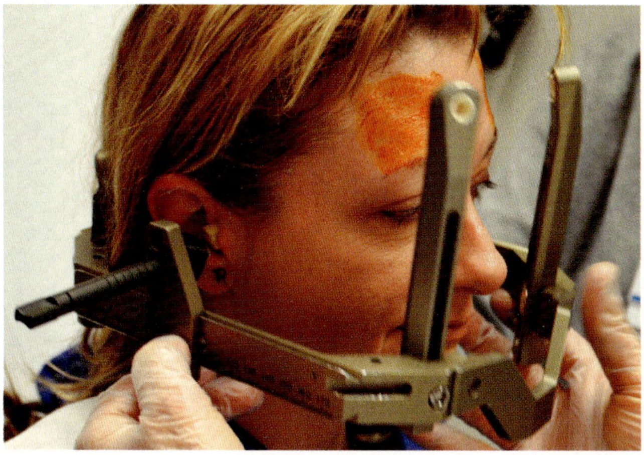

Fig. 17.6: Initial approximation of head frame.

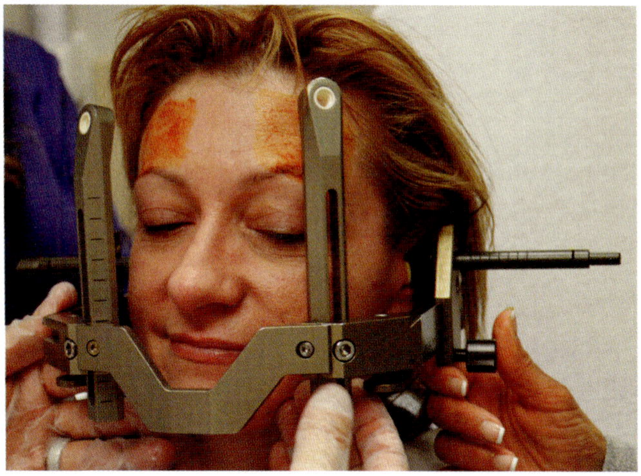

Fig. 17.7: Adjustment of anterior vertical bars.

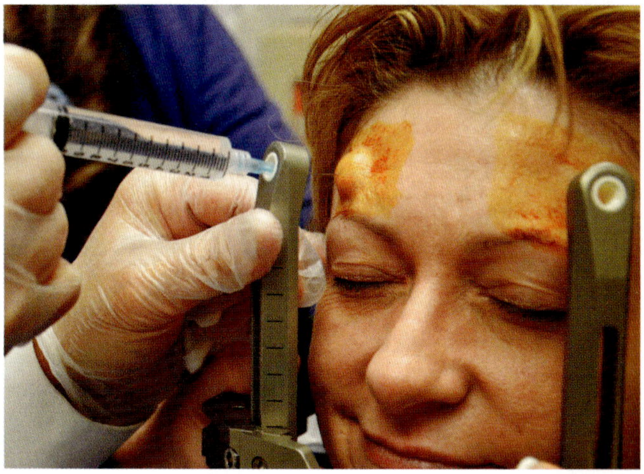

Fig. 17.8: Injection of local anesthetic.

Step 4: The anterior posts of the frame are adjusted for pin placement over the forehead above the orbital ridge (Fig. 17.7).
Step 5: Local anesthetic is injected where pins of the frame will enter (Fig. 17.8). Use of the local anesthetic needle allows estimation of pin size as well.
Step 6: The pins are placed in all four quadrants, by tightening of the diagonal pins (Fig. 17.9).
Step 7: The plastic mock collimating helmet, which allows for measurements is attached to the head frame (Fig. 17.10).
Step 8: Measurements of the distance from the skull to the plastic mock collimating helmet are taken and recorded (Fig. 17.11).
Step 9: The height of the anterior and posterior posts is also recorded (Fig. 17.12).
Step 10: The screw distance of each four screws extending outward from the post is measured (Fig. 17.13). Ideally the screws should not extend from the posts >5 mm, which minimizes collisions.
Step 11: In order to minimize accidental inverting of images and wrong-sided delivery of therapy, a vitamin E capsule is attached to the interior side of the frame base ring, which is visible on imaging indicating the correct side (Fig. 17.14).
Step 12: MRI (Fig. 17.15) and CT (Fig. 17.16) scans are performed with the fiducial box in place.

Treatment Planning and Radiation Delivery

The treatment team usually consists of a radiation oncologist, a neurosurgeon and/or neurotologist, and a medical physicist. The images obtained after placement of the frame are used.

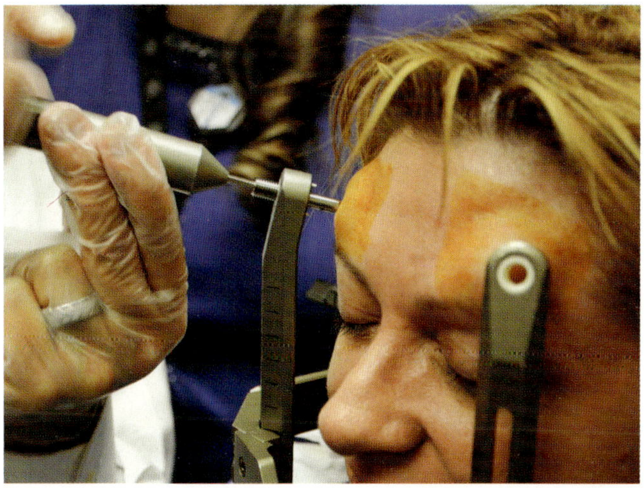

Fig. 17.9: Pin placement.

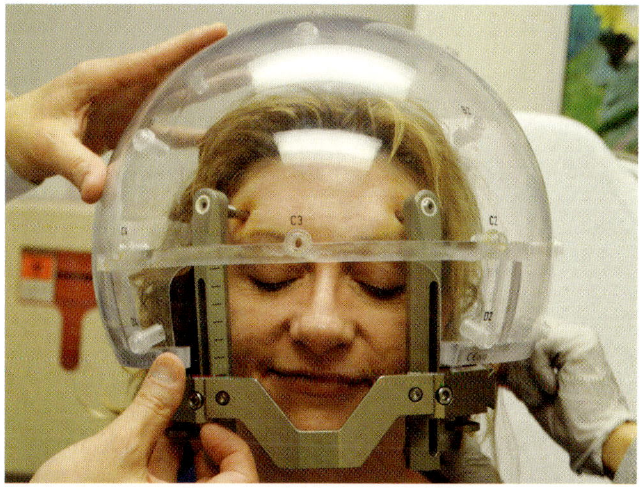

Fig. 17.10: Placement of plastic mock helmet for measuring.

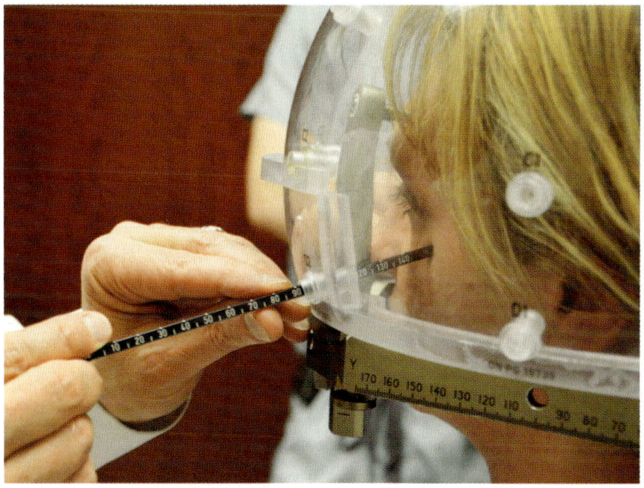

Fig. 17.11: Measurement of skull distance.

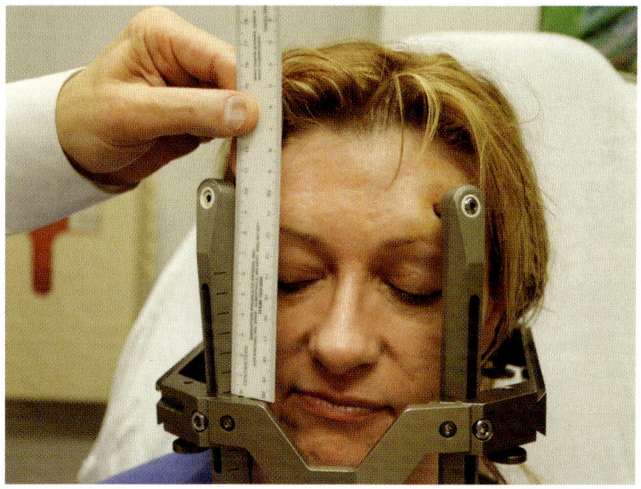

Fig. 17.12: Measurement of the height of the anterior vertical bar.

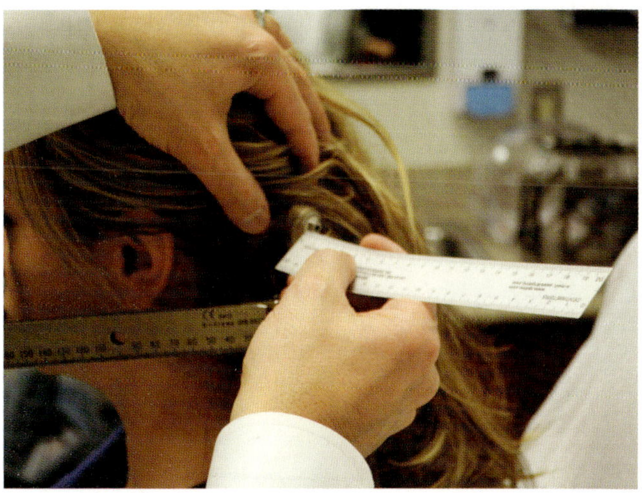

Fig. 17.13: Measurement of screw distance outside of frame.

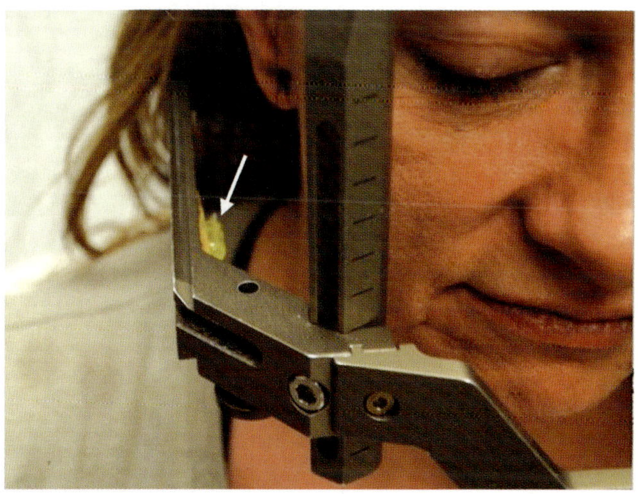

Fig. 17.14: Placement of vitamin E capsule (arrow) to denote sidedness on imaging.

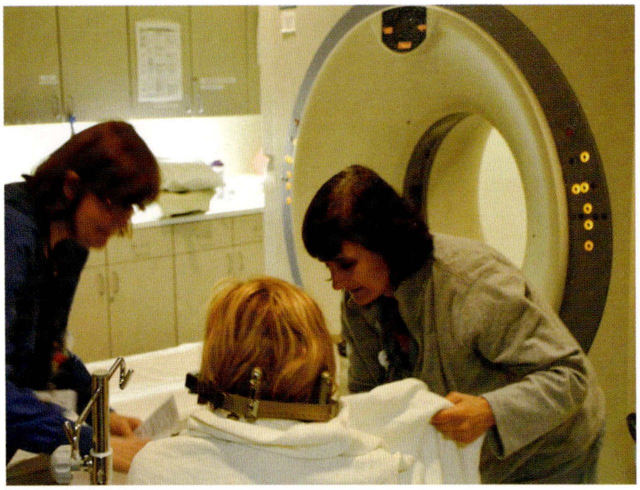

Fig. 17.15: MRI scanning.

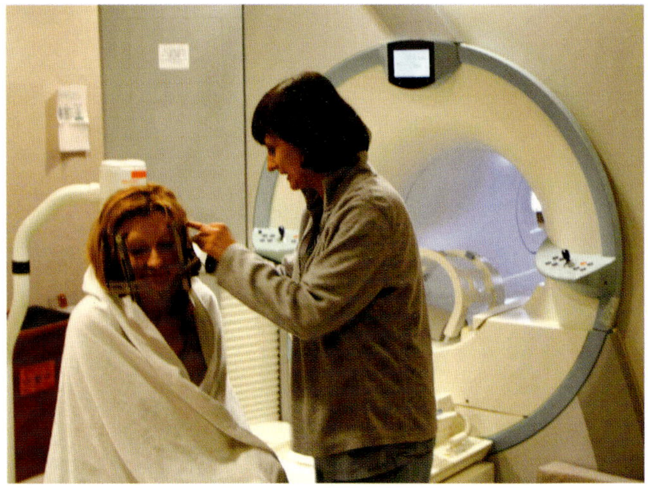

Fig. 17.16: CT scanning.

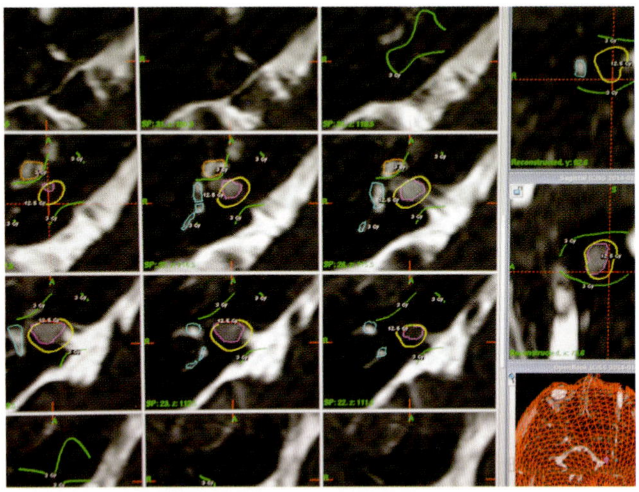

Fig. 17.17: Treatment planning and delineation of structures. Tumor is outlined (pink). Cochlea (orange) and labyrinth (blue) are also outlined. Dosing plan shown with 50% isodose line (yellow) and 3 Gy line (green). Exposure of <3 Gy to the inner ear is planned.

Step 1: Usually, the tumor is first outlined on MRI scans. For most tumors, a T1 1-mm slice thickness scan through the head in addition to a T2 sequence is performed. If the patient is postsurgery wherein fat has been placed, an additional fat-suppression sequence should be performed. A CT is also performed for several reasons: (1) checking the distortion in the MRI sequences, (2) using the skull outline in the treatment planning program for a more accurate calculation, and (3) outlining the cochlea and labyrinth. Likewise important structures such as major blood vessels, brain, and inner ear organs are also outlined. For a typical vestibular schwannoma case, this involves outlining the tumor, brainstem, cochlea, and vestibule (Fig. 17.17). Perception of what is tumor and what is normal adjacent tissue can sometimes be difficult. This is especially in the cases following prior surgery.

Step 2: Only then can the 50% isodose lines be effectively and safely placed. Fewer complications are expected when the marginal dose conforms to the tumor's edge. Radiation tolerance for the acoustic nerve, cochlea, and vestibular end organs are currently being investigated, but in general, less radiation exposure to these structures, if possible, is better.

Step 3: For the Gamma Knife system, the Leksell Planning System (GammaPlan) is used. The treatment plan consists of discrete shots, or isocenters. These shots are planned within the tumor outline previously drawn. Collimator size dictates the spread of the radiation. Tools within the Leksell GammaPlan program allow for efficient evaluation of a given plan. Fine tuning of the plan that builds from the original plan is performed if needed. This may include the occlusion (plugging) of some of the 201 collimators that decreases a dose to a certain area if needed (Fig. 17.18). The GammaPlan program then groups shots in the most efficient manner for radiation delivery, as changes in collimator size necessitate changing the collimator helmet.

Step 4: The treatment runs are then delivered to the patient (Fig. 17.19). While receiving the radiation, the patient is allowed to communicate to the team with a speaker system (Fig. 17.20).

Post-Treatment Care

Few acute problems arise with stereotactic radiosurgery. In larger tumors, signs and symptoms of hydrocephalus and edema, which rarely occur, should be reviewed with

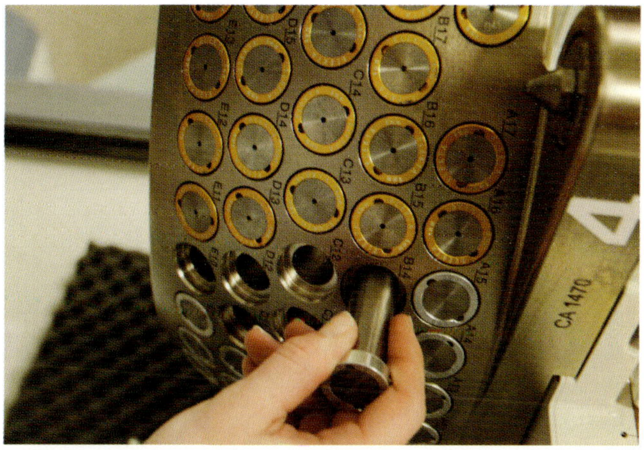

Fig. 17.18: Plugging of collimeters based on treatment plan.

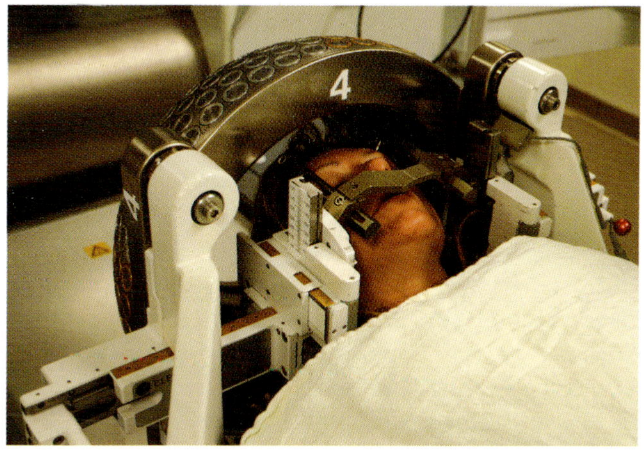

Fig. 17.19: Patient in helmet immediately prior to treatment.

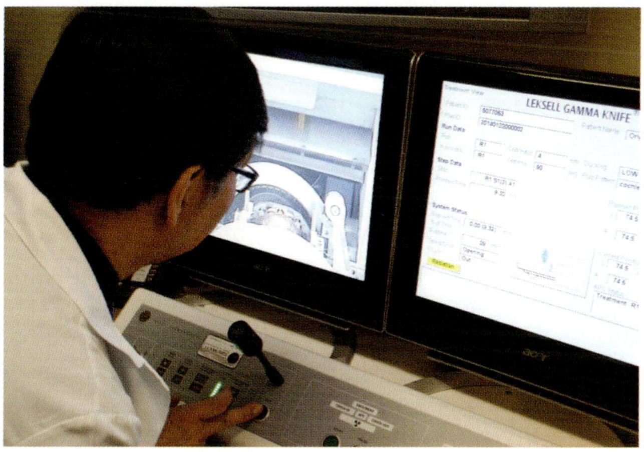

Fig. 17.20: Control station that allows communication and monitoring of the patient during treatment.

the patient. Usually, the patient is discharged from the treatment facility the same day and is treated with a short burst of steroids. In general, the patients are then followed with periodic MRI scans (6 months and then yearly intervals) to monitor the tumor. Audiograms and electronystagmography testing are routinely performed. It is not uncommon to find the tumor to increase in size during the first 6 months following treatment. It should be noted that this initial increase in size does not denote failure of tumor control in most cases. Four types of tumor change have been identified within the first couple of years: (1) tumor growth, (2) tumor stability, (3) tumor regression, and (4) tumor central necrosis.[3,4]

Outcomes

Gamma Knife

Radiosurgery has evolved rapidly over the last 30 years. The first large report on vestibular schwannomas was in 1993 by Norén using Gamma Knife technology.[5] An average marginal dose of 19.75 Gy was used. In unilateral tumor cases, 55% regressed, 33% were unchanged, and 12% continued to grow temporarily; the 1-year control rate was reported to be 94%. High facial nerve palsy (15%) and low hearing preservation (33%) were reported with this treatment plan.

In 1999, Miller et al. reported prospectively on 82 patients and found that marginal doses above 18 Gy were associated with facial nerve palsy.[6] Similarly, Flickinger noted high rates of facial nerve palsy with patients treated above 16 Gy, while those treated with 14 Gy or less had 0% weakness yet showed adequate tumor control. These, along with other studies, have guided the lower marginal doses seen today.

More recent data using lower marginal dosing have become available over the last decade, and outcomes are very favorable to date. Two large studies include Flickinger et al. (N = 190) and Lunsford et al. (N = 829) both from the University of Pittsburgh.[7,8] Flickinger et al. reported a 97% control rate at 5 years, while Lunsford et al. maintained a 97% control rate at mean of 10 years. Although the definition of control rates varies in studies, many smaller studies support these high (>95%) control rates. However, unlike the earlier studies, facial nerve palsy (<5%) was dramatically lowered with the lower marginal doses. It should be noted that "control" has not meant that the tumor is not growing, but instead, the patient is living without significant complications with their tumor. This definition has varied at different centers.

Hearing preservation rates are currently unreliable. Early studies using lower marginal doses had high rates of hearing preservation. Flickinger et al. reported hearing levels as stable (defined as testable hearing on the

Robertson-Gardner scale) in 73% of patients at a mean follow-up of 5 years.[9] It should be noted that "stable hearing" levels are ambiguous as some patients may not have serviceable hearing at the time of treatment, but their hearing remained "stable." Hearing improved in 7% of patients. Hasegawa et al. showed a 68% hearing preservation rate in those receiving <13 Gy as a marginal dose versus 13% in those receiving 13 Gy as the marginal dose at 7.8 years. In a later paper by Hasegawa et al., hearing preservation at 8 years was 34%, decreased from 55% at 3 years.[10] Similarly, Carlson et al. showed that serviceable hearing went from 80% at 1-year post-treatment to 23% at 10 years.[11] The marginal dose was between 12 Gy and 13 Gy. A systematic review of 4,234 patients demonstrated 51% of patients with serviceable hearing at a mean follow-up of 44 months.[12] Doses <3 Gy to the cochlea have been shown to have higher hearing preservation rates.[13]

OTHER FORMS OF STEREOTACTIC RADIOTHERAPY

Other forms of stereotactic radiotherapy have been used to treat lateral skull base tumors. These include LINAC-based technology. As these systems have evolved from standard radiation therapy regimens, a variety of protocols exist. In general, there are fewer studies reported with LINAC-based systems than studies with the Gamma Knife technology. Multiple studies have shown that 20-25 Gy given at weekly fractions of 3–5 Gy have >90% tumor control. Most studies have follow-up of 5 years or less.

CyberKnife and Trilogy are the LINAC-based technologies whose uses are becoming more widespread for the treatment of skull base tumors. A robotic arm is used to deliver the LINAC radiation. Chang et al. reported on 61 patients followed for 28 months with a margin dose of 18–21 Gy over 3 fractions, noting only a 2% progression rate.[14] Transient facial nerve palsy occurred in only two patients. Serviceable hearing was found in 74% of patients. Morimoto et al. reported on 26 patients receiving hypofractionated treatment with a marginal dose of 21 Gy on average.[15] The 7-year progression-free rate was 95%. In three patients, hydrocephalus occurred, and two patients had facial nerve palsies. Vivas et al. reported that 83% of patients had stable tumors (0–2 mm growth) over 40 months.[16] Serviceable hearing (based on the Gardner-Robinson scale) was preserved in 53% of patients who had serviceable hearing prior to treatment.

Stereotactic Radiation for Paragangliomas

Stereotactic radiation can also be used for paragangliomas of the head and neck. External beam radiation has been used in the past. Although the tumors cells themselves are thought to be radioresistant, tumor control rates of >70% have been reported with external beam radiation and is thought to be due to radiation effects to the vasculature of the tumor.[17,18] More recently, stereotactic radiosurgery has been applied to paragangliomas and tumor control rates of 90–95% have been observed.[19,20] However, pulsatile tinnitus, which is the most common and often only symptom of patients, is alleviated in only 49% of patients.[21] It should be noted that there are far fewer reports treating paragangliomas with stereotactic radiosurgery compared to vestibular schwannomas, with most having follow-up for <5 years. Furthermore, optimal doses have yet to be standardized.

COMPLICATIONS

With the use of modern planning techniques, complication rates have become very low with stereotactic radiosurgery. Facial nerve palsy has decreased markedly with current doses. With Gamma Knife, <4.5% of patients will have facial nerve weakness, with <1% having permanent weakness.[22] Hearing loss occurs in many patients and seems to be dependent on dose and time as hearing loss continues to progress in many patients years after treatment.[12] Dose to the cochlea also may play a role in hearing loss. Vertigo and imbalance are noted to occur in <2% of treated patients.[23] Trigeminal neuropathy is reported in up to 6% of patients and is often delayed when it does occur.[24] In a meta-analysis, hydrocephalus that required intervention happened in 0.85% of patients.[23] Malignant transformation of tumors occurs very rarely and has been estimated at 3 in 200,000 patients.[25] There have been only 14 cases of reported malignancy in vestibular schwannomas after radiotherapy, and interestingly four had NF2.[2] Tumors that continue to have growth progression are noted to be more difficult to surgically remove, often resulting in higher postoperative complications.[26]

REFERENCES

1. Hahn Y, Bojrab DI. Gamma Knife Radiosurgery Otology & Neurotology. San Diego: Plural Publishing; 2013.
2. Link MJ, Driscoll CL, Foote RL, et al. Radiation therapy and radiosurgery for vestibular schwannomas: indications,

techniques, and results. Otolaryngol Clin North Am. 2012; 45:353-66.
3. Pollock BE. Management of vestibular schwannomas that enlarge after stereotactic radiosurgery: treatment recommendations based on a 15 year experience. Neurosurgery. 2006;58(2):241-8; discussion 241-8.
4. Nagano O, Higuchi Y, Serizawa T, et al. Transient expansion of vestibular schwannoma following stereotactic radiosurgery. J Neurosurg. 2008;109:811-6.
5. Noren G, Greitz D, Hirsch A, et al. Gamma knife surgery in acoustic tumours. Acta Neurochir Suppl (Wien). 1993;58: 104-7.
6. Miller RC, Foote RL, Coffey RJ, et al. Decrease in cranial nerve complications after radiosurgery for acoustic neuromas: a prospective study of dose and volume. Int J Radiat Oncol Biol Phys. 1999;43:305-11.
7. Flickinger JC, Kondziolka D, Niranjan A, et al. Results of acoustic neuroma radiosurgery: an analysis of 5 years' experience using current methods. J Neurosurg. 2001;94:1-6.
8. Lunsford LD, Niranjan A, Flickinger JC, et al. Radiosurgery of vestibular schwannomas: summary of experience in 829 cases. J Neurosurg. 2005;102 (Suppl):195-9.
9. Hasegawa T, Fujitani S, Katsumata S, et al. Stereotactic radiosurgery for vestibular schwannomas: analysis of 317 patients followed more than 5 years. Neurosurgery. 2005; 57(2):257-65.
10. Hasegawa T, Kida Y, Kato T, et al. Factors associated with hearing preservation after Gamma Knife surgery for vestibular schwannomas in patients who retain serviceable hearing. J Neurosurg. 2011;115:1078-86.
11. Carlson ML, Jacob JT, Pollock BE, et al. Long-term hearing outcomes following stereotactic radiosurgery for vestibular schwannoma: patterns of hearing loss and variables influencing audiometric decline. J Neurosurg. 2013;118:579-87.
12. Yang I, Sughrue ME, Han SJ, et al. A comprehensive analysis of hearing preservation after radiosurgery for vestibular schwannoma. J Neurosurg. 2010;112:851-9.
13. Baschnagel AM, Chen PY, Bojrab D, et al. Hearing preservation in patients with vestibular schwannoma treated with Gamma Knife surgery. J Neurosurg. 2013;118:571-8.
14. Chang SD, Gibbs IC, Sakamoto GT, et al. Staged stereotactic irradiation for acoustic neuroma. Neurosurgery. 2005;56: 1254-61; discussion 61-3.
15. Morimoto M, Yoshioka Y, Kotsuma T, et al. Hypofractionated stereotactic radiation therapy in three to five fractions for vestibular schwannoma. Jpn J Clin Oncol. 2013;43(8): 805-12.
16. Vivas EX, Wegner R, Conley G, et al. Treatment Outcomes in Patients Treated With CyberKnife Radiosurgery for Vestibular Schwannoma. Otol Neurotol. 2014;35:162-70.
17. Spector GJ, Fierstein J, Ogura JH. A comparison of therapeutic modalities of glomus tumors in the temporal bone. Laryngoscope. 1976;86:690-6.
18. Mukherji SK, Kasper ME, Tart RP, et al. Irradiated paragangliomas of the head and neck: CT and MR appearance. AJNR Am J Neuroradiol. 1994;15:357-63.
19. Ivan ME, Sughrue ME, Clark AJ, et al. A meta-analysis of tumor control rates and treatment-related morbidity for patients with glomus jugulare tumors. J Neurosurg. 2011; 114:1299-305.
20. Chen PG, Nguyen JH, Payne SC, et al. Treatment of glomus jugulare tumors with gamma knife radiosurgery. Laryngoscope. 2010;120:1856-62.
21. Sheehan JP, Tanaka S, Link MJ, et al. Gamma Knife surgery for the management of glomus tumors: a multicenter study. J Neurosurg. 2012;117:246-54.
22. Roche PH, Noudel R, Regis J. Management of radiation/radiosurgical complications and failures. Otolaryngol Clin North Am. 2012;45:367-74, ix.
23. Sughrue ME, Yang I, Han SJ, et al. Non-audiofacial morbidity after Gamma Knife surgery for vestibular schwannoma. Neurosurg Focus. 2009;27:E4.
24. Ogunrinde OK, Lunsford LD, Flickinger JC, et al. Cranial nerve preservation after stereotactic radiosurgery for small acoustic tumors. Arch Neurol. 1995;52:73-9.
25. Ganz JC. Gamma knife radiosurgery and its possible relationship to malignancy: a review. J Neurosurg. 2002;97: 644-52.
26. Slattery WH, 3rd. Microsurgery after radiosurgery or radiotherapy for vestibular schwannomas. Otolaryngol Clin North Am. 2009;42:707-15.

Index

Note: Page numbers followed by *f* and *t* indicate figures and tables, respectively.

O

P

R

S

T